Pediatric Dermatologic Surgery

Pediatric Dermatologic Surgery

Edited by

Keyvan Nouri, MD
Professor of Dermatology, Ophthalmology, Otolaryngology & Surgery
Louis C. Skinner, Jr., M.D. Endowed Chair in Dermatology
Richard Helfman Professor of Dermatologic Surgery
Vice-Chairman of the University of Miami Medical Group
Director of Mohs, Dermatologic, & Laser Surgery
Director of Surgical Training
University of Miami Leonard M. Miller School of Medicine
Miami, FL, USA

Latanya Benjamin, MD, FAAD, FAAP
Associate Professor of Pediatric Dermatology, Florida Atlantic University
Boca Raton, FL, USA

Jasem Alshaiji, MD
Consultant Dermatologist, Head of Pediatric Dermatology Unit
Department of Dermatology, Amiri Hospital
Kuwait City, Kuwait

Jan Izakovic, MD
Voluntary Associate Professor, Department of Dermatology & Cutaneous Surgery
Division of Pediatric Dermatology
University of Miami Leonard M. Miller School of Medicine
Miami, FL, USA

WILEY Blackwell

This edition first published 2019

Registered Office(s)
John Wiley & Sons, Inc., 111 River Street, Hoboken, NJ 07030, USA
John Wiley & Sons Ltd, The Atrium, Southern Gate, Chichester, West Sussex, PO19 8SQ, UK

Editorial Office
9600 Garsington Road, Oxford, OX4 2DQ, UK

For details of our global editorial offices, customer services, and more information about Wiley products visit us at www.wiley.com.

Wiley also publishes its books in a variety of electronic formats and by print-on-demand. Some content that appears in standard print versions of this book may not be available in other formats.

Library of Congress Cataloging-in-Publication Data

Names: Nouri, Keyvan, editor. | Benjamin, Latanya, editor | Alshaiji, Jasem, editor. |
Izakovic, Jan, editor.
Title: Pediatric dermatologic surgery / edited by Keyvan Nouri, Latanya Benjamin,
Jasem Alshaiji, Jan Izakovic.
Description: Hoboken, NJ : Wiley-Blackwell, 2019. | Includes bibliographical
references and index. |
Identifiers: LCCN 2019003178 (print) | LCCN 2019004241 (ebook) | ISBN
9781118769713 (Adobe PDF) | ISBN 9781118769782 (ePub) | ISBN 9781118769850
(hardcover)
Subjects: | MESH: Dermatologic Surgical Procedures | Pediatrics–methods |
Laser Therapy–methods
Classification: LCC RJ511 (ebook) | LCC RJ511 (print) | NLM WS 265 | DDC
618.92/5–dc23
LC record available at https://lccn.loc.gov/2019003178

Cover Design: Wiley
Cover Image: © Baciu/Shutterstock

Set in 10/12pt Warnock by SPi Global, Pondicherry, India

Printed in the UK by Bell & Bain Ltd, Glasgow.

10 9 8 7 6 5 4 3 2 1

Contents

List of Contributors *vii*

1 The Embryogenesis of the Skin *1*
Jasem Alshaiji

2 Basic Structure and Function of the Neonatal, Infantile, and Childhood Skin *13*
Nawaf Almutairi

3 Approach to the Child as a Patient *23*
Nawaf Almutairi

4 Preoperative and Postoperative Care of Children Undergoing Pediatric Dermatology Procedures *31*
Alanna F. Bree

5 The Pediatric Surgical Tray *37*
V.M. Carlberg and J.L. Fewkes

6 Anesthesia for Children *49*
Marcia Hogeling

7 Skin Biopsy Techniques *63*
Grace Sun

8 Common Pediatric Dermatologic Surgery Procedures *73*
Meagan Barrett, Nicole Harter, and Ashley Wysong

9 Suturing Techniques *93*
Israel D. Andrews, Jennifer J. Schoch, and Kathryn Ann Potter

10 Wound Closure Technique *105*
Daniel Belkin and Ashley Wysong

11 Wound Closure Material *115*
V.M. Carlberg and J.L. Fewkes

12 Dressings *125*
Grace Sun

13 Nail Surgery *131*
Jane Sanders Bellet

14 Complications of Surgery and Invasive Procedures *143*
Yoon Cohen and Harper N. Price

15 Improving Scars *161*
Harper N. Price and Maria Princesa P. Curtis

16 Special Dermatologic Surgery *171*
Ramin Fathi, James William Behan, and Meena Julapalli

17 Lasers for Vascular Lesions *189*
Nawaf Almutairi and Jasem Alshaiji

18 Lasers for Scars and Striae *197*
Sebastian Verne, Robert Magno, Ariel Eber, Marina Perper, Ibrahim Alomair, Abdulkareem Alfuraih, Mana Alharbi, and Keyvan Nouri

19 Lasers for Acne *207*
Mohammad-Ali Yazdani Abyaneh, Robert D. Griffith, Leyre Falto-Aizpurua, Harleen Arora, and Keyvan Nouri

20 Laser for Verrucae *223*
Ariel Eber, Marina Perper, Sebastian Verne, Robert Magno, Mana Alharbi, Ibrahim Alomair, Abdulkareem Alfuraih, Ali Rajabi-Estarabadi, and Keyvan Nouri

21 Lasers and Lights for Onychomycosis *229*
Elizabeth Yim, Leyre A. Falto-Aizpurua, Jennifer Ledon, and Keyvan Nouri

22 Lasers for Pigmented Lesions *241*
Harleen Arora, Leyre Falto-Aizpurua, Ali Rajabi-Estarabadi, and Keyvan Nouri

23 Lasers for Tattoos *257*
Stephanie Mlacker, Leyre Falto-Aizpurua, Colin McNamara, and Keyvan Nouri

24 Lasers for Hair Removal *273*
Fleta Netter Bray, Leyre Falto-Aizpurua, Robert D. Griffith, Brian Simmons, Ali Rajabi-Estarabadi, and Keyvan Nouri

25 Lasers for Other Specific Dermatologic Disorders *289*
Leyre Falto-Aizpurua, Mohammad-Ali Yazdani Abyaneh, Harleen Arora, Robert D. Griffith, Ali Rajabi-Estarabadi, and Keyvan Nouri

26 Medical Ethics and Bioethics in Pediatric Dermatology *303*
Katlein França, Tulsie Narendra Patel, Shailee Bipin Patel, and Keyvan Nouri

Index *315*

List of Contributors

Abdulkareem Alfuraih MD
Al-Imam Mohammad Ibn Saud Islamic University (IMSIU), Riyadh, Saudi Arabia

Mana Alharbi MD
Al-Imam Mohammad Ibn Saud Islamic University (IMSIU), Riyadh, Saudi Arabia

Nawaf Almutairi MD
Faculty of Medicine, Department of Medicine, Dermatology Unit, Kuwait University, Kuwait City, Kuwait

Ibrahim Alomair MD
Al-Imam Mohammad Ibn Saud Islamic University (IMSIU), Riyadh, Saudi Arabia

Jasem Alshaiji MD
Consultant Dermatologist, Head of Pediatric Dermatology Unit, Department of Dermatology, Amiri Hospital, Kuwait City, Kuwait

Israel D. Andrews MD, FAAD
Associate Program Director, Department of Dermatology, Phoenix Children's Hospital, Phoenix, AZ, USA;
Assistant Professor – Pediatrics, Mayo College of Medicine, Rochester, MN, USA;
and
Clinical Assistant Professor, Department of Child Health, University of Arizona – College of Medicine, Tucson, AZ, USA

Harleen Arora MD
Undergraduate Student, University of Miami, Coral Gables, FL, USA

Meagan Barrett MD
The Keck School of Medicine of USC and LAC + USC Medical Center, Los Angeles, CA, USA

James William Behan MD
Staff Physician, Department of Dermatology, Kaiser Permanente, Pleasanton, CA, USA

Daniel Belkin MD
The Keck School of Medicine of USC and LAC + USC Medical Center, Los Angeles, CA, USA

Jane Sanders Bellet MD, FAAD
Associate Professor of Pediatrics and Dermatology, Duke University School of Medicine, Durham, NC, USA

Fleta Netter Bray BS
Clinical Research Fellow, Department of Dermatology & Cutaneous Surgery, University of Miami Miller School of Medicine, Miami, FL, USA

Alanna F. Bree MD
A Children's House for Pediatric Dermatology, Houston, TX, USA

V.M. Carlberg MA
Department of Dermatology, Massachusetts General Hospital;
and
Harvard Medical School, Boston, MA, USA

Yoon Cohen DO
Alta Dermatology, Phoenix, AZ, USA

Maria Princesa P. Curtis MD
Phoenix Children's Hospital, Phoenix
AZ, USA

Ariel Eber BS
Department of Dermatology & Cutaneous Surgery, University of Miami Miller School of Medicine, Miami, FL, USA

Leyre Falto-Aizpurua MD
Clinical Research Fellow, Department of Dermatology & Cutaneous Surgery, University of Miami Miller School of Medicine, Miami, FL, USA

Ramin Fathi MD
Fellow, Micrographic Surgery and Dermatologic Oncology, Department of Dermatology, University of Texas Southwestern Medical Center
Dallas, TX, USA

J.L. Fewkes MD
Department of Dermatology, Massachusetts General Hospital
Harvard Medical School;
and
Department of Otolaryngology, Massachusetts Eye and Ear Infirmary, Boston, MA, USA

Katlein França MD, MSc
Volunteer Faculty-Assistant Professor, Department of Dermatology & Cutaneous Surgery, University of Miami Miller School of Medicine, Miami, FL, USA

Robert D. Griffith MD
Clinical Research Fellow, Department of Dermatology & Cutaneous Surgery, University of Miami Miller School of Medicine, Miami, FL, USA

Nicole Harter MD
The Keck School of Medicine of USC and LAC + USC Medical Center, Los Angeles, CA, USA

Marcia Hogeling MD
Assistant Professor, Director of Pediatric Dermatology, David Geffen School of Medicine at UCLA, Los Angeles, CA, USA

Meena Julapalli MD
Assistant Professor, Department of Dermatology, Children's Hospital Colorado, University of Colorado School of Medicine, Aurora, CO, USA

Jennifer Ledon MD
Department of Dermatology & Cutaneous Surgery, University of Miami Miller School of Medicine, Miami
FL, USA

Robert Magno BS
Department of Dermatology & Cutaneous Surgery, University of Miami Miller School of Medicine, Miami, FL, USA

Colin McNamara MD
Charles E. Schmidt College of Medicine, Florida Atlantic University, Boca Raton
FL, USA

Stephanie Mlacker MD
Charles E. Schmidt College of Medicine, Florida Atlantic University, Boca Raton
FL, USA

Keyvan Nouri MD
Professor of Dermatology, Ophthalmology, Otolaryngology & Surgery, Louis C. Skinner, Jr., M.D. Endowed Chair in Dermatology, Richard Helfman Professor of Dermatologic Surgery, Vice-Chairman of the University of Miami Medical Group Director of Mohs, Dermatologic, & Laser Surgery, Director of Surgical Training University of Miami Leonard M. Miller School of Medicine, Miami, FL, USA

Tulsie Narendra Patel BS
Medical Student, University of Miami Miller School of Medicine, Miami
FL, USA

Shailee Bipin Patel BS
Research Fellow, Department of Dermatology & Cutaneous Surgery, University of Miami Miller School of Medicine, Miami, FL, USA

Marina Perper BS
Department of Dermatology & Cutaneous Surgery, University of Miami Miller School of Medicine, Miami, FL, USA

Kathryn Ann Potter MD, FAAD
Procedural Dermatology Fellow, Division of Dermatology, University of Vermont Medical Center, Burlington, VT, USA

Harper N. Price MD, FAAD, FAAP
Chief, Division of Dermatology
Pediatric Dermatology Fellowship Director
Phoenix Children's Hospital;
and
Clinical Assistant Professor, Department of Child Health
University of Arizona College of Medicine
Phoenix, AZ, USA

Ali Rajabi-Estarabadi MD
Department of Dermatology & Cutaneous Surgery, University of Miami Miller School of Medicine, Miami, FL, USA

Jennifer J. Schoch MD, FAAD
Assistant Professor, Department of Dermatology, University of Florida Gainesville, FL, USA

Brian Simmons, MD
Clinical Research Fellow, Department of Dermatology & Cutaneous Surgery, University of Miami Miller School of Medicine, Miami, FL, USA

Grace Sun MD
Pediatric Dermatologist, Dermatology Medical Group, Oxnard, CA, USA

Sebastian Verne BS
Department of Dermatology & Cutaneous Surgery, University of Miami Miller School of Medicine, Miami, FL, USA

Ashley Wysong MD, MS
Chair, Department of Dermatology, William W. Bruce, M.D. Distinguished Chair of Dermatology, University of Nebraska Medical Center (UNMC) College of Medicine, Nebraska Medical Center, Omaha, NE, USA

Mohammad-Ali Yazdani Abyaneh BS
Clinical Research Fellow, Department of Dermatology & Cutaneous Surgery, University of Miami Miller School of Medicine, Miami, FL, USA

Elizabeth Yim MD
Department of Dermatology & Cutaneous Surgery, University of Miami Miller School of Medicine, Miami, FL, USA

1

The Embryogenesis of the Skin

Jasem Alshaiji

Department of Dermatology, Amiri Hospital, Kuwait City, Kuwait

1.1 Introduction

The skin is complex tissue and is the biggest constantly renewable organ in the body. It has many different cell types and specialized structures (such as hair, nails, and glands) derived from both embryonic ectoderm and mesoderm. Skin cell types that originate from ectoderm include keratinocytes, neural crest-derived melanocytes, Merkel cells, and neurons, whereas skin cell types that originate from mesoderm include fibroblasts, endothelial cells, adipocytes and bone marrow-derived Langerhans cells [1].

There are two distinct dating systems, one refers to estimated gestational age (EGA) and is used in textbooks and by researchers, in which fertilization occurs on day 1 (first day of the last menstrual period (LMP)), whereas menstrual age, used by obstetricians and most clinicians, has fertilization occurring on day 14 [2, 3].

Fetal skin development can be divided into three temporally overlapping stages: organogenesis (specification), histogenesis (morphogenesis) and maturation (differentiation) [4]. These stages roughly correspond to the embryonic period (0–60 days), the early fetal period (2–5 months), and the late fetal period (5–9 months) of development. The first stage involves the specification of ectoderm lateral to the neural plate to become epidermis and the allocation of subsets of mesenchymal and neural crest cells to become dermis. The second stage is the process by which these committed tissues begin to form their specialized structures, including epidermal stratification, epidermal appendage formation, subdivision between the dermis and subcutis, and vascular formation. The third stage refers to the process by which these newly specialized tissues further differentiate and assume their mature forms [1].

Understanding the stages of normal human skin development allows the definition of critical periods when the skin may be more vulnerable to developmental errors; it provides an opportunity to study the evolution of skin function, establishing a background for understanding the natural history of expression of genetic skin disease in its earliest form; and it provides the essential information for the evaluation of skin samples used in the prenatal diagnosis of genodermatoses for which molecular methods are still not adaptable [5].

The timing at which sampling of the skin for various diagnostic procedures are performed should be recognized. Chorionic villus sampling for fetal DNA is sampled around 10 weeks EGA, amniotic fluid cells (amniocentesis) can be obtained at around

Pediatric Dermatologic Surgery, First Edition. Edited by Keyvan Nouri, Latanya Benjamin, Jasem Alshaiji, and Jan Izakovic.

14–16 weeks EGA, whereas fetal skin biopsy is performed typically at 19–21 weeks EGA [5–8].

1.2 Stages of Skin Development

1.2.1 Embryonic Stage (Specification)

During the third week after fertilization, the human embryo undergoes gastrulation, a complex process of involution and cell redistribution that results in the formation of the three primary embryonic germ layers: ectoderm, mesoderm, and endoderm. Shortly after gastrulation, ectoderm further subdivides into neuroectoderm and presumptive epidermis [1].

1.2.1.1 Epidermis

At six weeks EGA, the epidermis that covers most of the embryo are two-layered epithelium consisting of basal cells and periderm cells [9–11]. The basal cells are more columnar and have intercellular attachment mediated by E- and P-cadherin and they express keratins K5, K14, K8 and K19 [12–14]. The periderm cells are larger and flatter than underlying basal cells and they express K5, K14, K8, K18 and K19 [13–16]. Their apical surfaces are studded with microvilli and tight junctions attach them at their lateral surfaces [11]. Two of the immigrant cells, melanocytes and Langerhans cells, are present in the embryonic epidermis among basal cells. Melanocytes are dendritic as early as 50 days EGA in general body skin but there is no evidence of melanosomes in the cytoplasm [17]. Langerhans cells are recognized in embryonic skin as early as 42 days EGA and they have dendritic morphology and probably derived from yolk sac or fetal liver at this age [18–20]. The third immigrant cells, Merkel cells, can be seen in embryonic palmar skin as early as 55–60 days EGA and they express K8, K18, K10 and K20 [21–25]. K20 is the only keratin found exclusively in Merkel cells. They are distributed randomly and in a suprabasal position. They are neuroendocrine cells acting as slow-adapting mechanoreceptors. It is generally accepted that Merkel cells are derived from keratinocytes in situ [21, 23, 25–27].

1.2.1.2 Dermis

The embryonic dermis is highly cellular and amorphous, consisting of a loose network of mesenchymal cells (fibroblasts, mast cells and skin-derived precursor-SKP-cells) with little intervening fibrous connective tissue matrix, and its origin varies depend on the body site [28]. Dermal mesenchyme of the face and anterior scalp is derived from neural crest ectoderm; the limb and ventral body wall mesenchyme is derived from the lateral plate mesoderm, whereas the dorsal body wall mesenchyme derives from the dermomyotomes of the embryonic somite [29].

The cell migration is promoted through the high water content and hyaluronic-acid-rich environment of the dermal mesenchyme, whereas the exchange of signals between epidermis and dermis is achieved through the compact mesenchyme and is very important in stimulating the onset of appendage formation [5, 30].

Types I, III and VI collagen are distributed uniformly throughout the dermis whereas type V collagen is concentrated primarily along basement membranes and surrounding cells. The ratio of collagen III to collagen I is 3:1, the opposite what it is in the adult [31].

The embryonic dermis does not contain elastic fibers yet, but fibrillin and elastin proteins of the elastic fibers can be identified by immunohistochemistry and microfibrils can be seen by electron microscopy (EM) [11]. Blood vessels have been identified in fetal skin through the process of vasculogenesis (de novo) as early as nine weeks EGA and its pattern varies among different regions of the body [32]. Development of the cutaneous innervation closely parallels that of the vascular system in term of its pattern, rate of maturation, and organization. Cutaneous nerves are composed of somatic sensory fibers, which can be identified at seven weeks

EGA, and sympathetic autonomic fibers, which are not yet recognized [33].

1.2.1.3 Dermoepidermal Junction (DEJ)

The Dermoepidermal Junction (DEJ) connects the developing epidermis (the basal cells) to the dermis and it provides resistance against shearing forces on the skin. The embryonic DEJ is simple, flat, and generic basement membrane and consists of a lamina lucida and a lamina densa. It is composed of molecules that are common to all basement membranes zones (e.g. type IV collagen, laminin, heparin sulfate, proteoglycans, nidogen/entactin) [34]. The α6 and β4 integrin subunits are expressed quite early by embryonic basal cells, but they become localized to the basal surface until after 9.5 weeks EGA, at the same time as bullous pemphigoid antigens (BPA1 and BPA2) are first detected by immunohistochemistry and hemidesmosomes are recognized by EM [34, 35]. The anchoring filaments and anchoring fibrils are identified by nine weeks EGA [4, 36]. Collagen VII (the anchoring fibril protein) is seen slightly earlier at eight weeks EGA [36].

1.2.1.4 Subcutis (Hypodermis)

The subcutis can be first recognized at 50–60 days EGA through a plane of thin-walled vessels that separate the hypodermis from the overlying cellular dermis [4]. However, it is difficult distinguish it from dermis before this time due to similarities in the cells found in both structures and the fact that the adipose tissue is not yet synthesized. There is no morphologic evidence that epidermal appendages started to form in embryonic skin [37].

1.2.2 Embryonic-Fetal Transition (Morphogenesis)

The embryonic-fetal transition is regarded as the most remarkable time in skin development and occurs at around two months (eight weeks) EGA. During this time hematopoiesis has switched from the extraembryonic yolk sac to the bone marrow. The cells of the skin begin to express nearly every characteristic of adult skin. It is also the time that is more vulnerable to errors in development [5].

1.2.2.1 Epidermis

The most important change in the skin at this stage is stratification of the epidermis from two to three cell layers. Intermediate cells are both similar to and distinct from basal and periderm cells. Keratins are more abundant and distributed in a more specific manner than in other two cells. The expression of the major keratin pairs in both basal- and intermediate-layer keratinocytes is now identical to that seen in adult epidermis. The K5 and K14 basal cells keratins are downregulated in the intermediate cells and a new keratin pair, K1 and K10, is synthesized [13, 14]. Also, pemphigus antigen, cornified cell envelope proteins, blood group antigens and cell-surface glycoproteins are expressed in the cytoplasm or on the surface of intermediate-layer cells [38–41]. The cells of both basal and intermediate cell layers express epidermal growth factor (EGF) receptors respond to EGF and retain the ability to proliferate [42–44]. However, only basal cells express P-cadherin, which has a proliferative ability, by the end of the first trimester. Basal cells change in morphology and cell-surface properties after stratification. The cells of the periderm increase in size and begin to develop microvilli-covered blebs that extend from the outermost surface of the cells into the amniotic cavity. Melanocytes are easily recognized in sections of fetal epidermis at eight weeks EGA by their position along the basement membrane, dense cytoplasm, an absence of glycogen and a heterochromatic nucleus [45]. Langerhans cells are more abundant in the epidermis at this stage (~50/mm^2) and they express HLA-DR more than CD1a [46]. Merkel cells are located along the primary epidermal ridges of palmar skin in regular alignment relative to the sites of origin of the sweat duct primordial by the end of the first trimester. Merkel cells are also present in the dermis of both thick (palms and soles) and hairy skin (around developing hair follicles) where they play a role in attracting and organizing nerve fibers [47]. Epidermal Merkel cells lack nerve growth factor NGF receptors, whereas dermal and follicular Merkel cells are immunopositive [47]. Merkel cells decrease in number during the later stages of fetal development [47].

1.2.2.2 Dermis

Dermal mesenchymal cells still retain glycogen in the cytoplasm, assume a fibroblastic morphology and are responsible for the synthesis of all of the matrix molecules that are characteristic of adult dermis.

There is significantly greater accumulation of small bundles of fibrous proteins within the interstitial space. The papillary and reticular regions of the dermis are demarcated on the basis of increased cell density proximal to the epidermis (the papillary region) and larger collagen fibril diameter and fiber bundle size in the reticular region [31]. The position of the subpapillary vascular plexus of arterioles and postcapillary venules also forms an approximate boundary between these two dermal regions. The dermosubcutaeous vascular plexus demarcates the dermis from the subcutis. Vertically oriented vessels connect the two horizontal plexuses, and fine capillaries extend into the papillary dermis [11]. Nerves are also readily apparent in both regions.

1.2.2.3 Dermoepidermal Junction (DEJ)

The DEJ has acquired all of the adult features that are characteristic for this region. Hemidesmosomes, anchoring filaments and anchoring fibrils are structurally complete and the antigens related to them are also expressed [34–36]. The relative strength of this interface may not be too different from the adult. The dermoepidermal interface is still flat, although modifications of individual basal cells begin to alter the smoothness of this junction.

1.2.2.4 Subcutis

The dermis and hypodermis are distinguished on a morphological basis by differences in the organization and composition of the matrix. The subcutis appears to have markedly fewer cells and smaller bundles of fibrous matrix.

1.2.3 Fetal Stage (Differentiation)

The first stages of fetal skin development occur from the time of the embryonic-fetal transition at two months to the end of the first trimester at three months, when a template of the adult skin is established. During the second trimester, the fetal skin completes the formation of the lanugo hair follicle and synthesis of hair (~17–19 weeks EGA), nail formation (~20–22 weeks EGA) and keratinization of the interfollicular epidermis (~22–24 weeks EGA). During the third trimester, the skin appears structurally similar to postnatal skin, in which the epidermis is fully keratinized, the DEJ starts to have contours, the regions of the dermis are well defined, the adnexae are fully formed and reside deeply in the dermis, and large fat lobules fill the hypodermis [11].

1.2.3.1 Epidermis

The epidermis is now thicker, having more layers of intermediate cells (three by 100–110 days EGA), and the glycogen is still a major constituent of the cytoplasm compared to basal cells. The basal cells having smaller bundles of keratin filaments and the cytoplasm are more ribosome-rich, dense, and organelle-filled. A few layers of thin, flattened, keratinized cells mimicking stratum corneum are visible around 22–24 weeks EGA. With the presence of larger keratohyalin granules and less glycogen content of the cytoplasm, the granular cell layer is now more typical of an adult one. By 22–24 weeks EGA, 1700 Merkel cells/mm^2 can be measured in the epidermis and the number of Langerhans cells begins to increase (~200 cells/mm^2). Melanosomes are transferred to keratinocytes in the fifth month of gestation.

The epidermis is still a less effective barrier than the infant epidermis.

1.2.3.2 Dermis

After embryonic-fetal transition, the presumptive dermis is distinguishable from the underlying skeletal condensations. By 12–15 weeks, the fine interwoven mesh of the papillary dermis can be distinguished from deeper, more fibrillar reticular dermis [4, 31]. Large collagen fibers accumulate in the reticular dermis during the second and third trimester. Definitive elastin fibers first become detectable by EM around 22–24 weeks EGA [48]. By the end of gestation, the dermis is thick and well organized, but is still much thinner than in the adult and has higher water content. Increasing tensile strength and transition from a nonscarring to a scarring response after wounding marks maturation of the dermis. By three months, the distinct horizontal and vertical vascular networks have formed and by the fifth month vasculogenesis has largely ceased and the formation of the complex vascular plexus is initiated by angiogenesis (the budding and migration of endothelium from pre-existing vessels).

1.2.3.3 Dermoepidermal Junction (DEJ)

All the structures of the DEJ were formed in the first trimester, and only a few antigens of the DEJ (AF-1 and AF-2 associated with anchoring fibrils) remain to be recognized at this age [49]. By 19–21 weeks EGA, the hemidesmosomes are present at the basal keratinocytes plasma membrane with adult-like frequency and show a strong association with basal cell keratin filaments. Anchoring filaments and banded anchoring fibrils are well formed [11].

1.2.3.4 Subcutis

The hypodermis remains distinct from the dermis by its less dense matrix and cellularity. Around 15–16 weeks EGA, mesenchymal cells collect in globular arrays surrounded by a capsule-like assembly of matrix. By 18 weeks EGA, lipid droplets are evident within some of the mesenchymal cells, and by 20 weeks fat lobules are established [5].

1.3 Special Features of Developing Human Skin

1.3.1 Periderm

The periderm is the outermost, transient cellular layer of the developing skin of some mammals and birds. The periderm is released as single cells and as sheets of cells into the amniotic fluid at the end of the second trimester when the epidermis keratinizes [11]. The origin of the periderm is unknown, but there are many hypotheses. A reasonable hypothesis would be that the cells of the original, single ectodermal layer of the early embryo divide and give rise to a second cell layer that become superficial to the basal layer. Second, it is also possible that the periderm arises from the cells of the amnion that grow over the single-layered epidermis. A third possibility is that the periderm layer is the original ectodermal layer that covers the very early blastocyst and embryo. Periderm cells do not express the primary K5 and K14 proteins of basal keratinocytes (or the K1/K10 keratins of differentiated keratinocytes) but they do express other keratins in common with the fetal basal cells. The most remarkable features of the periderm are the morphological changes that the periderm cells undergo with progressive stages of development [9]. The periderm cells neither undergo the events of differentiation that are typical for the keratinocytes nor undergo keratinization. The presence of transglutaminase in periderm cells may have implications for the fate of these cells, as the presence of this enzyme is a feature of cells undergoing programmed cell death or apoptosis [50]. The structural properties of periderm cells may provide clues as to the function of the layer. The blebs and microvilli increase the surface area of the periderm as it faces the amniotic fluid, suggesting its role in the exchange of substances between the fetus and the amniotic fluid. They also have a role in regulating water transport, absorption of nicotine dissolved in amniotic fluid and as a secretory epithelium that adds material to the amniotic fluid [51, 52]. There are no genetic disorders that can affect the periderm cells unlike other cells in the epidermis. Toward the end of the second trimester, they are eventually sloughed and become a component of the vernix caseosa covering the newborn [1].

1.3.1.1 Regionalization in Developing Skin

Regional differences in properties of the skin are well documented in adult skin as well as in developing skin. Without a clear appreciation and accurate knowledge of differences in normal morphology at various sites, structural evaluation of skin samples that may be from unknown regions can be risky.

Also systematic studies of affected fetal skin from multiple regions are valuable to undertake when tissue becomes available, especially in situations where fetal biopsy remains the only current method available to diagnose a severe genetic disease in utero [5].

1.3.1.2 Keratinization

Keratinization of the nails, hair follicles, intraepidermal sweat duct, and the interfollicular epidermis occurs at different times during gestation. The nails are the earliest structures of the skin to keratinize in utero, as early as 11–12 weeks EGA, whereas the follicular epidermis keratinizes consistent with the cephalocaudal direction of follicle morphogenesis [53]. The interfollicular epidermis keratinizes first in thick skin and then in thin skin.

1.3.1.3 Appendage Formation

After the embryonic-fetal transition, around 10–11 weeks EGA, basal epidermal cells undergo proliferation at specifically patterned sites to form buds that grow down into the dermis as hair germs, sweat ducts, or as a nail fold. Nerves and vessels, cellular adhesion molecules (CAMs), soluble mediators and homeobox genes (homeoproteins) have been implicated in the pattern formation of certain appendages. The epithelial-mesenchymal interactions are thought to be responsible for initiation of appendage formation [5].

1.3.1.4 Nail Formation

The distal rays of the digit are evident on the hand of 50-day EGA embryo, and within the next seven days the digit separates. Formation of nail on the dorsal surface of the digits and the eccrine sweat glands on the ventral surface is initiated at about the same time after embryo-fetal transition. By 70 days EGA, proximal, lateral and distal folds establish the boundaries of the nail field externally and sections through the digit reveal a shallow nail fold. By 90 days EGA, the dorsal ridge is evident superficially. The nail fold has invaginated deeply into the dermis and organized into dorsal and ventral layers (the nail matrix) that are distinguished from one another morphologically and functionally. The earliest nail consists of several layers of keratinized cells. By 15 weeks EGA, a thick cornified layer covers the nail bed. This preliminary nail is composed of keratinized epidermal cells from the nail bed rather than from the nail matrix. The nail of a 19-week EGA fetus is established by both the nail matrix and the nail-bed epidermis.

The nail of the newborn is composed of layers derived from the dorsal nail fold (gives outermost layer), the nail matrix (gives the intermediate layer), and the distal nail bed (gives the inner layer).

1.3.1.5 Eccrine Sweat Gland Formation on the Digits

The sweat gland primordial are recognized around 13–14 weeks EGA at regular sites along the epidermal ridges (which first formed around 10–11 weeks EGA) as narrowed, solid, epithelial cords of cells that contain basal cell keratins and express classical carcinoembryonic antigen (CEA) on all cells [54]. As the cords of epithelial cells elongate into the dermis, a thickening at the terminus defines the glandular segment from the duct. Ductal, secretory, myoepithelial and acrosyringial cell types differentiate in the dermal and intraepidermal regions of the gland and duct [55]. The secretory cells border a central lumen within the gland; myoepithelial cells are evident at the periphery of the structure. Ductal and glandular cells are distinct from one another at 15 weeks EGA by their morphological properties and by differences in expression of keratins (duct) and vimentin (gland) and CAMs [55]. By 22–24 weeks EGA, the sweat glands on the palms and soles have attained the structure of the adult glands, with a coiled secretory segment positioned deeply within the dermis.

1.3.1.6 Eccrine Sweat Gland Formation on the General Body Surface

Eccrine sweat glands form on the general body surface at least four to six weeks later than on the palms and soles.

1.3.1.7 Pilosebaceous Apparatus Formation

It is best described as a composite epithelial-mesenchymal structure. Morphogenesis of the hair follicle begins on the head and face at around 70–80 days EGA, then proceeds in a cephalocaudal direction. The process is completed at around 19–20 weeks EGA. The description of the hair germ, hair peg, bulbous hair peg, and lanugo follicle stages of follicle formation are based on the appearance of vellus hairs on the trunk [5, 11]. Follicles form only during development and decline in numbers as a function of aging. Little is understood about the events that establish the patterns of human follicles or the molecular nature of the inductive messages that start the process. The sites of follicle formation can be recognized even before the hair germs are visible by immunostaining the tissue with an antibody that recognized tenascin [56].

Tenascin is expressed in tissue where there is evidence of matrix remodeling, cell migration, and proliferation. It is also associated with the formation of patterned structures and at sites of epithelial-mesenchymal interaction and mesenchymal condensation [5].

Many signaling molecules including Notch, Sonic hedgehog, Wnt (wingless-related), fibroblast growth factors (FGFs), and bone morphogenetic proteins (BMPs) as well as transcription factors such as HOXC13 AND FOXN1 are important in hair follicle development and cycling [57, 58]. Cells from the basal epidermal layer bud into the dermis at the tenascin-rich sites to become hair germs. Merkel cells, which may play a role in targeting nerve fibers toward the developing appendage, are recognized in some of the developing germs.

At around 13–14 weeks EGA, the hair germs elongate into the dermis as cords of cells called hair pegs. The hair peg consists of an inner core of cuboidal cells (contain intermediate cell keratins) and outer layer of columnar cells (contain same keratin as basal cells) that is associated with the basal lamina. Merkel cells are distributed among the outer root sheath keratinocytes. Early hair pegs are cylindrical, but as they elongate further they develop three regions: a constricted, neck-like connection with the epidermis (the presumptive infundibulum); a central, cylindrical region (the presumptive isthmus); and a terminal zone that becomes widened at its most distal end (the lower follicle and the presumptive bulb). Melanocytes aggregate in the matrix (the bulb) and produce melanin ahead of melanocytes in the general body skin. Between 15 and 17 weeks EGA, bulges of epithelial cells begin to grow out from the epithelial cord on the posterior surface of the follicle. Now the follicle is called a bulbous hair peg. The most superior bulge is the primordium of the sebaceous gland. The second bulge, the "true bulge", is thought to be the site of follicular stem cells and the point of attachment of the arrector pili muscle. A third bulge may form superior to the sebaceous gland as the primordium of the apocrine sweat gland at restricted sites (axilla, areola, scalp, external eyelid, auditory meatus and anogenital regions) [59]. Merkel cells also concentrate in the bulge at early stages of bulge formation and may play a role in stimulating proliferation or attracting nerve fibers and smooth muscle cells to the site. The first hairs of the fetus are in the anagen phase of the hair cycle. In some newborns, a significant number of them will enter telogen and be shed, creating alopecia that can last up to six months [5].

1.4 Conclusion

In conclusion, the understating of the skin development and embryogenesis is crucial for the diagnosis and management of various congenital or inherited skin diseases. There are many resources available for both diagnosis and treatment of those disorders. Data on genetic test availability are provided by GeneTest (www.genetests.org). Other useful websites include: www.omim.org, www.genedx.com, and www.rarediseases.org. Also, there is online textbook called GeneReviews, containing expert-authored, peer-reviewed disease descriptions ("chapters") presented in a standardized format and focused on clinically relevant and medically actionable information on the diagnosis, management, and genetic counseling of patients and families with specific inherited conditions.

Knowing the mechanisms controlling angiogenesis during intrauterine life holds promise for wound healing and creating new anticancer therapies [58]. Also, knowing the factors involved in wound healing in embryos may point to interventions that may decrease scarring in children and adults. Therefore, advancing the knowledge of skin embryology may lead to life-saving or life-enhancing therapies [58].

References

1 Loomis, C.A., Koss, T., and Chu, D. (2008). Fetal skin development. In: *Neonatal Dermatology* (ed. L.F. Eichenfield, I.J. Frieden and N.B. Esterly). Saunders-Elsevier.

2 Larsen, W.L. (1997). *Human Embryology*. New York: Churchill Livingstone.

3 Cunningham, F.G., MacDonald, P.C., Gant, N.F. et al. (1997). *Williams' Obstetrics*. Stanford, CT: Appleton & Lange.

4 Holbrook, K.A. (1998). Structural and biochemical organogenesis of skin and cutaneous appendages in the fetus and newborn. In: *Fetal and Neonatal Physiology* (ed. R.A. Polin and W.W. Fox), 729–752. Philadelphia, PA: WB Saunders.

5 Holbrook, K.A. (2011). Embryogenesis of the skin. In: *Harper's Textbook of Pediatric Dermatology* (ed. A.D. Irvine, P.H. Hoeger and A.C. Yan). Oxford: Wiley-Blackwell.

6 Regauer, S., Franke, W.W., and Virtanen, I. (1985). Intermediate filament cytoskeleton of amnion epithelium and cultured amnion epithelial cells: expression of epidermal cytokeratins in cells of a simple epithelium. *J. Cell Biol.* 100: 997–1009.

7 Nanbu, Y., Fujii, S., Konishi, I. et al. (1989). CA125 in the epithelium closely related to the embryonic ectoderm: the periderm and the amnion. *Am. J. Obstet. Gynecol.* 161: 462–467.

8 Lane, A.T., Negi, M., and Goldsmith, L.A. (1987). Human periderm: a monoclonal antibody marker. *Curr. Probl. Dermatol.* 16: 83–93.

9 Holbrook, K.A. and Odland, G.F. (1975). The fine structure of developing human epidermis: light, scanning, and transmission electron microscopy of the periderm. *J. Invest. Dermatol.* 65: 16–38.

10 Holbrook, K.A. and Odland, G.F. (1980). Regional development of the human epidermis in the first trimester embryo and the second trimester fetus (ages related to the timing of amniocentesis

and fetal biopsy). *J. Invest. Dermatol.* 74: 161–168.

11 Holbrook, K.A. (1991). Structure and function of the developing human skin. In: *Physiology, Biochemistry, and Molecular Biology of the Skin* (ed. L.A. Goldsmith), 63–110. New York: Oxford Press.

12 Furukawa, F., Fujii, K., Horiguchi, Y. et al. (1997). Roles of E- and P-cadherin in the human skin. *Microsc. Res. Tech.* 38: 343–352.

13 Dale, B.A., Holbrook, K.A., Kimball, J.R. et al. (1985). Expression of epidermal keratins and filaggrin during human fetal skin development. *J. Cell Biol.* 101: 1257–1269.

14 Moll, R., Moll, I., and Wiest, W. (1983). Changes in the pattern of cytokeratin polypeptides in epidermis and hair follicles during skin development in human fetuses. *Differentiation* 23: 170–178.

15 Lehtonen, E., Lehto, V.P., Vartio, T. et al. (1983). Expression of cytokeratin polypeptides in mouse oocytes and preimplantation embryos. *Dev. Biol.* 100: 158–165.

16 Jackson, B.W., Grund, C., Winter, S. et al. (1981). Formation of cytoskeletal elements during mouse embryogenesis. II. Epithelial differentiation and intermediate-sized filaments in early postimplantation embryos. *Differentiation* 20: 203–216.

17 Holbrook, K.A., Underwood, R.A., Vogel, A.M. et al. (1989). The appearance, density and distribution of melanocytes in human embryonic and fetal skin revealed by the anti-melanoma monoclonal antibody, HMB-45. *Anat. Embryol.* 180: 443–455.

18 Foster, C.A., Holbrook, K.A., and Farr, A.G. (1986). Ontogeny of Langerhans cells in human embryonic and fetal skin: expression of HLA-DR and OKT-6 determinants. *J. Invest. Dermatol.* 86: 240–243.

19 Drijkoningen, M., DeWolf-Peeters, C., VanDerSteen, K. et al. (1987). Epidermal Langerhans cells and dermal dendritic cells in human fetal and neonatal skin: an immunohistochemical study. *Pediatr. Dermatol.* 4: 11–17.

20 Foster, C.A. and Holbrook, K.A. (1989). Ontogeny of Langerhans cells in human embryonic and fetal skin: cell densities and phnotypic expression relative to epidermal growth. *Am. J. Anat.* 84: 157–164.

21 Moll, R., Moll, I., and Franke, W. (1984). Identification of Merkel cells in human skin by specific cytokeratin antibodies: changes in cell density and distribution in fetal and adult plantar epidermis. *Differentiation* 28: 136–154.

22 Moll, R. and Moll, I. (1992). Early development of human Merkel cells. *Exp. Dermatol.* 1: 180–184.

23 Moll, I., Moll, R., and Franke, W. (1986). Formation of epidermal and dermal Merkel cells during human fetal skin development. *J. Invest. Dermatol.* 87: 779–787.

24 Moll, R., Lowe, A., Laufer, J. et al. (1992). Cytokeratin 20 in human carcinomas: a new histodiagnostic marker detected by monoclonal antibodies. *Am. J. Pathol.* 140: 427–447.

25 Moll, I., Kuhn, C., and Moll, R. (1995). Cytokeratin 20 is a general marker of cutaneous Merkel cells while certain neuronal proteins are absent. *J. Invest. Dermatol.* 104: 910–915.

26 Moll, I., Lane, A.T., Franke, W.W. et al. (1990). Intraepidermal formation of Merkel cells in xenografts of human fetal skin. *J. Invest. Dermatol.* 94: 359–364.

27 Narisawa, Y. and Hashimoto, K. (1991). Immunohistochemical distribution of nerve-Merkel cell complex in fetal human skin. *J. Dermatol. Sci.* 2: 361–370.

28 Toma, J.G., Akhaven, M., Fernandes, K.J. et al. (2001). Isolation of multipotent adult stem cells from the dermis of mammalian skin. *Nat. Cell Biol.* 3: 778–784.

29 Chu, D.H. (2008). Development and structure of skin. In: *Fitzpatrick's Dermatology in General Medicine*, 7e (ed. K. Wolff, L. Goldsmith, S. Katz, et al.). New York: McGraw Hill.

30 Breen, M., Weinstein, H.G., Johnson, R.L. et al. (1970). Acid glycosaminoglycans in human skin during fetal development and in adult life. *Biochim. Biophys. Acta* 201: 54–60.

31 Smith, L.T., Holbrook, K.A., and Madri, J.A. (1986). Collagen types I, III, and V in human embryonic and fetal skin. *Am. J. Anat.* 175: 507–521.

32 Karelina, T.V., Goldberg, G.I., and Eisen, A.Z. (1995). Matrix metalloproteinases in blood vessel development in human fetal skin and in cutaneous tumors. *J. Invest. Dermatol.* 105: 411–417.

33 Terenghi, G., Sundaresan, M., Moscoso, G. et al. (1993). Neuropeptides and a neuronal marker in cutaneous innervation during human fetal development. *J. Comp. Neurol.* 328: 595–603.

34 Fine, J.D., Smith, L.T., Holbrook, K.A. et al. (1984). The appearance of four basement membrane zone antigens in developing human fetal skin. *J. Invest. Dermatol.* 83: 66–69.

35 Hertle, M.D., Adams, J.C., and Watt, F.M. (1991). Integrin expression during human epidermal development in vivo and in vitro. *Development* 112: 193–206.

36 Smith, L.T., Sakai, L.Y., Burgeson, R.E. et al. (1988). Ontogeny of structural components at the dermal-epidermal junction in human embryonic and fetal skin: the appearance of anchoring fibrils and type VII collagen. *J. Invest. Dermatol.* 90: 480–485.

37 Morasso, M.I., Chu, D.H., and Schwarz, T. (2011). Structure and function of the skin. In: *Pediatric Dermatology*, 4e (ed. L.A. Schachner and R.C. Hansen). Elsevier.

38 Holbrook, K.A., Underwood, R.A., Dale, B.A. et al. (1991). Formation of the cornified cell envelope in human fetal skin: presence of involucrin, keratolinin, loricrin and transglutaminase activity. *J. Invest. Dermatol.* 96: 542A.

39 Akiyama, M., Smith, L.T., Yoneda, K. et al. (1997). Expression of transglutaminase 1 (TG1) and cornified cell envelope (CCE) proteins during human epidermal development. *J. Invest. Dermatol.* 108: 598. (Abstract).

40 Dabelsteen, E., Holbrook, K.A., Clausen, H. et al. (1986). Cell surface carbohydrate changes during embryonic and fetal skin development. *J. Invest. Dermatol.* 87: 81–85.

41 Watt, F.M., Keeble, S., Fisher, C. et al. (1989). Onset of expression of peanut lectin binding glycoproteins is correlated with stratification of keratinocytes during human epidermal development in vivo and in vitro. *J. Cell Sci.* 94: 355–359.

42 Nanney, L.B., Stoscheck, C.M., King, L.E. et al. (1990). Immunolocalization of epidermal growth factor receptors in normal developing human skin. *J. Invest. Dermatol.* 94: 742–748.

43 Bickenbach, J.R. and Holbrook, K.A. (1986). Label retaining cells (LRCs) in human embryonic and fetal epidermis. *J. Invest. Dermatol.* 88: 42–46.

44 Bickenbach, J.R. and Holbrook, K.A. (1986). Proliferation of human embryonic and fetal epidermal cells in organ culture. *Am. J. Anat.* 177: 97–106.

45 Holbrook, K.A., Underwood, R.A., Vogel, A.M. et al. (1989). The appearance, density and distribution of melanocytes in human embryonic and fetal skin revealed by the anti-melanoma monoclonal antibody, HMB-45. *Anat. Embryol.* 180: 443–455.

46 Drijkoningen, M., DeWolf-Peeters, C., VanDerSteen, K. et al. (1987). Epidermal Langerhans cells and dermal dendritic cells in human fetal and neonatal skin: an immunohistochemical study. *Pediatr. Dermatol.* 4: 11–17.

47 Narisawa, Y., Hashimoto, K., and Pietruk, T. (1992). Biological significance of dermal Merkel cells in development of cutaneous nerves in human fetal skin. *J. Histochem. Cytochem.* 40: 65–71.

48 Deutsch, T.A. and Esterly, N.B. (1975). Elastic fibers in fetal dermis. *J. Invest. Dermatol.* 65: 320–323.

49 Lane, A.T., Helm, H.F., and Goldsmith, L.A. (1985). Identification of bullous pemphigoid, pemphigus, laminin and anchoring fibril antigens in human fetal skin. *J. Invest. Dermatol.* 84: 27–30.

50 Paus, R., Rosenbach, T., Haas, N. et al. (1993). Patterns of cell death: the significance of apoptosis for dermatology. *Exp. Dermatol.* 2: 3–11.

51 Riddle, C.V. (1985). Intramembrane response to cAMP in fetal epidermis. *Cell Tissue Res.* 241: 687–689.

52 Koren, G. (1995). Fetal toxicology of environmental tobacco smoke. *Curr. Opin. Pediatr.* 7: 128–131.

53 Pinkus, H. (1958). Embryology of hair. In: *The Hair Growth* (ed. W. Montagna and R.A. Ellis), 1–32. New York: Academic Press.

54 Metze, D., Bhardwaj, R., Amann, U. et al. (1966). Glycoproteins of the carcinoembryonic antigen (CEA) family are expressed in sweat and sebaceous glands of human fetal and adult skin. *J. Invest. Dermatol.* 106: 64–69.

55 Moll, I. and Moll, R. (1992). Changes of expression on intermediate filament proteins during ontogenesis of eccrine sweat glands. *J. Invest. Dermatol.* 98: 777–785.

56 Kaplan, E.D. and Holbrock, K.A. (1994). Dynamic expression patterns of tenascin, proteoglycans and cell adhesion molecules during human hair follicle morphogenesis. *Dev. Dyn.* 199: 141–155.

57 McGrath, J.A., Eady, R.A.J., and Pope, F.M. (2004). Anatomy and organization of human skin. In: *Rook's Textbook of Dermatology*, 7e (ed. T. Burns, S. Breathnach, N. Cox, et al.). Oxford: Blackwell Publishing.

58 Koster, M.I., Loomis, C.A., Koss, T., and Chu, D. (2012). Skin development and maintenance. In: *Dermatology*, 3e (ed. J.L. Bolognia, J.L. Jorizzo and J.V. Schaffer). Philadelphia, PA: Saunders-Elsevier.

59 Hashimoto, K. (1970). The ultrastructure of the skin of human embryos. VII. Formation of the apocrine gland. *Acta Dermatovenerol.* 50: 241–251.

2

Basic Structure and Function of the Neonatal, Infantile, and Childhood Skin

Nawaf Almutairi

Faculty of Medicine, Department of Medicine, Dermatology Unit, Kuwait University, Kuwait City, Kuwait

2.1 Introduction

Healthy skin of a child is often described as soft, supple and flawless; an ideal state aspired by adults too. At the same time it is also fragile and sensitive, rendering it prone to many dermatitides and infections. Skin being the largest organ of the body fulfills various vital functions. It serves as physical and immunological protection from harmful environmental elements including micro-organisms, ultraviolet radiation, humidity and temperature extremes; sensory perception of pain temperature and touch; water and electrolyte homeostasis; thermoregulation, metabolism, innate immunity communication and identification. These roles of the skin remain fundamentally the same throughout life, but there are several structural differences between the skin of a baby and that of an adult that help to explain the functional differences. In this chapter we discuss the unique structure, function and composition of pediatric skin in the three stages of neonatal, infantile and childhood skin to understand the various dermatological diseases affecting the pediatric population.

2.2 Neonatal Skin

2.2.1 Development

Skin development starts in utero from ectoderm during the first trimester of pregnancy. It achieves some function of maturation of the stratum corneum (SC) at around 24 weeks of gestation although it is not obviously visible before 34 weeks. As part of the barrier's maturation during the third trimester, the vernix caseosa forms a protective coating of the skin, derived from sebaceous secretions and dead corneocytes, composed mainly of water, lipids and proteins. Histologically epidermal maturation is considered largely complete before term, but full-term infants are not equipped with a fully mature skin at birth – for example neither sebaceous nor sweat glands are functioning maturely at term [1].

2.2.2 Adaptation at Birth

The time of birth marks a significant change for skin of the newborn as it transits from the warm, aqueous and mostly sterile intrauterine environment to a gaseous, cooler, arid and

Pediatric Dermatologic Surgery, First Edition. Edited by Keyvan Nouri, Latanya Benjamin, Jasem Alshaiji, and Jan Izakovic.

variable extrauterine environment with constant microbial interaction. To adapt to this environment the neonatal skin undergoes reduction in permeability to water measured as transepidermal water loss (TEWL) and skin pH and increase in its water content [2]. Sebaceous activity may still be present in neonates under the influence of maternal hormones but reduces drastically beyond the first few weeks of life.

2.2.3 Structure and Composition

Skin (Figure 2.1) is a dynamic tissue, engaged in a continuous process of keratinocyte proliferation in the basal layer of the epidermis and desquamation of corneocytes on the outermost layer of the epidermis, the SC (Figure 2.2). The organization of the SC has been illustrated as a brick and mortar model, with corneocytes representing the bricks embedded in the intercellular lipid matrix as the mortar [3]. Recent technical innovations like non-invasive *in vivo* techniques, such as evaporimetry, electrical impedance measurement, *in vivo* video and confocal microscopy and *in vivo* fiber-optic based spectroscopy have enlightened the field of *in vivo* infant skin physiology research.

Skin becomes functional and develops a protective barrier during late fetal period of 20 weeks to birth. As gestation increases, the number of cell layers of the epidermis and its thickness increase. Formation of an increasingly undulated dermoepidermal junction takes place and a histologically well-developed epidermis emerges at 34 weeks of gestation. The epidermal thickness of full-term neonates at birth is $43 \pm 7\,\mu m$ versus $31 \pm 7\,\mu m$ for preterm infant (24–30 weeks of gestation) [4]. The epidermis of full-term neonates at birth has been found to have 4.3 ± 0.7 cell layers, vertically stacked from the basal layer to the stratum granulosum, whereas the preterm neonates have only 2.9 ± 0.5 cell layers [4]. The suprapapillary epidermis and the SC has been found to be on average 20 and 30% thinner in infants than in adults.

2.2.4 Function

SC, the top layer of the epidermis, plays a vital role in skin barrier function. Skin barrier function is critical for the survival and preventing percutaneous entry of bacteria and other pathogens into neonatal skin. The skin barrier is competent at birth in healthy, full-term neonates

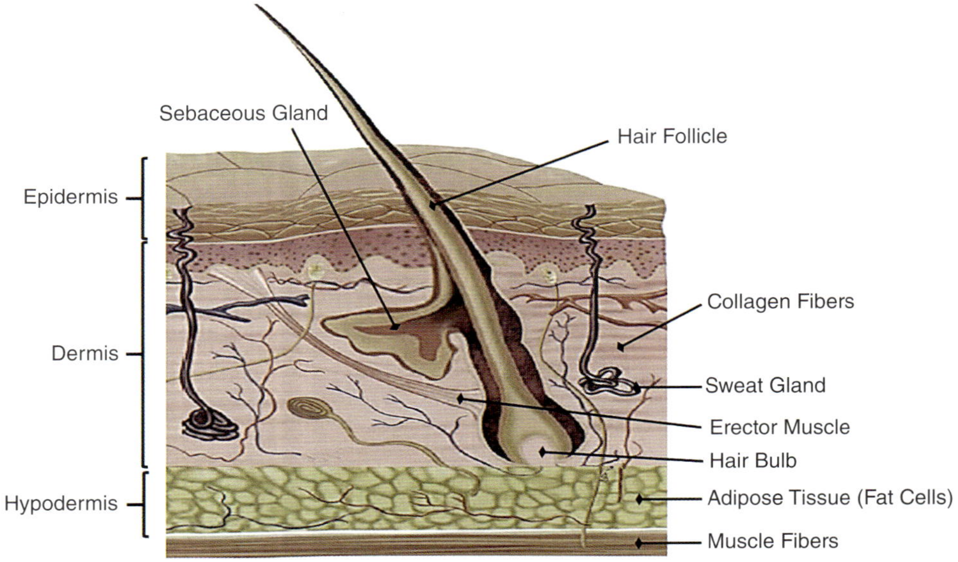

Figure 2.1 Structure of the skin.

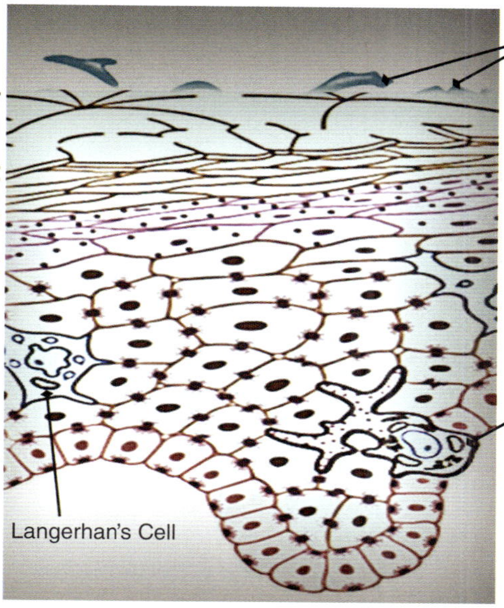

Figure 2.2 Layers of the epidermis.

to prevent organ dehydration, and their epidermis appears to be fully differentiated as compared to preterm infants, who have underdeveloped skin barrier. Newborn skin is drier and rougher because of lower skin surface hydration and increased water loss compared to older infants, in whom skin becomes considerably more hydrated and hence smoothens, especially during the first months of life.

The small corneocytes and relatively thin SC of neonates result in a weaker SC barrier compared to adults. Water loss through the neonatal skin contributes to their water balance. TEWL, considered a surrogate marker for the skin barrier, is higher in preterm infants compared to full term. The water-handling properties of neonatal skin are in a state of flux as the controlling mechanisms are still being developed. It is highly influenced by external parameters such as temperature, relative humidity and nutritional status at birth. These cutaneous changes on interaction with external microbial environment result in colonization of some microbial species and prohibition of others. Immediately after birth, bacterial communities on neonatal skin have been found to be undifferentiated across body sites. Firmicutes predominantly colonize the skin, with Stapholococci and Streptococci accounting for 40% of the total skin microbiome. The neonatal microbiome is unstable and evolves subsequently, giving an opportunity for aberrant development if the normal establishment of commensal microbiota goes awry. Early microbial colonization is expected to influence the evolution of infant skin microbiome during the first few years of life, which plays a role in skin barrier function and serves as a sentinel of innate immune defense.

2.3 Infantile Skin

Skin continues to mature after birth to adapt from life inside the womb to the terrestrial environment outside. Infant skin continues to mature through at least the first year of life. During this time of development the infantile skin differs from the adult skin in structure, function and biochemical composition (Table 2.1).

Table 2.1 Structure, composition and function of infantile skin.

Skin parameters	**Infantile skin**
Skin structure	
Cell Size – Corneocytes	Smaller
• Granular keratinocytes	Smaller
Cell density	Cells more densely packed
Skin thickness	
• SC	30% thinner
• Epidermis	20% thinner
Skin surface	
• Microrelief network	denser
• Glyphics	Smaller, rounder, plump
Dermis	
• Dermal papillae	More homogenous
• Collagen fibers	Less dense, less thick
• Transition	Gradual transition between papillary and reticular dermis
• Rete ridges	Undulations increased at dermo-epidermal junction
Skin composition	
Water content	Lower at birth (dry rough skin) Higher in older infants (smooth, hydrated skin)
NMF	Lower concentration
Melanin	Lower concentration
Skin Function	
Skin barrier function	Mature but weaker
TEWL	Lower at birth Variable in infancy
Water absorption	Higher
Water holding	Lower
Skin pH	Alkaline to neutral at birth Decreases during first 2 weeks of life Higher than adults during infancy
Cell proliferation	Higher proliferation and desquamation rate High cell turnover rate
Skin microbiome	Unstable Firmicutes predominate Site-specific evolution by 3 months of infancy

2.3.1 Infant Skin Structure

Corneocytes from the SC and keratinocytes of the granular layer in infants have smaller projected cell size, by 20 and 10% respectively as compared to adults. This is due to higher epidermal proliferation rate in infants, confirmed by using an intrinsic fluorescence marker of epidermal cell proliferation. This high cell turnover rate of infantile skin progressively decreases during the first year of life. SC thickness ranges from 5.6 to 35.4 µm for infants as compared to 15.2–35.4 µm for adults [2]. Infantile SC was found to be 30% thinner and infantile epidermis 20% thinner than in adults. This implies that the brick size as well as thickness of the wall is less in infants, according to the brick and mortar analogy. In contrast, infant corneocytes have been found to be thicker in height than adults.

The network of microrelief lines is denser and the intra-relief structures (glyphics) of the SC are smaller, though more rounded and plump in infants. The surface glyphics are matched one to one with the underlying dermal papillae, collagen structure containing nerve endings and capillary vessels at the dermo-epidermal junction, indicating a single structural unit relationship [5]. Thus there is a structural relationship between dermal papillae at the bottom of the epidermis and skin surface glyphics in infants which disappears later in life, pointing to the presence of a possible common precursor proliferative unit at the basal layer. The dermal papillae in infants are also more homogeneous in size, density and distribution than in adults, in whom they vary in size and are more irregular in shape. Morphologically there is increased epidermal cellularity and undulation of the rete ridges at dermo-epidermal junction in infants. The collagen fibers in the upper part of dermis in infants are less dense and not as thick as seen in adults. The transition between papillary and reticular dermis is more gradual and less clear in infants than in adults [6]. Thus infantile skin structure differs in cell size, epidermal and SC layer thickness, microglyph density, dermal structure and density of papillae.

2.3.2 Infant Skin Composition

Skin composition affects its barrier function against harmful substances, against water loss and its regenerative capacity in an interdependent manner. Water content of SC enables enzymatic activities leading to corneodesmolysis, lipid processing, and production of natural moisturizing factor (NMF). In response, corneodesmolysis by shedding outer skin layers maintains optimal hydration level, provided by the NMF and by the permeability barrier constituted by intercellular lamellar lipids. NMF acts as a humectant, with a role in water retention and moisturization. It is formed during the corneocyte maturation process from filaggrin proteolyzed into amino acids and other derivatives.

NMF concentration is significantly lower in infantile skin, affecting its water-handling properties. Skin hydration significantly increases during the first few months of infant, who were born with relatively dry skin. Infantile skin has higher water concentration on the skin surface as well as till the depth of outermost 26 µm, as assessed by Raman confocal spectroscopy [7]. Apart from increasing functional maturity of eccrine sweat glands, many other factors contribute to the reversal of SC hydration between infant and adult during the first few months of life, turning the rough and dry skin of newborn into a smooth hydrated skin of infant. Water content within the SC has a profound effect on its desquamation, epidermal expression of keratins and cornified envelope proteins in addition to skin surface morphology.

The skin water-handling process undergoes a maturation process over the first year of life, presenting a distinct local micro-environment in infants leading to differences in their skin microbiome. Infants are colonized predominantly by Firmicutes, followed in abundance by Actinobacteria, Proteobacteria, and Bacteriodetes [8]. Buttocks of infant have higher levels of clostridia, although the arm, and forehead show higher levels of the Bacilli class of Firmicutes. The forehead of infants has higher levels of the Actinobacteria, as seen in adult sebaceous sites [9]. Such site-specific evolution of skin microbiome appears to begin within the first three months of life. In contrast to an established and maintained adult skin microbiome, microflora of infants shows a measured increase in population evenness with age. This, coupled with site-specific evolution of microflora in infants, indicates that the infant skin microbiome is unstable. This instability may present the opportunity for infection and dermatitides if normal establishment of commensal microbiota goes awry. Evolution of the human skin microbiome during the first years of life also serves as a sentinel of innate immune defense.

The surface of infant skin contains significantly lower total lipids and lower sebum levels compared to adults. These reduced lipid levels on the infant skin contribute to the barrier function being not yet fully mature. Despite this impairment, the infantile skin is unique in having high water content compared to adult skin.

Infants have significantly lower concentration of melanin compared to adults in body sites exposed to the sun. Lower melanin concentration and thinner SC of the infantile skin, along with its increased SC hydration, lead to reduced light scattering by it, resulting in its increased sensitivity to the harmful effects of UV light. Increase in melanin concentration in sun-exposed skin of infants in the first year of exposure has been shown to follow UV-induced DNA damage [10]. Hence, sun exposure during infancy may contribute to cumulative effect and skin damage of UV light.

2.4 Infant Skin Function

Mature skin functions as a protective physical barrier as well as regulating biochemical processes within the epidermis by controlling hydration, water evaporation, pH, cell proliferation, and acting as a sentinel of innate immunity. The age at which functional maturity is attained may be different for each of these parameters.

2.4.1 Skin Barrier Function

Skin barrier function resides primarily within the SC, the top layer of the epidermis, but it also depends on other factors such as lipid organization, hydration level, SC structure, and hygroscopic properties. Although skin barrier is competent at birth in a healthy, full-term neonate, it is weaker compared to adults due to small corneocytes, relatively thin SC and lower levels of NMF in infants [11].

2.4.2 Water-Handling Properties

The most widely assessed infant skin parameter is TEWL, which is measured as the loss of water other than the sweat from the body via the epidermis. TEWL is higher in infants compared to adults, indicating a weak infantile skin barrier. The dynamics of water handling in an infant are still unstable as the controlling mechanisms are still being developed. By water sorption–desorption test, the infantile skin absorbs larger amounts of water and loses it more rapidly than adults during first 45 seconds after blotting [7]. This increased water absorption is accompanied by significantly higher water concentration in the top layers of the SC. The high desorption rate in infants is possibly related to the limited amount of NMF, which is crucial for binding and retaining water. Both skin hydration and TEWL values are highly variable in infants compared to children or adults, indicative of a fluctuating barrier function [7].

2.4.3 Skin pH

Skin pH in infants continues to decrease from near alkaline to neutral pH at birth to an acidic pH during the first month of life and then remains stable until three months. Despite this decrease, skin pH remains significantly higher throughout infancy compared to adults who have more acidic skin with pH in range of 4.5–6.7. In particular, the occlusive and humid environment of the diapered infantile skin, which is exposed to the activity of fecal enzymes, has higher pH. Skin pH plays a role in maintaining epidermal permeability barrier, the desquamation process and bacterial proliferation on the skin. Hence the near-neutral pH of infantile skin in diapered area can make it prone to skin irritation and secondary microbial invasion. Once the skin barrier is disrupted, infantile skin is possibly less able to promote skin repair.

2.4.4 Immune Regulation

Changes in skin barrier and water-handling functions together with high rates of surface expansion and epidermal cell proliferation continue throughout the infantile years. As the infant skin microbiome evolves, site-specific diversity and the relative abundance of the community (evenness) significantly increase over the first year of age. The skin barrier prevents percutaneous entry of pathogens into infantile skin. Keratinocytes produce antimicrobial peptides (AMPs) including human β-defensins 1–3 and cathelicidin-derived peptide. If the skin barrier is disturbed in the absence of AMPs, pathogenic microorganisms will gain access to living epidermal keratinocytes and can induce defensive immune responses. If overcome, this can lead to infection, or an imbalance of commensal flora versus pathogenic bacteria. Hence, development of skin innate immunity during the first years of life is another fascinating aspect of skin function.

2.4.5 Cell Proliferation

Keratinocyte proliferation rates at the basal layers of the epidermis and corneocyte desquamation on the outermost surface are balanced over the long term to ensure constant thickness of the skin. Epidermal cell turnover in healthy skin is linked to proliferation and desquamation rate, as an imbalance would lead to thinning or thickening of SC. The desquamation rate has been found to vary depending on the anatomical site during the first three months of life. While the facial and forearm area of an infant shows a significant increase, the buttocks area showed a significant decrease in desquamation rate. It can be due to an elevated hydration in buttocks area because of the occlusive environment. Epidermal cell proliferation decreases rapidly during the first year of life and reaches adult levels during the second year of life. This higher cell proliferation rate in infants explains the smaller cell size and higher cell density observed in this age group.

2.5 Childhood and Adolescent Skin

Progression from infancy to adulthood encompasses major biological changes with significant physiologic and endocrinologic skin alterations occurring during childhood and adolescence. Skin continues to undergo a maturation-dependent shift in structure, composition and function as the child steps into the stage of sexual maturation.

2.5.1 Structure and Composition

In a young child the skin structural parameters such as skin thickness, cell size, density, microrelief network, glyphics and dermis continue to gradually mature to reach the adult size and composition. The corneocytes in adolescents are larger than children and skin turnover is less frequent. Their skin still contains abundance of elastin and collagen in the dermis, giving it flexibility and suppleness.

The human body grows faster during puberty than at any other time – except for infancy. Major skin structural changes occur during puberty. Body hairs increase in density and thickness. Development of the sebaceous glands is closely linked to hair follicles and the epidermis. Although their number remains approximately the same throughout life, their size tends to increase with age. Sebum secretion, which peaked during the first week after birth and then subsided, takes a new rise at about 9 years with adrenarche and continues up to age 17 years, when the adult level is reached [12]. Apart from androgens and other hormonal influences, terminal sebocytes differentiation is assisted by peroxisomes proliferator-activated receptor ligands. Maturation of sebaceous glands and sebum secretions in early childhood may progress asynchronously across body sites. It occurs the earliest at typically sebaceous and proximal skin regions, including the face, back and chest. Transition into a more lipophilic microbiome at distal and less characteristically sebaceous regions may be delayed. Physiologically, Tanner stage 4 and 5 children closely resemble adults in terms of sebum production and skin surface lipids in the face. Even though Tanner stages 2 and 3 are considered early stages of puberty, their skin-surface lipids and microbial flora still trend more toward Tanner stage 1.

Sebaceous lipids are responsible for the three-dimensional skin surface lipid organization, contributing to the integrity of the skin barrier. They also exhibit strong innate antimicrobial activity, transport antioxidants to the skin surface and express pro-inflammatory and anti-inflammatory properties. Metabolism of these increased epidermal lipids reduces skin pH, which in turn modulates the skin microbiome in adolescents. During puberty there is also increased apocrine gland activity, especially in the pubic area and axillae, contributing to changes in microbial flora in these areas, leading to an altered body odor. On the other hand, areas such as toe webs which lack apocrine glands and hence fatty acids secretions but produce a lot of sweat due to abundant eccrine glands become prone to maceration and infection.

Significant shifts in the microbiota occur with progressive sexual maturation, influencing the host-microbiome relationship. Shifts in bacterial communities can enhance or impair their pathogenicity and may have significant implications regarding prevention and treatment of pediatric disorders involving microbial pathogens and colonization. Julia et al. [13] observed that a greater diversity of bacteria, like Streptococcus and gram-negative Moraxella, Haemophilus and Neisseria, dominated the microbiomes of Tanner stage 1 children. In contrast, lipophilic bacteria including Propionibacterium, Corynebacterium and Turicella, associated with sebaceous skin regions, dominated Tanner stage 4 and 5 individuals, without any significant gender-related differences. They found these dramatic differences in the skin and nares microbiomes, suggesting that even modest increase in lipid production during puberty may be sufficient to alter microbiome colonization and composition. It is particularly striking in the nares, which contributes to the age-related reduction in incidence and severity of the skin disorders that dominate during pediatric age.

Immune components in skin are less mature in younger children and may permit the colonization and growth of a wider range of bacteria. This microbial diversity decreases with increasing sexual maturity in adolescents, leading to a more stable and less diverse microbiome with increased colonization by diphtheroids in mature individuals. These evolutionary host-microbiome interactions may reduce the ability to harbor potential pathogens upon reaching reproductive age, relevant to significant differences in infections and inflammatory skin diseases between children and adults.

2.5.2 Function

The unique properties of skin in young children make them vulnerable to an increased risk of xerosis, atopic dermatitis, and UVR damage. Sun-protective measures, emollient use and pharmaco-cosmetic products should be stratified according to relevant setting and ethnicity of child, to maintain a healthy skin which is still tender.

During adolescence the skin thickens and toughens, imparting its resilience and maturity to protect from environmental agents such as invading microorganisms, chemicals and physical injury. In the process of sexual maturation, with an increase in body hair at different sites, sebum and apocrine secretions and significant physical changes in their body structure, adolescents experience a highly dynamic perception of body image. They become prone to disorders associated with these pubertal changes influencing their skin and its appendages. They also become more vigilant of their skin and associated diseases which, if present, significantly affect their psycho-social well-being. The health of their skin and hair influence their self-evaluated and externally evaluated standards of attractiveness and appearance, which in turn powerfully influence their self-esteem.

2.6 Conclusion

The structure, composition and function of skin undergo dynamic changes after birth, which continue into infancy. Passing through childhood, as the adolescent skin matures into adult skin it is further influenced by various hormonal and environmental factors. Knowledge of the basics of these structural and functional mechanisms will help to develop a better understanding of diseases and pathology of pediatric skin discussed further in the book.

References

1 Agache, P.B.D., Barrand, C., and Laurent, R. (1980). Sebum levels during the first year of life. *The British Journal of Dermatology* 103 (6): 643–649.

2 Chiou, Y.B. and Blume-Peytavi, U. (2004). Stratum corneum maturation. A review of neonatal skin function. *Skin Pharmacology and Physiology* 17 (2): 57–66.

3 Nemes, Z. and Steinert, P.M. (1999). Bricks and mortar of the epidermal barrier. *Experimental & Molecular Medicine* 31 (1): 5–19.

4 Evans, N.J. and Rutter, N. (1986). Development of the epidermis in the newborn. *Biology of the Neonate* 49 (2): 74–80.

5 Stamatas, G.N., Nikolovski, J., Luedtke, M.A. et al. (2010). Infant skin microstructure assessed in vivo differs from adult skin in organization and at the cellular level. *Pediatric Dermatology* 27 (2): 125–131.

6 Stamatas, G.N., Nikolovski, J., Mack, M.C. et al. (2011). Infant skin physiology and development during the first years of life: a review of recent findings based on in vivo studies. *International Journal of Cosmetic Science* 33 (1): 17–24.

7 Nikolovski, J., Stamatas, G.N., Kollias, N. et al. (2008). Barrier function and water-holding and transport properties of infant stratum corneum are different from adult and continue to develop through the first year of life. *The Journal of Investigative Dermatology* 128 (7): 1728–1736.

8 Capone, K.A., Dowd, S.E., Stamatas, G.N. et al. (2011). Diversity of the human skin microbiome early in life. *Journal of Investigative Dermatology* 131: 2026–2032.

9 Grice, E.A., Kong, H.H., Conlan, S. et al. (2009). Topographical and temporal diversity of the human skin microbiome. *Science* 324: 1190–1192.

10 Paller, A.S., Hawk, J.L., Honig, P. et al. (2011). New insights about infant and toddler skin: implications for sun protection. *Pediatrics* 128: 92–102.

11 Telofski, L.S., Morello, A.P. 3rd, Mack Correa, M.C. et al. (2012). The infant skin barrier: can we preserve, protect and enhance the barrier? Dermatology Research and Practice 198789. https://doi.org/10.1155/2012/198789.

12 Zouboulis, C.C. (2004). Acne and sebaceous gland function. *Clinics in Dermatology* 22 (5): 360–366.

13 Julia, O., Conlan, S., Polley, E.C. et al. (2012). Shifts in human skin and nares microbiota of healthy children. *Genome Medicine* 4: 77.

3

Approach to the Child as a Patient

Nawaf Almutairi

Faculty of Medicine, Department of Medicine, Dermatology Unit, Kuwait University, Kuwait City, Kuwait

3.1 Introduction

As is commonly said, "Pediatric cases are not just miniature adults." Hence, the examination of a child is also somewhat different from examining an adult. The pediatric examination is not as methodical and chronological as is seen in adult examination [1]. Pediatric patients have their own specific needs, which must be met by the attending physician. Also, there are many obvious differential features that make it necessary for the physicians to develop certain skills while dealing with kids because it is often difficult to follow a particular protocol. Also, a lot depends upon the mood of the child, their general health, and whether they are sleeping or awake and so on. We would suggest a few small but very important steps to make the child skin examination look like a "child's play" when otherwise it could seem like a daunting task.

3.2 Initial Consultation

One major difference between a pediatric dermatology consultation and an adult dermatology consultation is that a child is almost always accompanied by one or more parents. Parents are usually very much concerned about their child's skin problem, and thus a physician must respect the parental perception [2], and should try to correct any wrong ideas or misinformation they may be carrying very tactfully.

The examining physician should be well trained to establish a high level of confidence, both with the patient and also with the accompanying parents. He needs to exercise a higher degree of patience and be more sympathetic toward the attitudes of the patient as well as the parents. A friendly attitude, a little bit of trickery, and a lot of appreciation can make a huge difference in building trust with the patient, and thus accomplishing the goal with ease. Establishing trust early on is important, because for kids there is usually a very fine line separating fear from cooperation.

The attention span of a child is highly variable. However, in almost all the cases it is much shorter than that usually seen in adults. Also, the end of examination is almost always decided by the child. It would be very rare for the attending physician to complete the examination.

Hence, the examining physician has to be very quick, and try to collect the most important information needed to establish the further line of management.

The pediatric skin examination may not follow a predictable pattern, with lots depending upon the mood of the child. Hence the physician needs to be highly

Pediatric Dermatologic Surgery, First Edition. Edited by Keyvan Nouri, Latanya Benjamin, Jasem Alshaiji, and Jan Izakovic.

adaptable to the need of the hour and act accordingly, rather than sticking to a fixed, predetermined protocol.

The ambience of the consultation chamber goes a long way to allay the fears of the child. It should be well-lit, and be made as colorful as possible, with colorful toys and other gadgets to keep the child busy. The attending physician can also whistle, make funny noises, and frequently call the child by name during the examination, and use age-specific vocabulary to make sure that the child is having fun and continues to cooperate during the examination.

Before starting a skin examination, it is important to obtain a written consent from the parent. It is particularly important that the physician understands that although a grandparent or other relative bringing the child might well know the parents' views on the matter, and be happy to consent on their behalf, this is not acceptable legally as consent must be from someone with parental responsibility. Finally, it is important to remember that consent on one occasion does not imply consent on all occasions. The parents' and child's views can change over time.

3.3 Establishing a Correct Diagnosis

Accurate history, detailed examination, and bedside/laboratory examination are the three main pillars of making the correct diagnosis in any clinical discipline. All three of them may not be needed at all times. Having even one or two of them in any combination may sometimes be sufficient to make a diagnosis.

Unlike other specialties, as a dermatologist we are lucky to be able to have a thorough look at the target organ, i.e. skin, with most the skin lesions being visible to the naked eye. Hence, a complete and detailed skin examination including nails, hairs, and mucosa becomes much more important.

First, and foremost is the observation regarding the individual lesion, which in my view holds the greatest significance. It includes the morphology of the primary skin lesions, their pattern of arrangement and distribution. This in most cases helps to arrive at a suspected diagnosis. If not, it at least helps to generate a list of differentials. This list can then be narrowed down with the help of investigations or a therapeutic drug trial in most cases. However, when dealing with kids in most cases every effort has to be made to make use of non-invasive or at the most minimally invasive tests to arrive at a diagnosis, and to avoid invasive investigative procedures unless there is no other way to arrive at a conclusion.

However, for proper diagnosis and management, a complete clinical history is also important, though it may not be as significant as the clinical examination for arriving at the correct diagnosis as far as our specialty is concerned. Nevertheless, its importance cannot be discounted and it should be given comparable time and attention. The clinical history can be obtained before the dermatologic examination, as seen in other disciplines. Alternatively, the child's skin can be examined first, before taking the history. The latter method has an advantage of allowing specific and direct questions pertaining to the case to be asked, thus saving time by not asking about history not relevant to the particular case.

Pediatric dermatology deals with skin diseases and skin care requirements in patients from birth to adolescence. Although this is a relatively short period in the lifetime of an individual, it is associated with significant physiological, psychological and maturity changes that occur at a fast pace. Also, the picture of skin lesions changes may not only be because of its own age, but some of it may be associated to comparable growing size of the skin and also the pubertal changes going on in the skin. Thus, it is advisable to obtain clinical pictures of the lesions in as many cases as possible, after obtaining written informed consent from the accompanying parent. Parents must be informed about the importance of pictures in monitoring of the response during follow-up visits, as well as for teaching [3].

3.3.1 Neonatal Period

Since the skin of the child is constantly evolving, there are specific physiological and pathological events characteristic of each age group, which the attending physician has to be careful about. For example, the first month of life (neonatal period) is associated with certain transient benign skin conditions that never recur again during lifetime, such as neonatal cephalic pustulosis, sebaceous hyperplasia, and erythema toxicum neonatorum. In others, the neonatal skin may have certain significant pathological conditions including the diseases transmitted *in utero* or during delivery by mothers, like neonatal lupus erythematosus or neonatal pemphigus or infections like herpes, etc. Also, many genetic and developmental skin diseases can be seen during this period like epidermolysis bullosa, keratinization disorders, or vascular malformations or other birthmarks. Examining these cases is relatively easy, because most of the time the child is sleeping. Also, even if awake they do not develop stranger anxiety before the age of 8–10 months.

3.3.2 Infancy Period

After initial one month and up till the age of one year, the child undergoes significant physical, intellectual, socio-emotional, and motor development. During this period eczema is the most significant skin problem, especially atopic dermatitis. Diaper dermatitis with or without superadded Candida infection is also commonly encountered in this age group.

Also, during this period the kid is now prone to develop infectious conditions, because of fading levels of protective maternal antibodies after six months of age. The examination of these children is expected to be difficult due to growing stranger anxiety.

3.3.3 Childhood Period

During this stage atopic dermatitis is the most common dermatosis. Also, direct contact with other individuals and animals increases the risk of infections like warts, chickenpox, molluscum, tinea capitis, and pediculosis. Playing in open spaces also makes them more amenable to insect bites and photo-induced dermatosis. It is during this stage that specific dermatosis like vitiligo, psoriasis, and alopecia areata appear for the first time. At this age children have their own individual temperament, which, apart from being influenced by their social upbringing and level of education, is also based upon their previous experiences with doctors. It may help the physician to get better cooperation from the child if they engage them with direct questions. It is better to discuss and explain to the child properly, before performing any painful diagnostic or therapeutic procedure. During the consultation, the physician should intermittently encourage the child, and reward them for cooperation. Preschool and young school children are the most difficult to handle in terms of doing a medical procedure, so every care has to be taken by the physician in trust building, before moving on to the actual procedure.

3.3.4 Adolescence Period

During this stage the child experiences unparalleled growth in terms of the physical development. Also, changing hormonal levels associated with puberty lead to development of secondary sexual characteristics. These anatomic and physiological changes result in the occurrence of new skin diseases like acne and seborrheic dermatitis. Also, some infections like pityriasis versicolor, tinea pedis, onychomycosis and genodermatosis like Darier's disease are seen for the first time during this period. These children are also vulnerable to getting sexually transmitted diseases, because of their uncaring attitude and curiosity to experiment. The handling of these children is a little tricky at this stage. Not only do they have difficulty finding a good way to communicate their problems to the examining physicians, but at times parents may also add to the already complicated relationship by trying to influence some decisions or by criticizing their kids. Still worse, some parents may attribute their skin conditions to their behavior. Under these circumstances, the examining physician has to carefully balance their approach so as not to hurt the feelings of either of them. It is also important for the physician to sympathize and listen to the concerns of these teenagers, assuring them of full confidentiality and treating them as a free-thinking individuals.

The clinical examination of these young people may sometimes be difficult due to their reluctance to show certain body parts like genitalia. The physician should maintain deep respect for their feeling of shyness and shame.

3.4 Parent Education About the Nature of Skin Lesion

Most children, including some adolescents, are dependent on parents for most of their day-to-day activities, and are unable to take decisions on their own. They are highly unlikely to adhere to the physician's recommendations regarding management of their skin condition, and need parental support. Hence, it is important to make the parents aware of the nature of the skin condition to ensure better skin care. Moreover, especially in the case of newborns, the parents have a set of expectations for their unborn child regarding their skin and health in general. So, any aberrations in child's skin can cause anxiety and feelings of guilt in parents. They blame themselves for being responsible for the child's condition, and thus need to be provided with enough information about the actual cause of the condition and its likely future course. If the skin condition is infectious in nature, the source of infection has to be explained to the parents to prevent recurrence and also to prevent its spread to other family members, for example in cases of tinea capitis caused by pets, warts spread due to sharing of personal items, pediculosis from other siblings or schoolmates, and scabies due to close contacts. Also, in cases of certain inherited genetic disorders with one or both parents as silent carriers, proper counseling and prenatal testing can be of great help in preventing them from having another child with a similar skin condition in future. Other skin conditions like atopic eczema may not have a causative agent but do have multiple aggravating factors. Thus, informing the parents about these factors can go a long way to help to at least minimize recurrences, if not preventing them altogether.

3.5 Discussing Any Necessary Further Evaluations

Although in a large majority of cases the attending physicians are able to make a working clinical diagnosis with the help only of appropriate history and detailed clinical examination, there are few cases (about 20%) which require further evaluation to come to a fruitful conclusion to decide a further course of action. Depending upon the skin condition, these evaluations could be blood sampling, KOH scrapping, hair shaft examination, Wood's lamp examination, dermoscopy, patch testing, photo testing, radiological investigations, or even a skin biopsy. These evaluating tests are generally required to pinpoint the diagnosis of the skin lesion, to determine the internal involvement, to confirm or rule out the skin lesions as a sign of internal disease, or to obtain a baseline level for further evaluation. The attending physician should make the parents aware of any such requirement during the course of initial consultation, in the course of which the parents should be given full details of the procedures (including complications, if any), the reason for doing them, and also the likely benefits. This would help in allaying any fear and/or apprehension in the mind of the parent, and thus will make them more cooperative during the evaluation. This is also a mandatory legal requirement to obtain their consent before undertaking any procedure, and should be strictly followed to avoid any medico-legal issues in future.

3.6 Discussion of Different Treatment Modalities

Once the diagnosis of the skin condition has been established, depending upon the disease the treatment could vary from just observation (in cases of self-healing/transient dermatosis) to surgical excision (in cases of suspected melanoma/tumor). However, at times the physician has multiple treatment modalities to offer for same skin condition. For example, in cases of warts the treatment modalities could include topical drugs like salicylic acid preparations, cryotherapy, electrocautery, laser ablation, or surgical excision. Keeping in mind the age of the child, the number and location of lesions, and the availability of time, money and resources, the physician could suggest a particular modality to the parents. However, this has to be done after the parents have been made aware of the details of all the possible modalities along with their potential benefits and risks. The final decision to choose the modality should rest with the parents. The physician's role should be limited to explaining the details of all the modalities and suggesting what is best for the child under the given circumstances.

It needs to be emphasized here that the physician's approach to the therapy is tailored for every individual based on collective experience and available literature. However, the quantum of data available in literature for pediatric patients is meager in most situations because the majority of commercially available medications have never been studied in children, which could be for various reasons, including stricter regulatory parameters for their use with children. This is applicable more to the newer drugs being launched including biologics and other molecular products. It is for this reason that children have often been labeled as "therapeutic orphans".

3.7 Timing of Surgical Procedures

The decision regarding the timing of the surgical procedure is largely dependent on the purpose, more than anything else. If the procedure is being carried out as a diagnostic tool, it has to be done before starting the treatment. Keeping this in mind, as well as the level of anxiety of the parent and the patient, it can be done immediately after the initial consultation, or a little later. In any case, it should not be overly delayed. However, if the procedure is being considered as a therapeutic tool, that case the timing is largely determined by the type of skin lesion [4].

For therapeutic laser surgeries of vascular and pigmented lesions, the composition of many of these lesions changes as child grows, making them more resistant to laser therapy. Thus, in many cases, treating lesions at an early age results in faster clearing with less incidence of complications. For vascular lesions, the pulsed dye laser is considered the laser of choice for its efficacy and relatively low-risk profile, whereas the Q-switched pigment-specific lasers are ideal for most childhood pigmented lesions. Some issues encountered while dealing with pediatric patients include the determination of suitable anesthesia, the provision of size-appropriate safety equipment, and the assessment and management of patient and parent anxiety [5, 6].

3.8 Pediatric Procedures: Developmental Approach to Anxiety

Surgery and anesthesia are significant sources of anxiety for children. In the preoperative period, reducing anxiety helps to prevent the negative consequences that may occur after surgery. It is challenging for surgical preparation providers to recognize the major cognitive and emotional developments as children grow up, and to offer presurgical preparation in a developmentally sensitive and family-centered manner [4, 5]. We will now examine how children of different ages perceive hospitalization and surgery, and discuss how to best prepare these children for the experience [4].

3.8.1 Infants and Toddlers

During this stage, children develop relationships based on trust with their parents and other primary caregivers. They are completely dependent on them for all of their physical and emotional needs and largely demonstrate anxiety through crying. For this age group, separation from the primary caregiver is a critical issue. A surgical experience involving strangers wearing unfamiliar costumes in strange settings can be frightening to these children. It is generally believed that, since the youngest age for which preparation can be helpful is not known, any child who can comprehend spoken words should be prepared. Parents of children in this age group are critical to the preparation and can provide emotional and physical comfort and support through tone of voice and facial expression. Encouraging the caregiver to remain with the child whenever possible, including the induction of anesthesia with proper preparation, and suggesting that the adult comfortingly strokes or holds the patient helps in calming down the patient.

3.8.2 Preschool and School-Age Children

As children at this stage develop their language and social skills, they start to gain more autonomy and self-control. These children tend to be creative thinkers captivated by fantasy, and often interpret messages by integrating past experience with their imagination. These children often have misconceptions about surgery.

They commonly fear pain or mutilation as a result of the surgery, and are also anxious about separation from family and home. They may at times believe that their surgery is the result of punishment for wrongdoing, so they need a factual, understandable explanation of what caused the problem and why they are in the hospital. Photographs and other audiovisual aids are very effective in explaining the procedure to these kids. Using terms easily identified by these children helps them to better anticipate the hospital experience. It is essential that these patients be given the opportunity to act out their fears so they can be addressed directly by the team in a developmentally-appropriate manner. In general, school-aged children should receive preparation as close to the actual day of surgery as possible

3.8.3 Adolescents

Surgery or hospitalization can pose a direct challenge to adolescents' struggle for independence. They may react to being told what to wear, when to eat, or how to act by withdrawing or not cooperating with the treating physician. Also, due to increased concerns about their body image, they are often extremely worried about the resulting cosmetic effects of an operation. The treating physician should address these issues respectfully, fully acknowledging the patient's right to privacy and allowing them to exert as much independence as feasible during the hospitalization. This approach leads to a greater sense of control, and ultimately improves cooperation during procedures. Adolescents require a minimum of 7–10 days' advance preparation for the hospitalization, accompanied by a detailed explanation about their upcoming procedure.

3.9 Assessment and Management of Parental Anxiety

A surgical procedure on a child can be traumatic for the whole family. Parents are trying to cope with a disruption in their routine, as well as fears and anxieties they might have about the well-being of their child. Allowing families to actively participate in their child's preparation can enable them to master this new experience and decrease levels of stress. The health care team can provide exercises, literature, or activities that parents can share with their children. Encouraging parents to act as a liaison when relaying health care information to the child, and letting them remain with the child during procedures, are some of the ways the attending physician can enable parents to support their child.

3.10 Conclusion

Dealing with a pediatric patient is itself an art, and the treating physician has to master this art for maximum benefit, both for himself and for the patient and their family. Each stage in the pediatric age group has its own unique method of handling, whether it is a simple examination or some surgical intervention – unlike with adult patients, where the encounter with the physician is mainly the patient-doctor relationship.

In pediatric patients, there is a stakeholder in the form of parents, who have their own requirements and expectations from the treating physician, while taking care of their kids. Hence, the treating physician has to satisfy the needs of the parents, in addition to taking good care of the patient.

References

1. Irvine, A.D., Hoeger, P.H., and Yan, A.C. (eds.) (2011). *Harper's Textbook of Pediatric Dermatology, 2 Volume Set*, 3e. Oxford: Wiley-Blackwell.
2. Craze, J. and Hope, T. (2006). Teaching medical students to examine children. *Arch. Dis. Child.* 91 (12): 966–968.
3. Edward Wilson, M. (2009). The art and science of examining a child. In: *Pediatric Ophthalmology* (ed. M.E. Wilson et al.), 1–6. Berlin Heidelberg: Springer-Verlag.
4. Ahmed, M.I., Farrell, M.A., Parrish, K., and Karla, A. (2011). Preoperative anxiety in children risk factors and non-pharmacological management. *Middle East J. Anaesthesiol.* 21 (2): 153–167.
5. Panella, J.J. (2016). Preoperative care of children: strategies from a child life perspective. *AORN J.* 104 (1): 11–22.
6. Cantatore, J.L. and Kriegel, D.A. (2004). Laser surgery: an approach to the pediatric patient. *J. Am. Acad. Dermatol.* 50 (2): 165–184.

4

Preoperative and Postoperative Care of Children Undergoing Pediatric Dermatology Procedures

Alanna F. Bree

A Children's House for Pediatric Dermatology, Houston, TX, USA

4.1 Introduction

The preoperative evaluation and postoperative care of a patient undergoing a pediatric dermatologic procedure, while sometimes overlooked or considered of less importance, is vital to the outcome and success of that procedure. The preoperative evaluation is an essential time for the physician to obtain the necessary medical and developmental information to determine the best surgical plan for the individual patient to optimize the safety and final result. It is a time to fully explain the steps of the procedure and to answer questions, as well as set realistic expectations, so the patient and family can make informed decisions. It is also a time to review the necessary postoperative requirements and restrictions so that plans can be made accordingly. The preoperative evaluation is a crucial piece in the overall management of patients undergoing a pediatric dermatologic procedure and sets the stage for what is to come.

4.2 Preoperative Care

4.2.1 Approach to the Patient

As someone who cares for pediatric patients, it is imperative to remember that the patient is your primary concern. It is equally important to remember that the patient's family or caregiver is integral in the life of the patient and therefore they must be considered in the overall care of the patient and included in the discussion. It is also important to remember that children are not miniature adults and incorporating knowledge of developmental pediatrics will allow the physician to appropriately establish the surgical plan according to the needs of the individual patient based on their age and developmental status.

4.2.2 Medical Evaluation

Fortunately, most children who are undergoing a pediatric dermatologic procedure are healthy overall and have no significant medical problems, but this is not always the case. It is important to obtain a thorough history that includes all health issues, prior surgical and anesthetic history, medications, allergies and family history. Again, most children who undergo dermatologic procedures are healthy, but as the physician you do not want any unexpected surprises. A history of reactive airways or gastroesophageal reflux may alter the management by the anesthesiologist if general anesthesia is to be used. A history of attention deficit disorders or mental health issues may help determine if a patient is able to tolerate a procedure under local anesthesia or if they would be best treated under general anesthesia, and will also help determine if a

Pediatric Dermatologic Surgery, First Edition. Edited by Keyvan Nouri, Latanya Benjamin, Jasem Alshaiji, and Jan Izakovic.

preoperative anxiolytic medication may be necessary. A personal or family history of a bleeding disorder is also important to assess, and further diagnostic evaluation or treatment may be warranted before proceeding. It is also important to discuss any previous procedures or surgeries to assess how they were tolerated and if there were any complications related to the anesthesia, procedure or postoperative course. It is also important to assess any skin changes, especially keloids or scars the patient may have due to prior procedures or injuries. A history of herpes labialis is important to know in considering the need for prophylactic anti-viral medications for any laser or surgical procedures on the face. A complete medication list which includes over-the-counter medications and any supplements or herbals, as well as latex or medication allergies, is important to obtain. There are many medications and supplements which can affect bleeding and potentially impact the surgical outcome. In addition, some surgical facilities may require that a medical evaluation and clearance be obtained and documented by the patient's primary care physician before any procedures requiring general anesthesia. Most patients will not require any laboratory evaluations prior to their procedure, but some surgical centers or hospitals may require a pregnancy test for girls of child-bearing potential that is done at the facility on the day of the procedure.

4.2.3 Developmental Evaluation

Establishing an office setting that is pediatric-friendly helps both the patient and the family feel comfortable and more relaxed during the evaluation. The training of the care team with regard to appropriate interactions with infants, toddlers, children, adolescents and teens will also help make the encounter a positive one. The developmental evaluation of the patient, as well as the assessment of the patient-family interactions, begins as soon as the physician walks into the examination room. How the patient responds to the physician and family members during the initial moments of the encounter are often very telling. When evaluating and talking with the patient, it is best for the physician to be on an eye-to-eye level. If possible, it is best to leave infants on their parents' lap and to allow toddlers or young children to look at books or draw/color on the exam table during the examination. It is also best to have a discussion with an adolescent or teen once the exam is over and they are fully dressed. Including the child in the discussion during the evaluation is important, and it is often very helpful to ask the child why they are being evaluated and what they want to do with regard to treating their problem. This will not only assess their level of understanding, but will also help empower them in the decision-making process. It is equally important to assess the patient and family interactions, as these have implications on how well a patient will respond during a procedure. A well-informed, calm, rational parent is a physician's best ally and can significantly reduce the stress of the procedure for their child, while an anxious parent can often lead to increased stress for the patient and the physician.

4.2.4 Communicating the Plan with the Patient and Family

The potential need for a pediatric dermatologic procedure may be anxiety-provoking for the patient and the family members. Patience and understanding are keys in establishing rapport with the patient and family, and will also help assuage any undue apprehension. It is important to use clear, easy-to-understand terms when reviewing the procedure and it is helpful to share a detailed, step-by-step plan of what to expect, including postop care. There are many age-appropriate resources that are available to help families and patients prepare for surgery. Written information can be found on the Internet or provided by the facility. This will include information such as NPO guidelines, where to go the morning of surgery and what to expect. If further information is desired by the patient or family, most pediatric facilities have child life specialists on staff. Child life specialists are trained to help children and families understand and feel empowered with regard to their health care, and they are indispensable in their care of pediatric patients.

4.2.5 Preparation Before the Procedure

It is important for the physician to talk with the patient and family before the surgery and answer any questions that may arise. The child should understand that they are undergoing a necessary procedure but that they will be cared for in the best way possible. It is important to validate the child's feelings, but to reassure them that there is no reason for fear. Explaining the procedure and what to expect will also help alleviate the patient's fears, and they will be reassured if the physician is understanding and patient with them throughout the process. If there are questions that remain before the surgery, the family should be encouraged to reach out to the physician's office or the child life specialist to have them addressed.

It is also helpful to encourage the patient to bring their own personal comfort item along to the procedure. Bringing a pillow, blanket, or stuffed animal can be reassuring. For in-office procedures, it is also helpful to bring movies or music along that can be used as a distraction both before and during the procedure. Bubbles and books are also a great tool for distracting patients. Teaching quick relaxation techniques like deep breathing, wiggling your toes and blowing out candles can be helpful. Allow the child to use the restroom if needed before the start of the procedure, even if it is a tactic to delay the procedure due to nervousness. It is also important to establish boundaries and rules regarding your expectations of the child during the procedure. Let the child know that they can talk during the procedure but they cannot move unless they inform the physician and obtain permission to do so. It is also helpful to give the child permission to cry or scream if they must, but reinforce that they are not allowed to kick, hit or bite. Reassure the patient that everyone involved wants to make this a good experience for them, and that the process and procedure will go more quickly if they cooperate.

It is also important for the patient to discontinue any non-steroidal anti-inflammatory medications (i.e. ibuprofen, naproxen) or herbal medications (i.e. ginger, garlic, licorice root) that interfere with bleeding two weeks before the surgery. Preoperative antibiotics are typically not necessary, but these should be taken in the rare instances when they are required. Bathing and washing the hair the night before surgery is advised. The patient should be informed that no hair will need to be shaved before or during the surgery. Tell the patient to dress comfortably on the day of the procedure, and to leave any jewelry at home. If general anesthesia is necessary, the patient and family should be aware of the restrictions regarding eating and drinking before the procedure: no solid foods after midnight, no milk or formula for six hours before the procedure, and no clear fluids for four hours before the procedure. If local anesthesia is to be used, it is helpful to have the patient eat a light meal or snack before the procedure. It is also important to let the family know that if the child is ill or has a fever within 24 hours of the procedure, then the procedure will be rescheduled in the best interest of the child. It is also nice for the family to have the opportunity to purchase any necessary medications or dressings prior to the day of surgery so that they do not have to be distracted by these details following the procedure. Encouraging the family to have all of the necessary paperwork gathered before the day of the procedure will also help limit any last-minute stress.

4.2.6 Explanation of Anesthesia

There is much to consider when choosing appropriate anesthesia for a patient's procedure. It is important to consider the age and developmental stage of the patient, whether the procedure will be one-time or require multiple sessions, and how extensive or involved the procedure will be. The main goal of anesthesia is to be able to perform the necessary procedure in the safest possible setting with the least amount of risks and the best potential outcome. Recently, there has been much attention focused on the potential neurodevelopmental impact of general anesthesia on the developing brain of young children. While much more research is still needed to draw definitive conclusions, it has been shown that a single exposure to anesthesia before three years of age may increase the risk of long-term disabilities in language and abstract reasoning. While this is a potential concern, it is also important to realize that there may be other confounding variables impacting the results. Regardless, it is an important issue for pediatric dermatologic surgeons to be able to discuss reasonably with their patients and families, and the recent consensus statement is a good reference for parents: http://www.texaschildrensblog.org/wp-content/uploads/2012/12/Consensus-Statement-on-the-Use-of-Anesthetics-and-Sedatives-in-Children.pdf.

In some cases, general anesthesia will be preferred. In that case, it is important to detail this process with the child. In addition, a child life specialist can add valuable information to the discussion and often provide hands-on materials, such as the anesthetic mask, for the child to experience before the actual procedure. If it is deemed appropriate to proceed with a procedure in the clinic, the information about what to expect should be reviewed before the procedure. It is of utmost importance not to lie to a child, but it is also important to be sensitive and to describe what will happen with reasonable terms that will not elicit fear. It is best to avoid terms such as "shot" or "needle", but to use terms like "pinch". If possible, it is best to use a topical anesthetic before injecting the local anesthetic, which should be buffered and at room temperature, to limit pain with injection. The topical anesthetic can be applied at home to increase the efficiency on the day of the procedure. Otherwise, the topical anesthesia can be applied in the office 30–60 minutes prior to the procedure. At the time of injection, the use of a cooling spray or vibratory instrument applied to the skin, while injecting the local anesthesia using a 30-gauge needle at a 90° angle to the skin will also help limit any discomfort.

4.2.7 Explanation of the Procedure

To make an informed decision, it is important for the patient and family to understand the risks and benefits of the procedure and any alternative treatments or therapies. Therefore it is important to help the family understand all of the components of the procedure you are recommending, along with the expected outcome.

The steps leading up to the procedure are important to the child, and appropriate story boards that provide a detailed step-by-step explanation of the process are great resources. Explaining the preoperative procedure in the operating room and what the operating room will look like is often helpful. For a procedure in the office, tell the patient that everyone on the team will work to make them as comfortable as possible and that their family members will be with them, along with any personal items that they may choose to bring along. The patient undergoing general anesthesia can be reassured that nothing painful will be done while they are awake, and that once they wake up they will not remember the procedure and that they will have medicine that helps them feel comfortable. For patients who are undergoing a local procedure, it is nice to reassure them that they will not feel anything uncomfortable after the numbing medication is given, but they should be advised that they may feel movement of their skin during the procedure but again reassured that it will not be painful. It is also advisable to keep all of the instruments covered and to avoid the patient visualizing any of the blood-tinged materials during the procedure, which will also help keep the patient at ease. Keeping the patient occupied with conversation, movies, music or reading is also helpful and keeps them from becoming anxious during the procedure.

4.2.8 What to Do After the Surgery

During the preoperative evaluation of the patient, it is wise to fully review the expected postoperative course, limitations, and requirements. If the physician reviews the potential issues before the procedure, then the patient and family are not as alarmed or upset if common complications develop. Advise the patient regarding the dressing and any materials they will need to purchase beforehand. Advise them of any postoperative restrictions, which may be up to four weeks for any strenuous activities or sports. If they cannot comply and the procedure is elective in nature, then it is best to postpone the procedure until they are able to follow the postoperative instructions.

4.3 Postoperative Care

The preoperative evaluation is the time to begin stressing to the patient and family the importance of complying with postoperative instructions to optimize the surgical result. Advising the patient of the restrictions and how to care for the surgical site, along with providing written take-home instructions, is desirable.

Following a procedure, most children will be tired and sleep for the majority of the day. Most patients can return to school the following day without difficulty. Postoperative nausea can occur, but this is unusual. To avoid this, it is best to advance the diet slowly. The patient should start with clear fluids and then advance slowly as tolerated. Usually the child's appetite will return to normal the day following the procedure. Pain is typically not significant due to the use of local anesthetics at the surgical site, but if the child is uncomfortable, then over-the-counter acetaminophen is recommended. It is best to avoid ibuprofen or naproxen for 10 days following a procedure to reduce bleeding risk. If pain is not controlled, then it is important to call the physician. In addition, a small amount of bleeding on the surgical dressing is not uncommon, but if the dressing is blood-soaked then the physician should be contacted. To limit bleeding, as well as swelling and pain, it is important to rest on the day of surgery, with no strenuous activities.

For pulsed dye laser procedures, it is important for the patient and family to anticipate the associated laser-induced purpura and swelling that will occur. Advising that blistering and scarring, as well as post-inflammatory pigmentary changes, are also possible is appropriate. Avoiding strenuous activities until the purpura resolves is advised as the skin is more fragile and prone to injury during this period. For swelling, application of ice packs to the area is helpful. Bathing and gently patting the area is fine, but harsh cleansing and picking at the area should be avoided. Application of a petrolatum-based ointment to the treated area several times during the day until the purpura resolves is desirable. As well, strict UV protection is also advised.

For biopsies and excisions, reviewing the potential for the most common complications is required as part of the informed consent process. These include wound infection, wound dehiscence, bleeding and contact dermatitis. Fortunately, the risk of these complications is reduced by complying with the recommended post-operative instructions. To avoid wound infection, the patient should be encouraged to follow the instructions regarding the dressing and be advised that less manipulation of the surgical site is preferable. The outer pressure dressing should be kept in place for 48 hours. Then this can be removed, but the Steri-Strips should be left in place and reinforced with tape if necessary. The wound should be kept completely dry until the sutures are removed. Exceptions to this are wounds in the groin or on the extremities. These areas should be gently washed with soap and water daily. Wounds on the scalp should be treated with petrolatum-based ointment several times throughout the day. If skin glue is utilized, it is important to avoid petrolatum-based ointments to the site. To reduce the risk of contact dermatitis, other topical medications and bandages should not be utilized. It is also important to explain that the deeper sutures will resolve slowly, but that most wounds will have superficial sutures that need to be removed in the office. Advice regarding suture reactions is prudent, and the patient should have full understanding that the procedure will result in a permanent scar. This scarring will include pigmentary changes as well as hair loss if in a hair-bearing area.

To limit bleeding, as well as swelling and pain, it is important to avoid excessive activity in the postoperative period. The use of an ice pack periodically to the site for the first 24 hours following the procedure is advisable to help limit swelling. To prevent wound dehiscence and excessive scarring, postoperative activity restriction is necessary. It is advisable that all strenuous physical and sports activities be avoided for four weeks to optimize the surgical results. Wounds over a joint should also be immobilized.

To improve the appearance of the scar, it is also important to begin scar massage to the site once the sutures have been removed. Silicone-based scar dressings can also be helpful. In addition, strict UV protection of the site is recommended for one year following the procedure. Patients and families should be advised that scars actively remodel for up to one year following the procedure and will continue to improve in appearance over that time if they adhere to the postoperative instructions.

The physician should evaluate the patient and remove the sutures from the surgical site when it is appropriate. Typically, facial wounds should be evaluated at 5–7 days, wounds on the trunk or extremities at 10–12 days and scalp wounds at 12–14 days. At that time, review the postoperative recommendations again and request a follow-up evaluation to assess the scar at three months.

4.4 Conclusion

Appropriate preoperative and postoperative care of a child is of the utmost importance not only in the outcome of the procedure, but also in the overall experience for the patient undergoing the procedure and the family member or caregiver who supports the child. The approach and actions of the physician during these critical times can help alleviate any undue stress or apprehension for the patient or family. It is important to remember that the procedure not only treats the skin, but is also an opportunity for a child to establish a positive relationship with the medical community that has the potential to impact their future attitudes and compliance regarding their health care. Helping the patient have a sense of control throughout the process, respecting them by listening to and answering their questions, and praising them for their cooperation and courage following the procedure truly empowers the child long after the procedure is over.

5

The Pediatric Surgical Tray

V.M. Carlberg[1,2] and J.L. Fewkes[1,2,3]

[1] Department of Dermatology, Massachusetts General Hospital, Boston, MA, USA
[2] Harvard Medical School, Boston, MA, USA
[3] Department of Otolaryngology, Massachusetts Eye and Ear Infirmary, Boston, MA, USA

5.1 Introduction

To perform efficient, high-quality, and safe surgical procedures in infants, children, and adolescents, thoughtful assembly of the surgical tray is a vital pre-procedural step. This chapter outlines the essential surgical tools required for successful biopsy, local excision, suture removal, and nail procedures. Special considerations for pediatric patients and review of several specialty tools have been highlighted throughout this chapter.

5.2 The Biopsy Tray

Key Points

- Biopsies are useful and often indispensable in providing histologic correlation to clinical diagnoses and may be performed in both inpatient and outpatient settings.
- Biopsies may be punch, shave, incisional or excisional depending on the lesion and patient characteristics.
- The skin biopsy is typically a clean procedure, not sterile, with a very low risk of infection.

Similar to adult dermatology, skin biopsies are employed in pediatric dermatology to aid in the diagnosis of inflammatory and neoplastic processes. Punch, shave, incisional, or excisional biopsy may be performed depending on lesion type, depth, and location [1, 2]. For example, a punch biopsy may be utilized for an inflammatory condition when involvement of the deeper dermis or fat is suspected. Conversely, a shave biopsy may be utilized when superficial inflammation or a superficial neoplasm is suspected, or when the biopsy site is overlying an important anatomic structure, such as a motor nerve or large vessel. Incisional biopsies take a small sample of a larger lesion. Excisional biopsies remove solitary lesions completely and are helpful in assessing the histologic architecture of melanocytic lesions. They also reduce sampling error and may provide definitive treatment, making it unnecessary to do a second procedure.

In children, one must also consider how the biopsy procedure, post-procedure wound care, and follow-up will be tolerated. Although punch biopsies allow evaluation of the superficial and deep tissues and are often preferred, they require more steps to remove the specimen and close the wound, thus taking slightly longer than shave biopsies. Depending on the size of a punch biopsy, it may be closed with suture or left to heal via secondary intention using surgical sponge, tissue adhesive, or aluminum chloride and

Pediatric Dermatologic Surgery, First Edition. Edited by Keyvan Nouri, Latanya Benjamin, Jasem Alshaiji, and Jan Izakovic.

petrolatum jelly [3]. Of these methods, suturing is slightly more time-consuming and may require that the pediatric patient follow up in clinic for suture removal unless absorbable or self-removable sutures are used.

Both punch and shave biopsies are performed using clean, not sterile, technique given the low risk for infection [1, 4]. In both cases, the trays should include a skin marker, antiseptic, anesthesia, gauze, pathology specimen container and a wound dressing. In addition, a punch biopsy tray should include a punch, forceps, scissors, a needle driver, and suture (see Figure 5.1). A shave biopsy tray should include the same preparatory and wound dressing materials as well as a blade, forceps, aluminum chloride, and electrocautery, if needed (see Figure 5.2). Additional specialized tools, such as the chalazion clamp or curette, may be added to the tray for removal in certain body locations (see Figures 5.3a,b and 5.4a,b) [1, 5]. Biopsies of the nail will be discussed later on in this chapter. Depending on the practice setting, pre-assembled and easily transported biopsy kits may be useful when there is a need for biopsies in both the clinical and hospital setting.

Components of the punch biopsy tray:

Punch. The punch may be disposable or reusable and is available in various sizes, ranging from less than 1 mm to greater than 10 mm [1, 2]. Disposable punches tend to have sharper blades and are conveniently single-use, making them preferable. Neonates and infants may have thinner skin; thus, one must be mindful while performing a punch biopsy, as the depth of the punch barrel may penetrate beyond the subcutaneous fat. Conversely, if a deeper specimen is desired, a telescoping

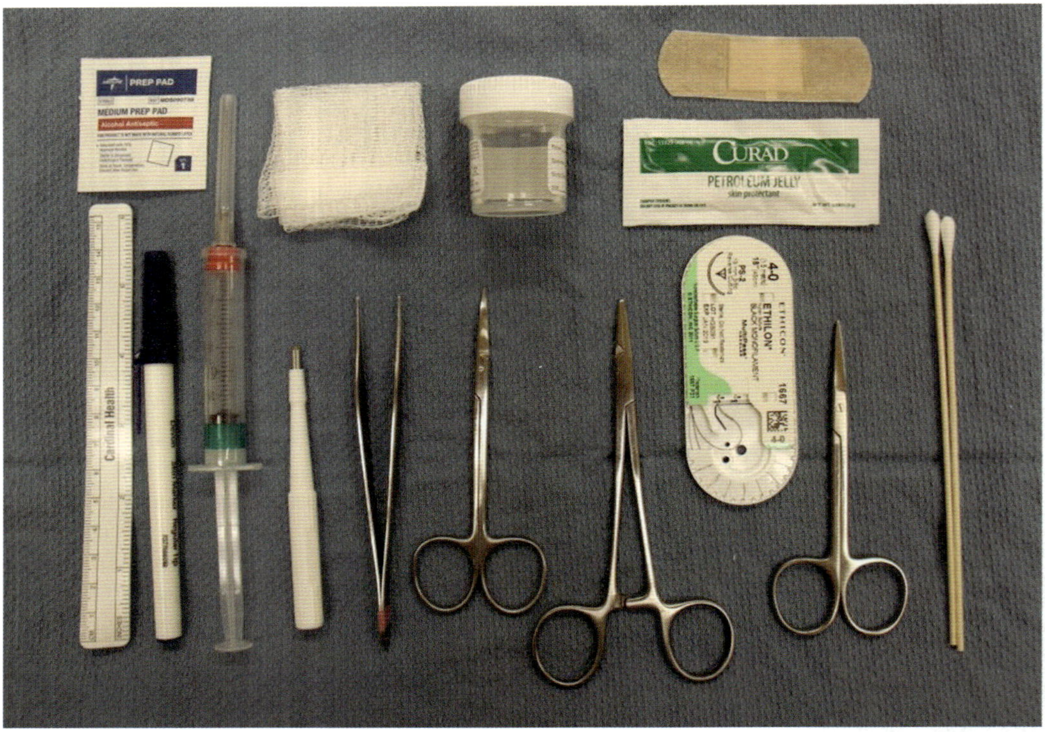

Figure 5.1 The punch biopsy tray: (top row, left to right) antiseptic, gauze, specimen bottle with formalin, petrolatum, bandage, (bottom row, left to right) ruler, skin marker, anesthesia, punch, forceps, tissue scissors, needle driver, suture, suture scissors, cotton-tipped applicators.

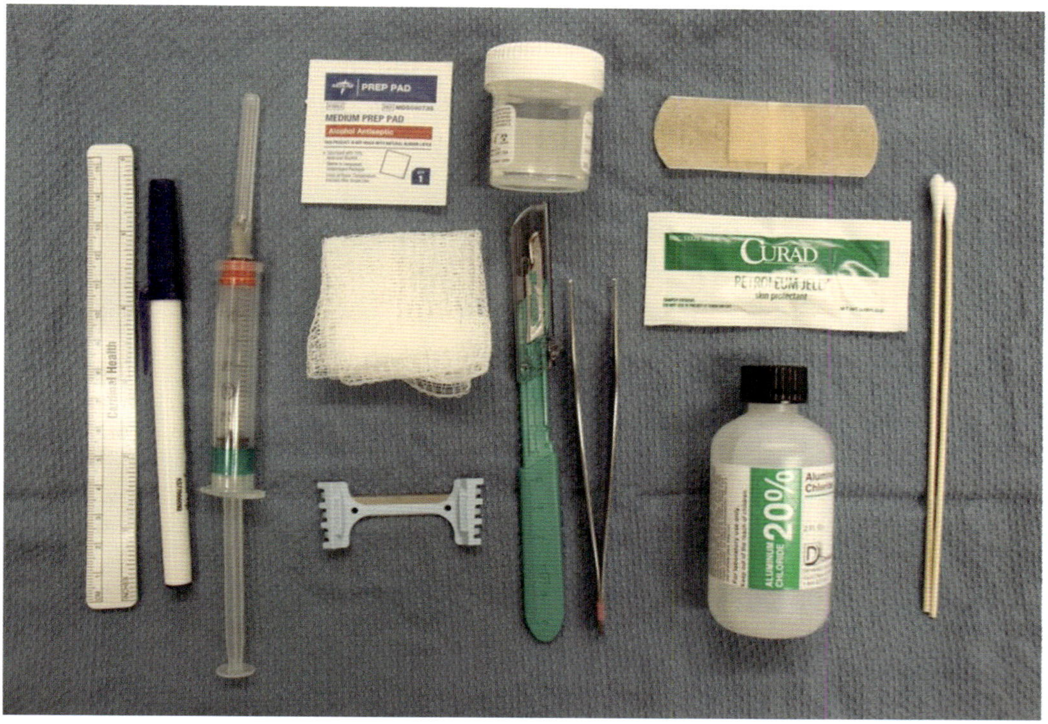

Figure 5.2 The shave biopsy tray: (top row, left to right) antiseptic, gauze, specimen container with formalin, bandage, petrolatum, (bottom row, left to right) ruler, skin marker, anesthesia, DermaBlade, disposable scalpel, forceps, aluminum chloride, cotton-tipped applicators.

(a) (b)

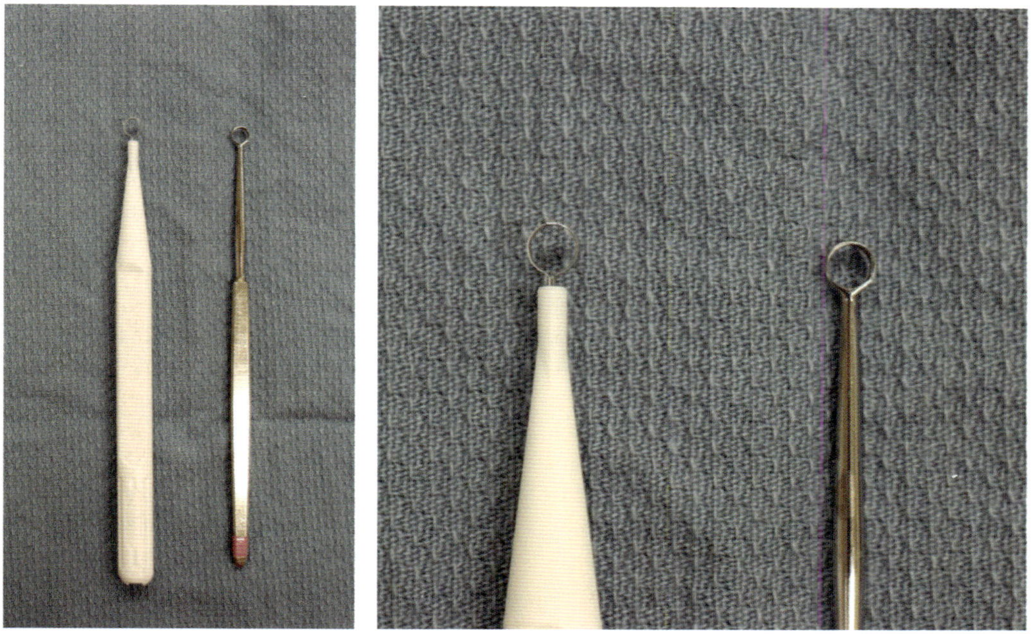

Figure 5.3 Curettes. (a): (left to right) disposable and reusable curettes. (b): magnified.

(a)

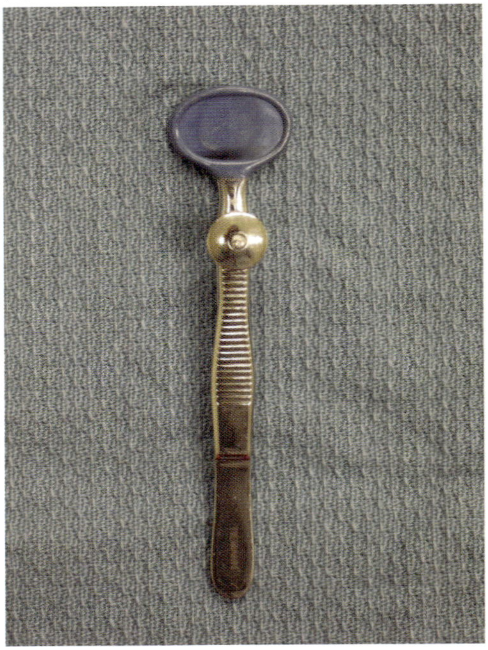

(b)

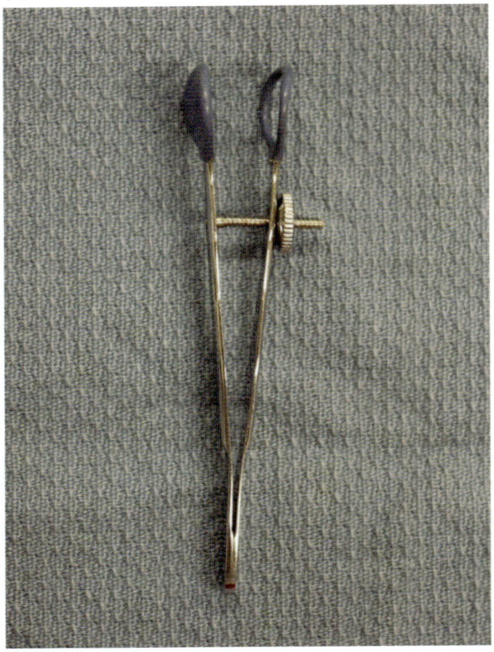

Figure 5.4 The chalazion clamp. (a and b) rotated views.

biopsy can be performed using two punches of differing size [6].

Forceps. Toothed forceps, such as Adson forceps or Brown-Adson forceps, may be used to gently grasp the biopsy specimen while avoiding crushing the sample [7]. Smooth forceps may also be used. However, there is greater risk of crush artifact if the operator is not careful. Lastly, forceps with a serrated platform make grasping sutures easier during the biopsy closure.

Scissors. If disposable scissors are used, there is often one pair on the tray, utilized for cutting the base of the tissue biopsy as well as cutting the sutures. When reusable scissors are used, fine-tipped scissors, such as the iris, Gradle or Westcott, are best suited for a punch biopsy, as the tip is able to reach and release the base of the punch specimen [7, 8]. These tissue scissors should not be used for suture cutting, if possible, as it dulls the blade. Instead, distinct suture-cutting scissors, such as the Northbent or standard operating scissors, should be included [7].

Needle driver. Needle drivers vary in size and are chosen, typically, to match the size of the suture. Smaller needle drivers, such as the Webster, are used for smaller sutures and larger needle drivers, such as the Halsey, are used for larger sutures [7, 8]. The jaws of the needle driver may also be smooth or fine-toothed. While smooth needle drivers incur less damage to the suture, fine-toothed jaws offer additional grip. Either choice is suitable given most skin biopsies are 4 mm in diameter or smaller and only require 1 to 2 sutures.

Suture. Suture selection is largely guided by absorbability as well as location on the body (see Chapter 11). Though non-absorbable sutures are often used to close a biopsy wound, absorbable sutures may be considered in children to obviate the need for suture removal. Nylon (Ethilon®, Dermalon®, Surgilon®, Nurolon®), polybutester (Novafil®), and polypropylene

(Prolene®, Surgilene®, Surgipro®) are all appropriate choices for the face, trunk, and extremities. Both silk and polyester (Ethibond®, Dacron®, Mersilene®) are soft, making them appropriate choices for mucosal, intertriginous surfaces, and scalp. Some absorbable sutures, such as fast-absorbing gut and partially hydrolyzed polyglactin 910 (Vicryl Rapide®), spontaneously dissolve within 7–14 days, thus avoiding the need for suture removal all together.

Alternative wound repair. According to at least one study [3], punch biopsies 8 mm in size that healed via secondary intention had equivalent cosmesis to similarly sized wounds that were sutured. Thus, when suture removal would like to be avoided, or in cumbersome areas such as the scalp, one might consider use of a cyanoacrylate tissue adhesive (Dermabond®), surgical sponge (Gelfoam®), or aluminum chloride and plain petrolatum jelly.

Components of the shave biopsy tray:

DermaBlade®. The most commonly employed shave biopsy tool, the DermaBlade, is a sterile, flexible, disposable sharp with protective handles.

Scalpel. Disposable scalpels are often used for biopsies, given the ease of one-time use. When reusable scalpels are used, selection of the handle is dependent on surgeon preference as well as the site of the lesion. The handle can be flat or round, long or thin [5, 7, 8]. The most commonly used handle, the No. 3 stainless steel, is flat and has an imprinted ruler. The No. 7 and Beaver handles will be discussed later, in the local excision tray. Regardless of handle choice, a No. 15 blade is most commonly employed for shave biopsies.

Forceps. These are similar to those used in a punch biopsy.

Aluminum chloride. To achieve hemostasis, aluminum chloride is applied via a cotton-tipped applicator to the base of the wound, rolling back and forth until there is no active bleeding.

Electrocautery. If a patient has a bleeding diathesis for any reason, it may be necessary to use light cautery for hemostasis.

Specialized biopsy tools:

Curette. Curettes are available as disposable or reusable instruments. Disposable curettes are typically sharper. They are available in a variety of sizes from 1 to 9 mm and they may be used for biopsies of soft, exophytic lesions that exhibit a plane of cleavage between the lesion and the underlying dermis [1, 4].

Chalazion clamp. A specialized instrument primarily used for procedures involving the eyelid, lip, or earlobe, the chalazion clamp consists of two limbs, similar to forceps. The flat end of one limb opposes the ring-shaped end of the other limb. These may be clamped together and fixed in place with a screw, thereby immobilizing the surgical site while also providing hemostasis [5].

5.3 The Local Excision Tray

Key Points

- Excisions are performed using sterile technique.
- Fine tools are preferred for procedures on the face or in young infants and children.

In children, indications for excision include removal of cysts, atypical nevi, and skin malignancies. The procedure should be done sterilely to minimize risk for infection.

Preparation of the wound for excision is best done using a separate tray or set-up that includes a skin marker, ruler, camera (optional), antiseptic, anesthesia, gauze, and surgical gloves. Another clean tray/setup may hold the wound dressing. Once the surgical site has been marked, photographed, prepped, and anesthetized, the surgeon can put on sterile gloves and begin using the sterile equipment, avoiding contamination.

The sterile local excision tray should include: sterile towels and towel clamps or

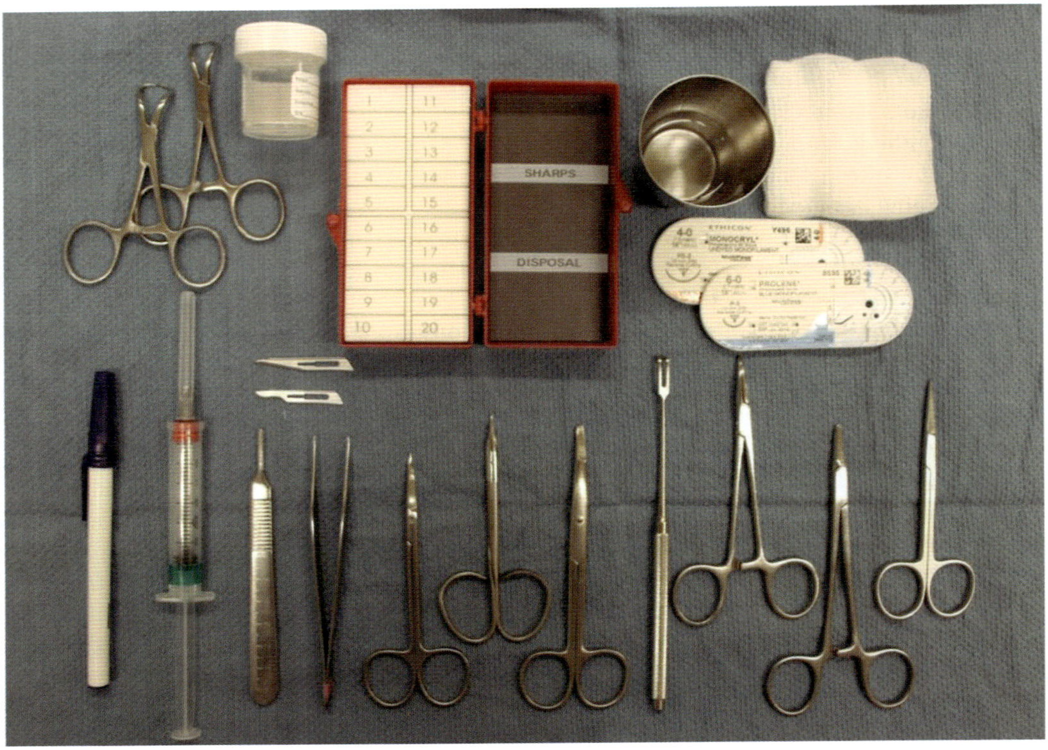

Figure 5.5 The local excision tray: (top row, left to right) towel clamps, specimen container with formalin, sharps container, cup with saline, sutures, guaze, (bottom row, left to right) skin marker, additional anesthesia, scalpel handle, surgical blades No. 11 and No. 15, forceps, tissue scissors, Gradle scissors, Mayo scissors, skin hook(s), hemostat, needle driver, suture scissors. Not pictured: sterile drape.

sterile drape, additional anesthesia, scalpel handle, surgical blade, forceps, skin hook(s), tissue scissors, gauze or cotton-tipped applicators, electrocautery, needle driver, suture, suture scissors, and a sharps container (if not available in the room) (see Figure 5.5). When working on the face, finer-caliber tools are utilized compared to those for the trunk or extremities [8]. In infants and small children, delicate tools may also be used, as their skin and subcutaneous tissues are not as thick as their adult counterparts. Additional specialized tools, such as the chalazion clamp, may be added to the tray as needed.

Components of the sterile local excision tray:

Sterile draping. Sterile towels offer flexibility when creating the surgical field, but must usually be secured with towel clamps. The clamps may also be used to secure cautery equipment. Alternatively, a sterile paper drape with a central cutout and adhesive backing may be used. In children, this latter option may be a better choice if there is unanticipated subtle movement by the patient, as the drape is less likely to fall. When working on hair-bearing areas, such as the scalp, keep in mind that the adhesive will stick to hair, causing discomfort with removal. In these instances, it may be useful to expose some or none of the adhesive backing when applying it, or to only use sterile towels.

Anesthesia. It is important to provide adequate anesthesia initially as children may be uncooperative and unforgiving if they experience any pain during the procedure. There should always be additional anesthesia ready at hand to be quickly accessed.

Scalpel. As previously mentioned, scalpel handles are determined based on surgical site as well as the personal preference of the surgeon. The most common type is the No. 3 handle, which is flat and has a ruler imprinted on the handle. The No. 7 handle and Siegel are rounded, offering more comfort and controlled movement via rolling of the handle with the fingers and hand rather than movement of the wrist to accomplish the same task with a flat handle [5, 7, 8]. For very delicate procedures or narrow surgical sites with rounded contour, such as the ear and nose, a Beaver blade handle, which is hexagonal or round, may be very helpful [8].

Surgical blade. Three main blades are used in dermatologic surgery: the No. 15, No. 11, and No. 10 [5, 7, 8]. Beaver blades are smaller and reserved for accessing small areas such as the ear canal. The No. 15 blade is the most commonly utilized and has a gentle curve, making it the most versatile [5]. The No. 10 blade is a larger version of the No. 15 blade and is used primarily on the back where the skin is thick. In children, this should be reserved for adolescents or those with larger body habitus. The No. 11 blade is sharp and pointed. It is primarily useful for incision and drainage, for extraction of milia, or for through-and-through excisions [8].

Forceps. The qualities of forceps were briefly reviewed earlier while discussing the biopsy tray. For excision, forceps should be lightweight and have fine tips. Toothed forceps are optimal for grasping tissue and avoiding crush injury [7]. Bishop-Harmon forceps are very lightweight and fine-tipped, making them ideal for work on the face or with delicate tissues. Adson forceps are the standard for excisions on the trunk and extremities [8]. Another helpful microsurgical instrument to utilize in the pediatric population is the Castroviejo forceps. Forceps such as these, with a smooth tying platform, may be useful when suturing.

Skin hooks. Skin hooks are useful for elevation and reflection of the skin during undermining, increase visualization of the operative field, and may also be used to reduce tissue injury while suturing. They are available as single-, double-, or multi-prong and the surgeon must be careful to avoid an accidental stick injury to self or others when using them [8].

Tissue scissors. Scissors are designed for various functions: cutting tissue, undermining, cutting sutures, and manipulating wound dressings. Tissue scissors, such as the iris, have sharp tips and are used for sharp dissection and for trimming grafts [8]. Other fine-tipped tissue scissors, such as the Gradle or Westcott, are used for delicate areas or for intricate dissection [7]. Blunt scissors, such as Metzenbaum scissors, are used for blunt dissection [5]. Tissue scissors should not be used for suture cutting, as they are more finely honed, more expensive, and easily blunted by cutting sutures.

Hemostat. A hemostat may be helpful for grasping cyst walls or small blood vessels while achieving hemostasis.

Chalazion clamp. As discussed earlier, this specialized tool immobilizes the surgical site (eyelid, lip, earlobe) while also providing hemostasis [5].

Electrocautery. Either monopolar or bipolar generators may be utilized and will be reviewed in further detail in Chapter 8.

Needle driver. When working on delicate skin and with smaller sutures, a Webster needle holder is the best option [8]. When working on thicker tissues or with larger suture, a Halsey needle holder is an appropriate choice.

Suture. As previously mentioned, suture selection depends on the surgical location as well as an understanding of suture material (see Chapter 11) [8–11]. The first distinction is between absorbable and non-absorbable suture. Absorbable sutures are most often utilized for buried deep stitches to close the wound and reduce wound tension. Non-absorbable sutures are used to approximate epidermal wound edges. The most commonly used absorbable sutures in dermatology include polyglactin 910 (Vicryl®), polydioxanone (PDS®), poliglecaprone (Monocryl®), surgical gut, and polycyclocolic acid (Dexon®). The most commonly used non-absorbable sutures include nylon (Ethilon, Surgilon), polypropylene (Prolene, Surgilene), polyester (Ethibond, Dacron), polybutester (Novafil), and silk. Additional features, such as tensile strength, degradation time, suture configuration (monofilament versus polyfilament), ease of handling, and tissue reactivity further guide suture selection (see Chapter 11).

Suture scissors. Tissue scissors should not be used for suture cutting, as the scissors will dull. Standard operating scissors or suture-cutting scissors, such as the Northbent or Iris stitch scissor, can be designated for this purpose [7, 8].

Sharps container. Safety is paramount when working with sharp tools. Keeping the surgical tray well organized and making use of sharps-designated storage helps avoid injury. Sharps-designated boxes, magnetic plate, or cups may be utilized. With boxes, the lid may be secured, further reducing risk of injury. With magnetic strips and cups, one must be careful not to dislodge the sharps.

Ruler. At the conclusion of the excision, the final repair should be measured and documented. Sometimes the ruler is imprinted on the scalpel handle, such as with the No. 3 handle. If not, a sterile ruler or disposable paper ruler can be added to the tray.

5.4 The Suture Removal Tray

Key Points

- Patients and their parents should receive clear information regarding the appropriate time for suture removal.
- Early suture removal may lead to wound dehiscence.
- Late suture removal may result in track marks.

The suture removal tray is clean, not sterile, and includes a cleansing agent, gauze, scissors or scalpel blade, and forceps (see Figure 5.6).

Components of the suture removal tray:

Cleansing agent. Saline-soaked gauze, an alcohol pad, or hydrogen peroxide-soaked gauze can be used to gently remove hemorrhagic crust.

Scissors. Typically, disposable scissors are utilized for suture removal. If reusable scissors are used, it is best to use ones specifically designated for suture-cutting, such as the Northbent, O'Brien, or standard operating scissors, and to avoid using tissue-cutting scissors, which may become dull [7, 8]. For the smaller pediatric patient, the Spencer stitch scissor with hook is recommended. The advantages for using this scissor are that it allows for removal of small sutures, aids in the agility needed to quickly remove sutures in moving children, and offers a safer blunt tip.

Scalpel blade. Alternatively to using suture scissors, one can use a No. 11 scalpel blade to release the sutures, being careful to always cut away from the patient and oneself. This is more suitable for adolescent patients who can cooperate with sitting still. This instrument is less advisable for use in the younger pediatric population.

Forceps. Disposable forceps may also be utilized for suture removal; however, they vary in quality. The reusable forceps best suited for suture removal are those with smooth or serrated tips [8], such as the Healy. Suture can readily pass through toothed forceps, making suture removal difficult. The 3.5″ Bishop-Harmon forceps is recommended when working with pediatric patients.

Special considerations. If needed, wound adhesive strips (Steri-Strips™) can be applied for reinforcement after suture removal, particularly in high-tension areas and in the setting of very active children [9].

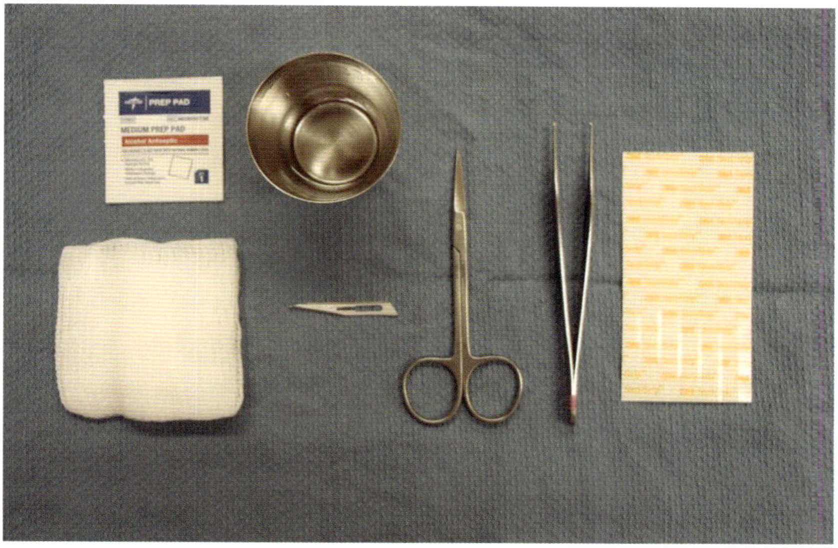

Figure 5.6 The suture removal tray: (left to right) cleansing agent (alcohol pad or saline), gauze, scalpel blade, suture scissors, forceps, adhesive strips (optional).

5.5 The Nail Tray

Key Points

- Nail surgery includes biopsies, avulsion, and matrixectomy.
- A thorough understanding of nail anatomy is essential to ensure successful surgery and decrease the risk for permanent nail dystrophy.
- Nail procedures should be done in a sterile fashion to reduce risk of infection.

Nail procedures can be performed efficiently when the surgeon has thorough understanding of nail anatomy, when the patient is appropriately prepped, and when the proper instruments are available. The proximal matrix produces the dorsal (superficial) surface of the nail plate. Large wounds involving the proximal matrix will therefore likely result in visible nail defects [12]. The distal matrix produces the ventral (inferior) surface of the nail plate. Wounds involving the distal matrix are less likely to produce visible defects. The biopsy selected should be sufficient to accomplish the task, yet should be as small as possible to reduce the risk of permanent nail dystrophy.

The nail tray may vary based on procedure, though nail avulsion, biopsy, and matrixectomy utilize several similar tools [13, 14]. A comprehensive nail tray includes a tourniquet, nail elevator, nail splitter, double-action nail splitter, hemostat or nail-pulling forceps, skin hook, scalpel or punch, scissors, phenol, urethral swabs, suture, and needle driver in addition to the standard antiseptic, anesthesia, hemostatic agents, and wound dressing (see Figure 5.7). Nail procedures are performed using sterile technique to minimize risk for infection.

Components of the nail tray:

Nail elevator. A nail elevator, such as a Freer septum, is used to separate the nail plate from the nail bed [12, 13].

Nail splitter. The English nail splitter has one sharp blade and an opposing flat blade and is utilized during partial longitudinal nail avulsions [14].

Double-action nail splitter. Double-action nail splitters are essential for cutting thickened nail plates [14].

Nail-pulling forceps. Nail-pulling forceps are generally flat or serrated and are used to remove the nail plate from the nail bed.

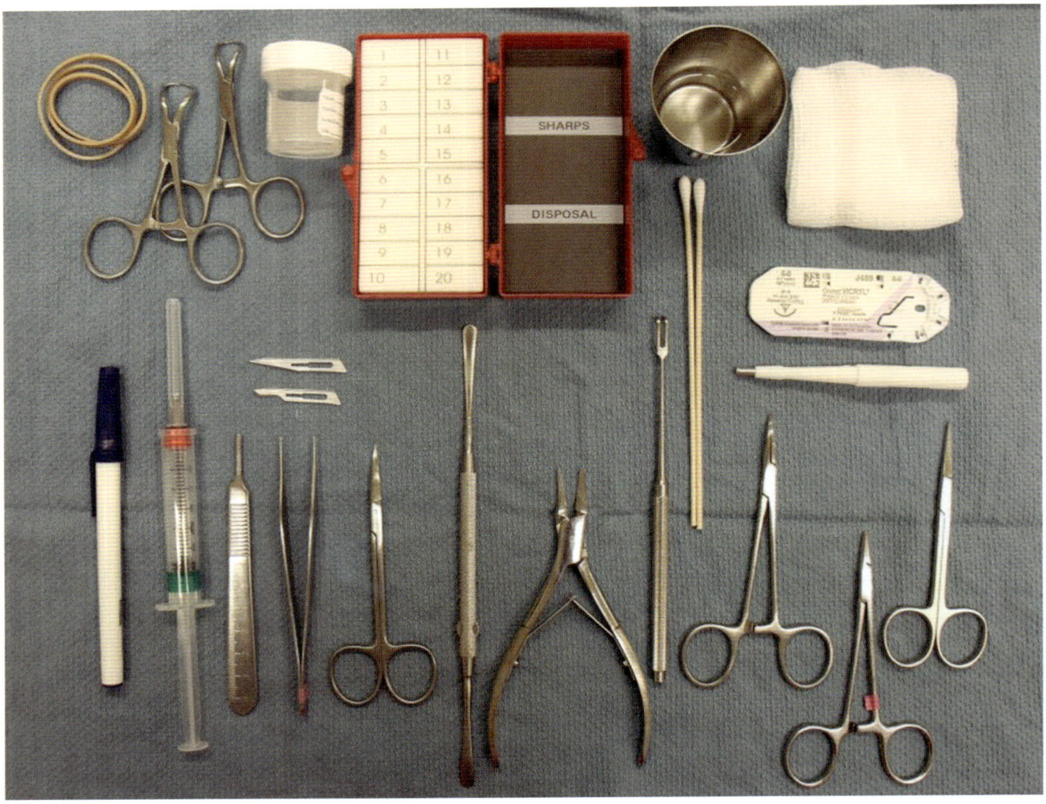

Figure 5.7 The nail tray: (top row, left to right) rubber band,[1] towel clamps, specimen container with formalin, sharps container, cup with saline, cotton-tipped applicators,[2] gauze, suture, punch, (bottom row, left to right) skin marker, anesthesia, scalpel handle, surgical blades No. 11 and No. 15, forceps, scissors, nail elevator, nail splitter, skin hook, hemostat[3], needle driver, suture scissors. Not pictured: sterile drape, double-action nail splitter, phenol. Alternatives: [1]tourniquet, [2]urethral swabs, [3]nail-pulling forceps.

Hemostat. If nail forceps are not available, a hemostat or a needle driver can be substituted.

Skin hook. Using the skin hook, the proximal nail fold can be reflected to permit exposure and biopsy of the proximal nail matrix.

Scalpel. As previously discussed for the local excision tray, scalpel handle and blade selection depends on surgeon preference as well as type and location of the procedure. For nail procedures, any combination of handle or blade may be used, with a primary goal of keeping the biopsy small.

Punch. A punch can be used to biopsy through the nail plate or after the nail plate is partially removed or avulsed. A maximum diameter of 3 mm is recommended to reduce the risk for nail dystrophy or need for suture [12, 13, 15]. When a punch is performed through the nail plate, telescopic technique may be utilized or the punch can be used to remove a small portion of the nail plate, followed by biopsy using the narrow No. 11 scalpel blade [14].

Scissors. Similar to those used for the local excision tray, fine-tipped scissors may be used for specimen removal.

Suture. For larger biopsies or excisions, suture may be necessary. Essentially any suture may be used, though some recommend absorbable 6–0 polyglactin sutures (i.e. Vicryl) [13–15].

Needle driver. If sutures are required, a small needle driver, such as the Webster, works well.

Phenol. Chemical matrixectomy can be achieved when phenol is applied to the nail matrix.

Urethral swabs. Very narrow swabs, urethral swabs, are used to apply phenol with precision [12].

Tourniquet. A clamped Penrose drain, a finger cut from a pair of gloves, Tourni-Cot™, or a rubber band can be used as a tourniquet for hemostasis in larger procedures [13].

Hemostatic agents. Surgical sponge (Gelfoam), aluminum chloride, and electrocautery may all be used for hemostasis, as discussed previously in this chapter. A good pressure dressing with finger immobilization is useful in pediatric surgery.

5.6 Conclusion

Many of the surgical tools utilized in pediatric dermatologic surgery are similar to those utilized in adult dermatology. In children, the dermatologic surgeon must be mindful of how the patient will tolerate the procedure, how pediatric anatomy may dictate use of finer tools, and how post-operative wound care may influence the choice of hemostasis and wound closure. Well-planned surgical trays enhance the efficiency, quality, and safety of dermatologic procedures.

References

1. Olbricht, S. (2012). Biopsy techniques and basic excisions. In: *Dermatology*, 3e, vol. 2 (ed. J.L. Bolognia, J.L. Jorizzo and J.V. Schaffer), 2381–2397. Philadelphia, PA: Elsevier Saunders.
2. Campbell, L.B. and Marks, V.J. (2009). Biopsy techniques. In: *Dermatologic Surgery* (ed. A.T. Vidimos, C.T. Ammirati and C. Poblete-Lopez), 117–122. Edinburgh: Saunders Elsevier.
3. Christenson, L.J., Phillips, P.K., Weaver, A.L. et al. (2005). Primary closure vs second-intention treatment of skin punch biopsy sites: a randomized trial. *Arch. Dermatol.* 141 (9): 1093–1099.
4. Affleck, A.G. and Colver, G. (2010). Skin biopsy techniques. In: *Surgery of the Skin: Procedural Dermatology*, 2e (ed. J.K. Robinson, C.W. Hanke, D.M. Siegel, et al.), 167–176. Philadelphia, PA: Elsevier Mosby.
5. Bhatia, A.C. and Taneja, A. (2009). Surgical instruments. In: *Dermatologic Surgery* (ed. A.T. Vidimos, C.T. Ammirati and C. Poblete-Lopez), 59–71. Edinburgh: Saunders Elsevier.
6. Ha, C.T. and Nousari, H.C. (2003). Surgical pearl: double-trephine punch biopsy technique for sampling subcutaneous tissue. 48: 609–610.
7. Bogle, M.A., Fisher, V.T. and Joseph, A.K. (2010). Instruments and materials. In: *Surgery of the Skin: Procedural Dermatology*, 2e (ed. J.K. Robinson, C.W. Hanke, D.M. Siegel, et al.), 65–72. Philadelphia, PA: Elsevier Mosby.
8. Ammirati, C.T. and Goldman, G. (2012). Wound closure materials and instruments. In: *Dermatology*, 3e, vol. 2 (ed. J.L. Bolognia, J.L. Jorizzo and J.V. Schaffer), 2353–2363. Philadelphia, PA: Elsevier Saunders.
9. Weitzul, S. and Taylor S. (2010). Suturing technique and other closure materials. In: *Surgery of the Skin: Procedural Dermatology*, 2e (ed. J.K. Robinson, C.W. Hanke, D.M. Siegel, et al.), 65–72. Philadelphia, PA: Elsevier Mosby.
10. Ethicon (2016) http://www.ethicon.com/healthcare-professionals/products/wound-closure (accessed 17 May 2016).
11. Medtronic (2016) http://www.medtronic.com/covidien/products/wound-closure (accessed 17 May 2016).

12 Billingsley (2009). Nail surgery. In: *Dermatologic Surgery* (ed. A.T. Vidimos, C.T. Ammirati and C. Poblete-Lopez), 189–197. Edinburgh: Saunders Elsevier.
13 Rich, P. (2001). Nail biopsy: indications and methods. *Dermatol. Surg.* 27 (3): 229–234.
14 Rich, P. (2012). Nail surgery. In: *Dermatology*, 3e, vol. 2 (ed. J.L. Bolognia, J.L. Jorizzo and J.V. Schaffer), 2435–2444. Philadelphia, PA: Elsevier Saunders.
15 Haneke, E. (2010). Nail surgery. In: *Surgery of the Skin: Procedural Dermatology*, 2e (ed. J.K. Robinson, C.W. Hanke, D.M. Siegel, et al.), 755–780. Philadelphia, PA: Elsevier Mosby.

6

Anesthesia for Children

Marcia Hogeling

David Geffen School of Medicine at UCLA, Los Angeles, CA, USA

Historically, procedural pain in young children has been undertreated as it was believed that children's pain pathways were undeveloped, and that they would forget painful procedures. However, it is now recognized that neonates experience pain. Intensely painful physical experiences in childhood can have persisting physiological and psychological consequences. Therefore, the management of acute pain with local or general anesthesia is essential. This chapter will discuss anesthetic options for pediatric patients undergoing dermatologic surgery.

6.1 Indications for Local Anesthesia

There are no specific guidelines for when children can have procedures performed under local anesthesia. The location of the lesion, type of procedure, and patient age are all considerations. Most skin biopsies and quick procedures such as shave and cautery of pyogenic granuloma, or intralesional injections can be done under local anesthesia at any age. Toddler wraps or swaddle can be useful techniques to hold infants still while performing a quick procedure. Older children benefit from distraction techniques such as watching a DVD or playing on a tablet device.

Generally adolescents and middle school-aged children can have excisions performed on the trunk or extremity under local anesthesia. Adolescents can usually tolerate excisions on the face and scalp under local anesthesia. In general, girls can tolerate procedures under local anesthesia at around age 8 or 9, and boys may be ready by 10 or 11 years [1]. Due to variability in development and personality, each child must be evaluated individually by the pediatric dermatologic surgeon to determine the appropriate type of anesthesia [2].

Elective procedures can often be delayed until preadolescent or adolescent years to avoid risks of general anesthesia. For example, a small nevus sebaceous on the scalp can wait to be excised under local anesthesia around puberty. However, general anesthesia should be considered when a procedure is necessary but a child is too young to fully cooperate with local anesthesia. General anesthesia is also recommended for lengthy and repeated procedures such as pulsed dye laser treatments of hemi-facial port-wine stains.

6.2 Topical Anesthetics

The use of topical anesthetics can help minimize the pain and anxiety associated with injectable anesthetics and laser treatments. Many types of topical anesthetics exist, providing choice for clinicians for different clinical situations.

Pediatric Dermatologic Surgery, First Edition. Edited by Keyvan Nouri, Latanya Benjamin, Jasem Alshaiji, and Jan Izakovic.

6.3 EMLA Cream

The most commonly used topical anesthetics are those in cream formulations. Eutectic mixture of local anesthetics (EMLA) is a mixture of lidocaine 2.5% and prilocaine 2.5%. Although the eutectic preparation melts at a lower temperature than its individual components, the mixture remains stable at room temperature. EMLA is available with a prescription, and should be applied under occlusion, one hour before the procedure. Tegaderm polyurethane film or simple plastic wrap with enough adhesive tape to ensure occlusion without extrusion can be used to cover EMLA. Longer application times can increase depth of anesthesia as both the duration and depth of pain blockage are related to application time. Shorter application times are indicated for certain sites, such as broken skin, genitalia, eyelids, and mucosal surfaces, due to faster absorption rates [3].

EMLA, originally proven effective for minimizing the pain of venipuncture, is commonly used as a local anesthetic for numerous dermatologic procedures including laser therapy for port-wine stains, intralesional injections for keloids and cysts, and in the paring of verruca vulgaris lesions. While EMLA alone does not provide adequate anesthesia for more invasive procedures such as skin biopsies and excisions in children, it is useful as a "prenumbing" agent, prior to the infiltration of local injectable anesthetics [4, 5].

Methemoglobinemia is a well-documented potential complication of prilocaine-containing creams. EMLA should only be applied to small areas, and should be used with caution in children younger than three years because of the incomplete maturation of the NADH-methemoglobin reductase system [6].

Significant risk of methemoglobinemia from EMLA in children is <6 months of age, and such use is controversial and cannot be recommended [7]. EMLA should be avoided in children with G6PD deficiency. Infants taking medications that can exacerbate methemoglobinemia such as sulphonamides, benzocaine, dapsone, and chloroquine should not receive EMLA cream [8].

Signs of methemoglobinemia are mottling and pallor of the skin, perioral cyanosis, and acral cyanosis which can occur hours after EMLA has been wiped off the skin. If symptomatic, drug induced methemoglobinemia can be treated with IV methylene blue or ascorbic acid [9].

EMLA may cause local side effects such as temporary erythema, edema, allergic contact dermatitis, and eye irritation (especially with periorbital application). Local purpura may also develop, and is thought to involve toxicity to the capillary endothelium. EMLA may cause blanching or vasoconstriction, which may be undesirable when using pulsed dye laser. As with any topical lidocaine toxicity due to systemic absorption, seizures may occur with extensive and prolonged EMLA application under occlusion.

Dose: To attain adequate anesthesia, 1–2 g of EMLA cream should be applied per 10 sq. cm of skin and covered with an occlusive dressing for 45–60 minutes. The maximum application areas recommended for children are [10]:

- less than 10 kg: 100 sq. cm
- 10–20 kg: 600 sq. cm
- greater than 20 kg: 2000 sq. cm

6.4 Topical Lidocaine

Liposomal 4% lidocaine cream (LMX – formerly known as ELA-Max) is available over the counter. LMX may be followed by a numeral, such as LMX4 or LMX5, which indicates the percent strength of lidocaine in the preparation. In comparative studies, LMX4 and EMLA cream were found to be equally effective in minimizing pain associated with simple dermatologic procedures [11, 12]. The recommended application time is 30 minutes prior to the procedure. Although occlusion is not required for maximum effect, LMX is also usually applied under occlusion to avoid causing a mess or being ingested by younger children. LMX can be dosed similarly to EMLA cream with 1–2 g of LMX per 10 sq. cm of skin. LMX is FDA-approved for children ages two and up. LMX does not contain prilocaine, and therefore has no risk of causing methemoglobinemia. Although LMX is safe and effective, topical anesthetics should be used with caution. Children have a lower body mass to surface area ratio and are at higher risk for cutaneous absorption and toxicity than adults. Seven deaths were reported by the American Association of Poison Control Centers from exposure to topical anesthetics, including OTC lidocaine preparations, between 1983 and 2003 [13].

6.5 Tetracaine Formulations

Liposome-encapsulated tetracaine (LET) consists of a combination of lidocaine (4%), epinephrine (0.1%), and tetracaine (0.5%) available as an aqueous solution or methylcellulose-based gel. LET is the topical anesthetic most frequently used for laceration repair, with either tissue adhesive or suture closures [14]. Many pediatric emergency departments have standing orders for application of LET in triage to avoid delays in laceration care in children, and are indicated in simple lacerations <5 cm in length. Based on several trials, it provides adequate local anesthesia for wound closure for most scalp and facial lacerations, similar to tetracaine, adrenaline, cocaine (TAC) topical solution. LET is less effective on extremity or truncal wounds. LET also reduces the pain of lidocaine injection. Generally LET is used for anesthesia for laceration repair on the face or scalp, and is not appropriate for large wounds and should be used with caution on mucous membranes. LET in a dose of 1–3 ml is applied to an open wound for 20–30 minutes. The gel formulation is preferred because it maintains better contact with the wound and is easier to apply. Additional buffered 1% lidocaine may need to be infiltrated to achieve complete analgesia. LET should be used with caution in infants younger than one month of age due to higher potential for systemic absorption of topical agents in neonates and the theoretical risk of methemoglobinemia posed by the tetracaine component.

Tetracaine gel is a topical anesthetic widely used in Europe, Canada, Australia and New Zealand, but is not currently FDA-approved in the USA. Amethocaine, a 4% tetracaine gel, has a more rapid onset (40 minutes) and longer duration of action than EMLA cream [15]. Topical amethocaine may be superior to EMLA cream based on a Cochrane review, particularly with regard to needle procedures [16].

TAC is a combination of tetracaine (0.25–0.5%), adrenaline (epinephrine 0.025–0.05%), and cocaine (4–11.8%). It is available as a solution or gel. TAC was among the first topical anesthetics developed. Misapplication or mucous membrane exposure may result in serious systemic toxicity such as hyperexcitability, seizures, stroke, cerebral hemorrhage, tachycardia, arrhythmias, malignant hypertension, and cardiac arrest. As a result, TAC has been replaced by other topical anesthetics with similar efficacy, primarily LET [17].

6.6 Iontophoresis

Iontophoresis is a novel technique for transdermal administration of lidocaine. It uses an electric current from two externally placed electrodes to move ionized lidocaine across the stratum corneum barrier to the dermis. It provides effective pain relief for venous catheter placement or venipuncture within 10–20 minutes. However, several drawbacks include discomfort associated with the procedure, local skin reactions (including burns), and the frightening appearance of the device with many wires that may scare an already apprehensive child [18].

6.7 Topical Anesthesia for Mucosal Surface

Topical anesthetics for mucous membranes have a rapid onset of action, as the stratum corneum barrier is absent. EMLA, lidocaine jelly, viscous lidocaine, and benzocaine preparations may be used. Topical intraoral anesthesia can be helpful in minimizing pain with nerve blocks via the intra-oral route. When using EMLA, cetacaine (combination of benzocaine/tetracaine/butamen) or benzocaine in neonates and young infants, the amount applied should be carefully monitored, to avoid the risk of methemoglobinemia [19, 20].

6.8 Limitations of Topical Anesthetics

Limitations of topical anesthesia in the pediatric dermatology clinic include their delayed onset of action, inadequate depth of penetration, and toxicity when applied to large surface areas. The delayed onset of topical anesthetics can limit their use in the busy dermatology clinic setting. Newer products are being developed to enhance the delivery of topical anesthetics and shorten time to onset of action. For example, needle-free jet injection of 1% buffered lidocaine using a J-tip has been shown to be as effective as a 30-minute application of LMX for reducing the pain of IV catheter placement and is used routinely at children's hospitals [21].

Other limitations are inadequate depth of penetration of topical anesthetics, necessitating use of additional injected local anesthesia to achieve adequate anesthesia.

Body surface area limitations, particularly in young children, limit the quantity of topical anesthetic that may be applied. There are many reports in the dermatology literature detailing adverse events when topical anesthetics are applied to large areas for laser procedures [22]. General anesthesia should be considered for laser procedures in children.

6.9 Types of Injectable Local Anesthetics

Most local anesthetics are classified as amides or esters. Local anesthetics in the amide class include lidocaine (the most commonly used), bupivacaine, mepivacaine, etidocaine, prilocaine, ropivacaine, and levobupivacaine. Ester local anesthetics include procaine, 2-chloroprocaine, tetracaine, cocaine, and benzocaine. Due to toxicity and allergic reactions the ester agents have limited indications for local infiltration, except in patients with allergy to amide agents.

Lidocaine, bupivacaine, mepivacaine, and procaine are the most commonly used agents for infiltration of local anesthesia.

6.10 Lidocaine

Lidocaine, the most commonly used anesthetic for local infiltration, is usually given as a 1% solution (10 mg/ml). Higher concentrations of lidocaine beyond 1% do not promote improved onset and duration of analgesia and may increase the risk of toxicity. Buffering of lidocaine decreases pain of injection, especially when using lidocaine with epinephrine, and may shorten the time to anesthetic effect [23]. Utilizing lidocaine with epinephrine (at concentrations of 1:100000 or 1:200000) is helpful by inducing vasoconstriction, which decreases bleeding, prolongs the duration of anesthesia (up to three hours), and reduces systemic lidocaine absorption. The maximum dose of lidocaine without epinephrine is 4 mg/kg (0.4 ml/kg), and the maximum dose of lidocaine with epinephrine is 7 mg/kg (0.7 ml/kg). It is important to calculate the maximum dose, particularly in small children [24]. Since amide anesthetics are metabolized by the liver and excreted by the kidneys, the total dose of lidocaine should be decreased by approximately 50% in children with severe liver or kidney disease.

6.11 Bupivacaine

Bupivacaine is an amide anesthetic that is more potent and has a longer duration of action than lidocaine, mepivacaine, or procaine. If systemically absorbed, bupivacaine has the highest risk of major toxicity (seizures, intractable cardiac arrhythmias) of lidocaine and most other local anesthetics [25]. Bupivacaine is contraindicated for local infiltration in pregnant women. Since injection with bupivacaine is painful, it is not usually used for in-office procedures. However, it may be useful as an adjunctive local anesthetic agent when a child is sedated or under general anesthesia. Bupivacaine can be useful for longer procedures, certain nerve blocks, situations where prolonged post-procedure pain control is preferred, or in the rare event where there will be a delay between infiltration of local anesthetic and the procedure.

The maximum dose of bupivacaine without epinephrine is 2 mg/kg (0.8 ml/kg of bupivacaine 0.25%), and the maximum dose of bupivacaine with epinephrine is 3 mg/kg (1.2 ml/kg of bupivacaine 0.25%) [26]. The onset of action of bupivacaine is five to ten minutes and the duration of effect is up to six to eight hours. The addition of epinephrine does not increase the duration of anesthetic effect but may decrease systemic absorption, and may be useful to help decrease bleeding.

6.12 Side Effects of Local Anesthetics

Side effects of injectable local anesthetics include allergy, systemic toxicity, vasovagal syncope, and local side effects. Complications from local anesthetics are rare, particularly when care is taken to avoid intravascular injection into major vessels, and the maximum dosage is avoided.

Allergic contact dermatitis to local anesthetics has been reported, and true allergy with urticaria and anaphylaxis is rare, and data is limited to case reports. True allergy with urticaria and anaphylaxis to a local anesthetic is a contraindication for use of that anesthetic and to other agents in the same amide or ester class. If a patient has a suspected allergy, it would be ideal to have them evaluated by an allergist prior to an elective procedure, to determine whether the allergy is to the anesthetic or to a preservative [27, 28].

Systemic toxicity, such as central nervous system and cardiovascular symptoms, are unusual but may occur with an overdose, intravascular injection, or as an idiosyncratic response. Central nervous system effects include metallic taste, tinnitus, tingling of the lips, agitation, and seizures. Seizures are dose-dependent, and more likely to occur in patients with predisposing underlying conditions, hypercarbia, or hypoxemia [24]. Patients with lidocaine toxicity typically have initial CNS findings of altered taste, paresthesias, or agitation, whereas those with bupivacaine toxicity often have seizures as the first manifestation of toxicity. Seizures due to local anesthetic toxicity are usually brief. Initial treatment consists of oxygenation, airway support, and administration of a benzodiazepine (e.g. lorazepam 0.05 mg/kg). Cardiovascular side effects include bradycardia, decreased myocardial contractility, atrioventricular block, vasodilation, ventricular arrhythmias, and cardiac arrest.

Vasovagal syncope is usually associated with dizziness, diaphoresis, pallor, and bradycardia. To avoid vasovagal reactions, children should be lying down during the injection. If vasovagal symptoms develop, they can be alleviated by placing the patient in the Trendelenburg position.

Local side effects include bruising and edema. Transient motor nerve paralysis sometimes occurs. Sensory nerve paresthesia may develop if a sensory nerve is injured by an intraneural injection. This is a potential complication with nerve blocks, and can be minimized by avoiding intraneural injection and by using small-gauge needles for injection.

6.13 Techniques to Decrease Injection Pain

Techniques to decrease the pain of injection of local anesthetics include patient preparation, sodium bicarbonate buffering of lidocaine, warming of lidocaine, rate of injection, and size of the needle [29, 30].

The lidocaine injection is usually the most painful part of the procedure for the patient. The physician first can explain the technique to the child. It is important not to lie about the pain associated with injection. Avoid using words like "needle" or "shot", and explain that they may feel a pinch and then warmth, and afterwards the skin will go to sleep and they will not feel anything. Distraction techniques can be useful: watching a DVD or playing on a tablet computer. Pretending to blow out birthday candles, blowing bubbles, or blowing on a pinwheel can be useful distraction measures. Rubbing on the skin prior to the injection, a vibratory device, pinching the skin, or using ice, may lessen the pain of injection.

Oral sucrose solution is helpful for infants: a 24% solution of sucrose can be administered two minutes before a procedure, by placing it on the anterior tip of the tongue or dipping a pacifier in the solution. The sucrose may work through activation of sites in the brain that decrease pain perception, or it may cause the release of chemicals that cause babies to have less feeling of pain. Oral sucrose solution can be used by dermatologists for biopsies, injections, and laser treatments in infants younger than one year [31]. Sucrose solution has been shown to be more effective than liposomal lidocaine in diminishing pain associated with venipuncture in newborns [32].

Child life specialists, if available, are also extremely helpful with minimizing anxiety and providing distraction for pediatric procedures.

The pain associated with the injection of buffered lidocaine has been shown to be less painful than injection with unbuffered lidocaine, in many studies [23]. Most local anesthetics are acidic with pH of 5.0–7.0. The anesthetic is more stable in this pH range and has a shelf life of three to four years at room temperature. If the pH of the anesthetic solution is increased to 7.2–7.4 (physiologic pH) by the addition of sodium bicarbonate, the pain of injection is decreased. The concentrations of both lidocaine and epinephrine decrease once sodium bicarbonate is added. The buffered lidocaine is also more susceptible to photodegradation, aldehyde formation, and other denaturing reactions, leading to a shelf life of one to three weeks at room temperature. To make up buffered lidocaine: mix 1 ml of 8.4% sodium bicarbonate (1 mEq/ml) per 10 ml of 1% lidocaine. Proper refrigeration permits batch buffering of lidocaine with epinephrine. This buffering approach cannot be used for agents such as bupivacaine because precipitation occurs at physiologic pH.

Since infiltration of cold lidocaine is more painful, the buffered lidocaine should be warmed prior to injection. This can be accomplished by placing the syringe in warm water immediately before injection, or by having several syringes removed from the fridge at the beginning of each clinic and allowed to come to room temperature.

A small needle (30-gauge, 0.5 in., silicon-coated) should be used, with a small volume syringe (1–3 ml) to reduce pressure of injection. Injection technique should ideally have the needle inserted through the skin into a follicular orifice at 90° to the skin surface [33]. This minimizes the number of nerves that are encountered during the needle entry into the skin. The needle should then be directed to the subcutaneous layer, which is less painful than intradermal injection. Slow injection into fat with continued injection during withdrawal, and intradermal injection done last, is the most effective method to gain rapid anesthetic with minimal discomfort.

In children the local anesthetic injection can be done prior to prepping and draping the skin to allow more time for anesthetic onset of action, and time for the epinephrine to cause vasoconstriction. For sites of thick skin such as the back of an older adolescent, a one-inch 30-gauge needle may be used.

6.14 Limitations of Injectable Local Anesthesia

The size of the lesion is a limitation of local anesthesia, where the volume of local anesthesia is close to, or exceeds the maximum safe dose. For certain large procedures, a regional nerve block may be preferable.

Due to tissue distortion from injection of local anesthesia, a regional block might be for surgery in certain locations that require precise alignment such as the vermilion border of the lip.

Lidocaine with epinephrine is safe to use on the face, nose, ear, digits and penis. However, patients with peripheral artery disease should not have lidocaine with epinephrine injected for digital anesthesia. The total volume of lidocaine reaching the maximum dosage is of greater concern than the historic concerns of the epinephrine causing vasoconstriction and ultimately digital necrosis/ischemia [34]. (Sample references: Digital anesthesia with epinephrine: an old myth revisited J Am Acad Dermatol. 2004 / A comprehensive review of epinephrine in the finger: to do or not to do. Plast Reconstru Surg. 2001 Jul;108(1):114–24).

6.15 Nerve Blocks

Nerve blocks are frequently utilized for regional anesthesia in anatomic locations such as the face, scalp, fingers, toes or feet. Advantages of nerve blocks include better and longer pain control with smaller amounts of anesthetic.

The digital nerve block to numb fingers and toes is one of the most common nerve blocks in dermatology. It is a myth that epinephrine should not be used for digital blocks, and large studies and reviews of the literature have shown that lidocaine with epinephrine does not cause ischemic complications [34]. Using a 0.5 in. 30-gauge needle, approximately 1 ml of anesthetic is injected into the webspace on both sides of the proximal digit, at the superior aspect of the interphalangeal crease. The needle is directed both dorsally and ventrally, and injection proceeds slowly with constant movement to minimize the risk of injecting the artery. The areas of injection are then softly massaged in an attempt to diffuse the anesthetic throughout the soft tissue. Adequate anesthesia for the thumb requires either a ring block or three separate injections including an injection into the thenar eminence at the branching point of the median nerve. Complete anesthesia is usually obtained within minutes. However, if incomplete anesthesia is present after that interval, additional local anesthetic can be infiltrated in the surgical field [35].

Facial lesions can be adequately anesthetized by blocking four separate nerves that share a common anatomic position. The mental nerve, infraorbital nerve, supraorbital nerve, and supratrochlear nerves are responsible for providing sensation to the central chin and lower lip, upper lip and medial cheek, and mid-forehead and the upper forehead and scalp to the coronal suture, respectively. These four nerves all lie along a vertical line that crosses the mid-pupil, approximately 2.5 cm from the midline. If the various bony foramina cannot be palpated, using these anatomic reference points can usually result in performing successful nerve blocks [36]. Facial nerve blocks may be useful for older teens having laser surgery.

For a nerve block of the forehead, both the supraorbital and supratrochlear nerves must be blocked. Using a 0.5 in. 30-gauge needle, a small intradermal wheal is raised overlying the supraorbital notch. This is massaged with the finger for one to two minutes; the needle is then advanced in a vertical fashion through this zone of anesthesia down to the frontal periosteum and 1.5 ml of anesthetic is injected to anesthetize the supraorbital nerve. The needle is then withdrawn halfway and redirected toward the tip of the nose to anesthetize the supratrochlear nerve. Then 1–2 ml of 1% plain lidocaine is injected. Again, after four to five minutes, complete anesthesia of the ipsilateral forehead can be expected. With practice, these blocks can be used to reduce the pain of injection.

A similar approach is used to inject the infraorbital nerve to obtain anesthesia of the medial cheek. Topical anesthetic is applied to the labial sulcus superior to the canine fossa. After several minutes, a 1 in. 30-gauge needle can be painlessly advanced superiorly 1–2 cm to the infraorbital foramen, where 1–2 ml of 1% plain lidocaine is injected.

The mental nerve block is not commonly used in pediatric dermatology but may prove beneficial for surgical procedures on the lower lip or chin. Pretreating the mucosa with benzocaine or viscous lidocaine can help with the discomfort of this block. Using a cotton-tipped applicator, a small quantity of anesthetic agent is applied to the sulcus of the mandibular-buccal junction at the bases of the first and second lower premolars. After several minutes, a 1-inch 30-gauge needle can be painlessly introduced through this zone of anesthesia and advanced to the depth of the mandibular periosteum. Then, 1–2 ml of 1% plain lidocaine is injected near the mental foramen. To prevent prolonged anesthesia, the anesthetic should not be injected directly into the nerve itself. Within five minutes, the effect of the nerve block should be complete.

The posterior scalp can be anesthetized with a regional block by blocking the greater occipital nerve, which innervates the scalp posterior to the coronal suture. With the patient supine, the head is turned to one side and the occipital artery is palpated at the base of the occipital protuberance on the posterior scalp. A total of 2 ml of 0.25% bupivacaine with 1:200000 epinephrine is injected just medial to the artery to anesthetize the greater occipital nerve [37].

6.16 Indications for General Anesthesia

General anesthesia should be considered when a procedure is necessary but a child is too young to cooperate with local anesthesia.

Situations where general anesthesia is recommended include multiple laser treatments for extensive vascular malformations.

Lesions that favor excision during infancy such as medium or large congenital nevi on the trunk or limbs, a large nevus sebaceous on the scalp, and lesions located in cosmetically sensitive areas are indications for general anesthesia.

Other situations where general anesthesia may be considered include difficult anatomic locations such as nail surgery in younger children or a lesion located on the eyelid. General anesthesia may be indicated for children at any age with extreme anxiety, behavioral or developmental problems that would prevent a procedure being carried out safely using local anesthesia.

6.17 Types of Anesthesia Used in Pediatric Patients

Anxious children may receive pre-operative sedatives such as oral midazolam dosed at 0.3–0.5 mg/kg given 20–30 minutes prior to the procedure.

A general anesthetic can be divided into three distinct phases: induction, maintenance, and emergence. Induction of general anesthesia for children generally involves inhalation via a mask. The masks can be scented, such as with a strawberry scent, that makes them more pleasant to inhale for children. Many children's hospitals allow parents to come into the operating room while the child goes to sleep, making it a more comfortable experience for the child. Typically halogenated volatile anesthetics, such as sevoflurane and desflurane, are utilized in the United States as inhalational anesthetics. Volatile anesthetics are a popular choice because of their ease of delivery, reliable recovery, excellent safety profile, and modest cost. Nitrous oxide is often used in combination with volatile anesthetic agents. Once asleep with the inhalation anesthetic, an Laryngeal Mask Airway (LMA) can be placed to maintain the airway patency during general anesthesia and allow continued delivery of inhalational anesthesia. The LMA is a supraglottic airway that does not prevent aspiration. Complications associated with LMA placement include sore throat, oropharyngeal trauma, and an estimated 2 in 10 000 risk of aspiration.

Once asleep, a peripheral intravenous catheter can be placed to allow administration of IV medications and or IV fluids. Veins of the dorsal hand and upper limbs are the most common cannulation sites used by anesthesiologists.

For teenagers and adults, induction of anesthesia is generally achieved with intravenous anesthesia. The disadvantage is that an IV needs to be placed while the child is awake. The most commonly used induction agent in the United States is propofol because of its favorable recovery profile and short elimination half-life (resulting in less prolonged sedation and less nausea) [38]. This is ideal for short procedures commonly performed in dermatology.

Maintenance of anesthesia can be achieved with volatile or intravenous anesthesia. Pain medications are generally administered concurrently.

Emergence or "waking up" from general anesthesia is a crucial time where the anesthesiologist welcomes the patient back to a restored state of consciousness. With this return of consciousness there is a short period of time in which the patient's body is aware of the emergence without a full return to consciousness. This may result in autonomic hyper-responsiveness where certain medications such as short-acting narcotics, beta-blockers or lidocaine may sometimes be used to blunt these responses.

6.18 Safety

The American Society of Anesthesiologists states that the risk of an anesthetic complication for a healthy child is 1:20 000 to 80 000 or less.

Utilizing a pediatric anesthesiologist is essential. A French survey found an increased morbidity associated with pediatric surgical cases attended by anesthesiologists who cared for fewer than 200 children a year, supporting improved outcomes when anesthesia was performed by pediatric anesthesiologists [39].

Several factors determine the risk of anesthesia in pediatric patients, including age. The highest risk period is the first month of life. Several studies extend this to the first year of life. At most institutions the pediatric anesthesiologists are comfortable using general anesthesia for elective procedures starting at six months of age. The nature of the procedure is also a consideration. Emergency procedures have an approximately threefold increase in risk versus elective procedures. A 2005 retrospective study of 881 procedures performed on 269 patients by six pediatric dermatologic surgeons or laser surgeons at two institutions evaluated the risks of general anesthesia specifically for pediatric dermatologic procedures. Approximately 5% of patients experienced nausea or emesis. Otherwise, no serious adverse events occurred [40]. A 2010 study of 681 procedures in 226 patients undergoing pediatric dermatologic surgery reported no anesthesia-related complications [41]. A Spanish study evaluated the risk of pediatric dermatologic surgery in 210 children and found that general anesthesia is safe in the hands of experienced pediatric anesthetists, and the most common complication was scar stretching [42]. The following factors likely contribute to the safety of general anesthesia for pediatric dermatologic procedures: short procedure duration, elective basis, healthy patients, anesthesiologists trained in pediatric anesthesia, anesthesia administered in children's hospitals.

Newer data on general anesthesia and the developing brain are causing anesthesiologists and surgeons to investigate the effects of general anesthesia on children more thoroughly. The concern arises from animal studies suggesting that anesthetic drugs may cause apoptosis, and that if this occurs during a critical period of brain development, it may correlate with later behavioral disturbances. This data raise concerns that general anesthesia given to infants and young children may induce similar problems [43]. The available clinical data are based on largely retrospective studies that are inconclusive, mainly due to confounding variables inherent in these observational epidemiologic methods.

The largest study in children is a cohort study of 5357 children: 4764 with no anesthesia exposure and 593 with exposure before age four years. Results showed no difference in the incidence of learning disabilities between children who had a single anesthesia exposure early in life and those who had none, but children with two or three exposures to anesthesia were more likely to have a learning disability. However, these results do not conclusively prove that the anesthesia exposures were the cause of the learning disabilities, because it is highly possible that children who need multiple procedures may have other illnesses that confound the results [44].

Several retrospective sibling studies have been done. One study compared identical twins younger than three years and classified them as concordant exposed, concordant not exposed, or discordant (one exposed, one not exposed). The incidence of learning disability was not different in the discordant twins [45]. Another study compared 304 siblings that were exposed to anesthesia prior to three years of age to 10 146 siblings that did not have surgical procedures under age three years, and found that the risk of being subsequently diagnosed with developmental and behavioral disorders was increased, though they admit that the extent that the risk is causally attributable to anesthesia remains to be determined [46].

An additional study evaluated neurobehavioral development in a retrospective cohort of 314 pediatric patients under the age of six years who underwent a general anesthetic for a urologic procedure. A slight but not statistically significant difference in the frequency of behavioral disturbances was noted in children who had their procedure at <24 months [47].

Several ongoing prospective studies such as "General Anesthesia and Apoptosis Study", "Pediatric Anesthesia NeuroDevelopment Assessment" and "Mayo Safety in Kids" trial are further evaluating the effects of anesthesia on children. The relevance of animal data to humans remains unknown, but a panel of experts, convened by the US Food and Drug Administration in March 2011, concluded that "at this time, the evidence is not yet conclusive enough to support warning parents of potential risk" [48]. Several recent review articles have explained that the available evidence on anesthesia and the developing brain currently does not support a change in practice in the anesthetic management of infants and children [49–51].

When counseling parents regarding the risks of general anesthesia for pediatric dermatologic procedures reassurance can be provided regarding the short procedure duration, elective nature of the procedure, good baseline health, and availability of pediatric anesthesiologists. General anesthetic use for elective pediatric dermatologic procedures is typically associated with few comorbid factors, making it relatively safe, especially when administered by physicians trained in pediatric anesthesia.

6.19 Conclusion

Performing dermatologic procedure in pediatric patients presents many challenges. The use of topical anesthetics and careful attention to injection technique can minimize injection-related pain. With proper preparation, using a few special techniques, pediatric dermatologists can create a more pleasant experience for the child and family undergoing a procedure. Nerve blocks can be helpful in certain situations. Knowledge of the risks and benefits of general anesthesia can help physicians determine when a procedure is best performed under local or general anesthesia

References

1 Cunningham, B. and Wagner, A.M. (2011). Surgical techniques. In: *Pediatric Dermatology* (ed. L.A. Schachner and R.C. Hansen). Philadelphia, PA: Elsevier Mosby.

2 Buckley, M.M. and Benfield, P. (1993). Eutectic lidocaine/prilocaine cream. A review of the topical anaesthetic/analgesic efficacy of a eutectic mixture of local anaesthetics (EMLA). *Drugs* 46 (1): 126–151.

3 Choy, L., Collier, J., and Watson, A.R. (1999). Comparison of lidocaine-prilocaine cream and amethocaine gel for local analgesia before venipuncture in children. *Acta Paediatr.* 88 (9): 961–964.

4 De Waard-van der Spek, F.B., Mulder, P.G., and Oranje, A.P. (1997). Prilocaine/lidocaine patch as local premedication for skin biopsy in children. *J. Am. Acad. Dermatol.* 37: 418–421.

5 Raso, S.M., Fernandez, J.B., Beobide, E.A. et al. (2006). Methemoglobinemia and CNS toxicity after topical application of EMLA to a 4-year-old girl with molluscum contagiosum. *Pediatr. Dermatol.* 23 (6): 592–593.

6 Guay, J. (2009). Methemoglobinemia related to local anesthetics: a summary of 242 episodes. *Anesth. Analg.* 108: 699–701.

7 Rincon, E., Baker, R.L., Iglesias, A.J. et al. (2000). CNS toxicity after topical application of EMLA cream on a toddler with molluscum contagiosum. *Pediatr. Emerg. Care* 16: 252–254.

8 Hall, A.H., Kulig, K.W., and Rumack, B.H. (1986). Drug and chemical induced methaemoglobinaemia. Clinical features and management. *Toxicology* 1: 253–260.

9 Gajraj, N.M., Pennant, J.H., and Watcha, M.F. (1994). Eutectic mixture of local anesthetics (EMLA) cream. *Anesth. Analg.* 73 (3): 574.

10 Eichenfield, L.F., Funk, A., Fallon-Friedlander, S. et al. (2002). A clinical study to evaluate the efficacy of ELA-Max (4% liposomal lidocaine) as compared with eutectic mixture of local anesthetics cream for pain reduction of venipuncture in children. *Pediatrics* 109: 1093–1099.

11 Eidelman, A., Weiss, J.M., Lau, J. et al. (2005). Topical anesthetics for dermal instrumentation: a systematic review of randomized, controlled trials. *Ann. Emerg. Med.* 46 (4): 343–351.

12 Curtis, L.A., Dolan, T.S., and Seibert, H.E. (2009). Are one or two dangerous? Lidocaine and topical anesthetic exposure in children. *J. Emerg. Med.* 37: 32–39.

13 Harman, S., Zemek, R., Duncan, M.J. et al. (2013). Efficacy of pain control with topical lidocaine-epinephrine-tetracaine during laceration repair with tissue adhesive in children: a randomized controlled trial. *Can. Med. Assoc. J.* 185 (13): E629–E634.

14 Huang, W. and Vidimos, A. (2000). Topical anesthetics in dermatology. *J. Am. Acad. Dermatol.* 43: 286–298.

15 Lander, J., Hodgins, M., Nazarali, S. et al. (1996). Determinants of success and failure of EMLA. *Pain* 64: 89.

16 Schilling, C.G., Bank, D.E., Borchert, B.A. et al. (1995). Tetracaine, epinephrine(adrenalin), and cocaine (TAC) versus lidocaine, epinephrine, and tetracaine (LET) for anesthesia of lacerations in children. *Ann. Emerg. Med.* 25 (2): 203.

17 Galinkin, J.L., Rose, J.B., Harris, K. et al. (2002). Lidocaine iontophoresis versus eutectic mixture of local anesthetics (EMLA) for IV placement in children. *Anesth. Analg.* 94 (6): 1484.

18 So, T.Y. and Farrington, E. (2008). Topical benzocaine-induced methemoglobinemia in the pediatric population. *J. Pediatr. Health Care* 22: 335–339.

19 Bong, C.L., Hilliard, J., and Seefelder, C. (2009). Severe methemoglobinemia from topical benzocaine 7.5% (baby Oragel) use for teething pain in a toddler. *Clin. Pediatr.* 48: 209–211.

20 Spanos, S., Booth, R., Koenig, H. et al. (2008). Jet injection of 1% buffered lidocaine versus topical ELA-Max for anesthesia before peripheral intravenous catheterization in children: a randomized controlled trial. *Pediatr. Emerg. Care* 24: 511–515.

21 Sobanko, J.F., Miller, C.J., and Alster, T.S. (2012). Topical anesthetics for dermatologic procedures: a review. *Dermatol. Surg.* 38 (5): 701–721.

22 Cepeda, M.S., Tzortzopoulou, A., Thackrey, M. et al. (2010). Adjusting the pH of lidocaine for reducing pain on injection. *Cochrane Database Syst. Rev.* (12): CD006581.

23 Berde, C.B. (1993). Toxicity of local anesthetics in infants and children. *J. Pediatr.* 122 (5 Pt 2): S14.

24 Smith, T., Moratin, P., and Wulf, H. (1996). Smaller children have greater bupivacaine plasma concentrations after inguinal block. *Br. J. Anaesth.* 76: 452–455.

25 Tetzlaff, J.E. (2000). The pharmacology of local anesthetics. *Anesthesiol. Clin. North Am.* 18: 217.

26 Glinert, R.J. and Zachary, C.B. (1991). Local anesthetic allergy. Its recognition and avoidance. *J. Dermatol. Surg. Oncol.* 17: 491–496.

27 Bhole, M.V., Manson, A.L., Seneviratne, S.L. et al. (2012). IgE-mediated allergy to local anaesthetics: separating fact from perception: a UK perspective. *Br. J. Anaesth.* 108: 903–911.

28 Metz, B.J. (2013). Procedural pediatric dermatology. *Dermatol. Clin.* 31 (2): 337–346.

29 Yeo, L.F., Eichenfield, L.F., and Chan, Y.C. (2007). Skin surgery in children: local anaesthesia and sedation techniques. *Expert. Opin. Pharmacother.* 8 (3): 317–327.

30 Sorell, J., Carmichael, C., and Chamlin, S. (2010). Oral sucrose for pain relief in young infants with hemangiomas treated with intralesional steroids. *Pediatr. Dermatol.* 27 (2): 154–155.

31 Taddio, A., Shah, V., Stephens, D. et al. (2011). Effect of liposomal lidocaine and sucrose alone and in combination for venipuncture pain in newborns. *Pediatrics* 127 (4): e940–e947.

32 Martires, K.J., Malbasa, C.L., and Bordeaux, J.S. (2011). A randomized controlled crossover trial: lidocaine injected at a 90-degree angle causes less pain than lidocaine injected at a 45-degree angle. *J. Am. Acad. Dermal.* 65: 1231.

33 Krunic, A.L., Wang, L.C., Soltani, K. et al. (2004). Digital anesthesia with epinephrine: an old myth revisited. *J. Am. Acad. Dermatol.* 51 (5): 755.

34 Scarff, C.E. and Scarff, C.W. (2007). Digital nerve blocks: more gain with less pain. *Australas. J. Dermatol.* 48: 60–61.

35 Moskovitz, J.B. and Sabatino, F. (2013). Regional nerve blocks of the face. *Emerg. Med. Clin. North Am.* 31: 517–527.

36 Suresh, S. and Wagner, A.M. (2001). Scalp excisions: getting "ahead" of pain. *Pediatr. Dermatol.* 18: 74–76.

37 Rigby-Jones, A.E. and Sneyd, J.R. (2011). Propofol and children-what we know and what we do not know. *Paediatr. Anaesth.* 21 (3): 247–254.

38 Auroy, Y., Ecoffey, C., Messiah, A. et al. (1997). Relationship between complications of pediatric anesthesia and volume of pediatric anesthetics. *Anesth. Analg.* 84 (1): 234–235.

39 Cunningham, B.B., Gigler, V., Wang, K. et al. (2005). General anesthesia for pediatric dermatologic procedures: risks and complications. *Arch. Dermatol.* 141 (5): 573–576.

40 Juern, A.M., Cassidy, L.D., and Lyon, V.B. (2010). More evidence confirming the safety of general anesthesia in pediatric dermatologic surgery. *Pediatr. Dermatol.* 27 (4): 355–360.

41 Alfageme Roldan, F., Ciudad Blanco, C., Campos Dominguez, M. et al. (2009). Risk factors in pediatric dermatologic surgery. *Dermatol. Online J.* 15 (9): 2.

42 Hays, S.R. and Deshpande, J.L. (2011). Newly postulated neurodevelopmental risks of pediatric anesthesia. *Curr. Neurol. Neurosci. Rep.* 11 (2): 205–210.

43 Wilder, R.T., Flick, R.P., Sprung, J. et al. (2009). Early exposure to anesthesia and learning disabilities in a population based birth cohort. *Anesthesiology* 110 (4): 796–804.

44 Bartels, M., Althoff, R.R., and Boomsma, D.I. (2009). Anesthesia and cognitive performance in children: no evidence for a causal relationship. *Twin Res. Hum. Genet.* 12 (3): 246–253.

45 DiMaggio, C., Sun, L.S., and Li, G. (2011). Early childhood exposure to anesthesia and risk of developmental and behavioral disorders in a sibling birth cohort. *Anesth. Analg.* 113 (5): 1143–1151.

46 Kalkman, C.J., Peelen, L., Moons, K.G. et al. (2009). Behavior and development in children and age at the time of first anesthetic exposure. *Anesthesiology* 110: 805–812.

47 Kuehn, B.M. (2011). FDA considers data on potential risks of anesthesia use in infants, children. *JAMA* 305 (17): 1749–1750, 1753.

48 Olsen, E.A. and Brambrink, A.M. (2013). Anesthesia for the young child undergoing ambulatory procedures: current concerns regarding harm to the developing brain. *Curr. Opin. Anaesthesiol.* 26 (6): 677–684.

49 Gleich, S., Nemergut, M., and Flick, R. (2013). Anesthetic-related neurotoxicity in young children: an update. *Curr. Opin. Anaesthesiol.* 26 (3): 340–347.

50 Vlisides, P. and Xie, Z. (2012). Neurotoxicity of general anesthetics: an update. *Curr. Pharm. Des.* 18 (38): 6232–6240.

7

Skin Biopsy Techniques

Grace Sun

Dermatology Medical Group, Oxnard, CA, USA

7.1 Introduction

Many different situations necessitate removal or sampling of a skin lesion, including concern for malignancy, histopathological identification, tissue culture (bacterial, viral, fungal, mycobacterial) and cosmesis. There are multiple biopsy techniques, each with distinct advantages and disadvantages, that need to be considered when choosing a method. In this chapter, we review the different skin biopsy techniques and give examples of when they should be utilized.

7.1.1 Preparation for a Procedure

The first key to a successful biopsy experience for both the patient and the provider is a comfortable, safe procedural environment. Infants and young children should be restrained adequately with a sheet wrap and assistant(s). The ability of the parents to act as an assistant depends on the parent's level of comfort with the procedure. In most cases it is best for the parent to remain a spectator and act in the role of post-procedural comforter. Rarely, a parent may experience such anxiety that it is prudent to have them wait outside the room during the actual procedure. Young children may be bundled and wrapped with a sheet for safe restraint in a fashion that leaves the biopsy site exposed. School-age children will often be able to cooperate with the assistance of distraction. Handheld gaming consoles, tablets, child-friendly internet videos or movie DVDs and conversation are all potential helpful distraction methods. For extremely anxious patients 1 mg/kg of diphenhydramine or 0.2 mg/kg of diazepam prior to the procedure may be beneficial as well.

All the tools needed for the skin biopsy should be organized on a tray before entering the room so the patient and parents do not observe the instruments being set up, which can increase anxiety levels. Specimen containers should be labeled, top loosened, ready to receive the tissue or alternatively an assistant may open the containers during the procedure. For histopathology, use 10% formalin jars for routine H & E, for tissue culture, use a sterile urine cup with saline-soaked gauze to prevent specimen desiccation, and for direct immunofluorescence specimens, use Zeus or Michel's medium.

The biopsy site is cleaned first with an isopropyl alcohol 77% pad or chlorhexidine gluconate 4% and anesthetized with lidocaine 1% with epinephrine mix 1:100000 with a 30-gauge needle. Distraction with conversation, a vibrating device (e.g. Buzzy®), pinching the adjacent skin before inserting the needle and using lidocaine buffered with

Pediatric Dermatologic Surgery, First Edition. Edited by Keyvan Nouri, Latanya Benjamin, Jasem Alshaiji, and Jan Izakovic.

sodium bicarbonate may also decrease the noxious sensation. Infiltrating the lidocaine slowly, entering the skin at an angle, and inserting the needle with the bevel directed upward are helpful as well. For many children topical anesthetics, such as liposomal lidocaine 4 or 5% cream and a combination of lidocaine 2.5% and prilocaine 2.5% cream, applied 20–60 minutes prior to injection of local anesthesia, make the process more bearable. Mucosal sites will absorb the topical creams more rapidly and will be anesthetized in 5–15 minutes (see Chapter 6 for more on anesthetics).

7.2 Punch Biopsy

The punch biopsy is the ideal procedure for obtaining small specimens containing the epidermis and dermis extending to the fat. Small discrete lesions, melanocytic, non-melanocytic and papulosquamous eruptions are commonly biopsied in this fashion. Subcutaneous lesions including panniculitis or tumors can be sampled by using the punch tool to remove a plug of epidermis and dermis and open a window into which forceps and scissors are inserted to dissect out a piece of the lesion in question. For firm deep nodules, a "punch in a punch" or "double punch" method obtains a deep cylinder of tissue using two punch trephines of differing sizes. In the same way, the punch tool can be used superficially by gently scoring the epidermis and superficial dermis to make a window to dissect out superficial lesions like a follicular cyst. This superficial punch technique is also utilized in areas with thin skin overlying sensitive structures such as the dorsal hands and feet.

7.2.1 Supplies

Punch biopsies require a plastic and surgical steel disposable punch instrument (Figure 7.1), although in the past reusable stainless-steel instruments were sterilized and reused. Circular punch instruments come in sizes ranging from 1 to 12 mm in diameter and are executed with a twisting motion. Elliptical punch biopsy tools are also available but a rocking motion is used instead to enter the skin. A pair of toothed forceps, iris scissors, a needle holder, and a non-absorbable suture such as nylon or polypropylene will be needed.

7.2.2 Procedure

When performing a punch biopsy, the punch biopsy instrument is inserted into the skin and twisted in one direction to the level of the fat. Twisting the instrument back and forth may cause the epidermis to shear and detach from the specimen. Spreading the skin perpendicular to the natural skin lines at the biopsy site is a nice technique that results in an elliptical defect once the skin is relaxed, thereby preventing the "dog ear" or "standing cone" phenomenon during closure. Next, the isolated plug of tissue is gently lifted with the toothed forceps, taking care not to crush the tissue, and the base detached from the surrounding fat with the scissors. The depth to which the punch is twisted depends on the depth needed and it is not necessary to bury the punch tool to the hub unless the skin is very thick at the biopsy site. Once the dermis has been penetrated there is a change in resistance felt as the firm dermis gives way to soft subcutaneous fat. When performing a "double punch" a larger punch is first performed; a smaller punch trephine is then inserted into this space to remove a smaller, deeper core of tissue. For example, a 6 mm punch would be done first and then a 4 mm punch used to obtain the deep sample. Because the hub of the punch is larger in diameter than the trephine, the larger first punch allows the hub of the second to pass through without obstruction to the deep tissue. Once the specimen has been safely deposited in the appropriate container, any biopsy site greater than 3 mm should be closed with either simple interrupted stitches, a horizontal mattress, or a figure of eight stitch.

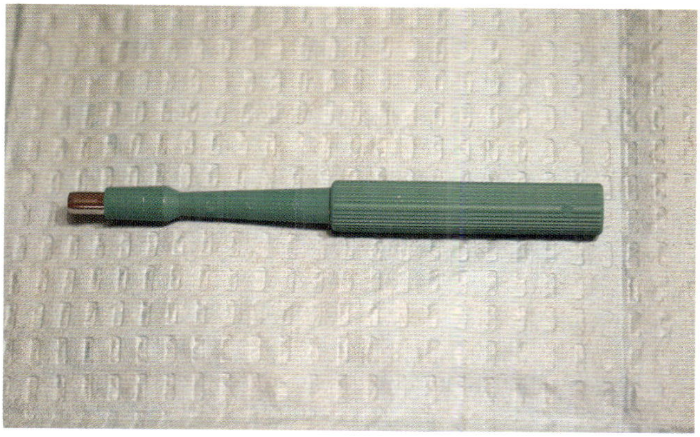

Figure 7.1 Punch biopsy instrument.

Small punch biopsies (2–3 mm) can be left to heal via secondary intention. A dermal suture(s) is often required for punch biopsies 6 mm and greater in diameter.

7.3 Shave Biopsy

The shave biopsy is an adaptable technique ideal for lesions that do not extend to the fat. Because the depth of the shave can be simply adjusted with user-technique, very superficial small samples with the "tangential shave" can be obtained for cosmetically sensitive areas while "saucerization shave" of larger lesions that extend deeper into the dermis can also be accomplished. This technique is most commonly used for suspected non-melanoma skin cancer as well as larger melanocytic lesions in which submitting the entire piece is preferable to a portion sample [1].

7.3.1 Supplies

Shave biopsies can be performed with a variety of tools including the flexible plastic and stainless steel DermaBlade®, double-edged razor (these can be easily snapped in half to eliminate the sharp edge facing the fourth and fifth fingers for safety purposes) (Figures 7.2 and 7.3) or a 15 blade scalpel. Sometimes a pair of forceps or a Q-tip is used to stabilize the specimen if it is particularly fragile or large.

7.3.2 Procedure

The lidocaine used for anesthesia should be injected into the superficial dermis, causing a distinct wheal of raised skin that will facilitate the biopsy. Both the double-edged razor and DermaBlades are utilized in the same manner, with the thumb and third finger on the short ends of the blade. Place the fifth finger against a firm surface or the patient to stabilize the entire hand (Figure 7.4). The curvature of the blade can be adjusted based upon the amount of pressure placed on either end, thereby determining the width of the biopsy. The depth of the biopsy is determined by the angle of the blade entering the skin and scooping under the lesion being sampled. The blade is pressed to the skin at the edge of the lesion to be biopsied and with a gentle back and forth motion, passed into the skin to the desired depth and continued horizontally beneath the lesion and then re-angled to exit on the other side of the lesion. The versatility of the blade allows one to remove lesions in a very exact manner (Figure 7.5). In areas of little traction or with a fragile specimen, the non-dominant hand may employ forceps or a cotton-tipped applicator to stabilize the specimen. Another option is to use the index finger of the dominant hand as the thumb and third finger are holding the blade. The main difference between the DermaBlade and double-edged razor is the length of the blade, as the DermaBlades are longer and can easily remove very large specimens.

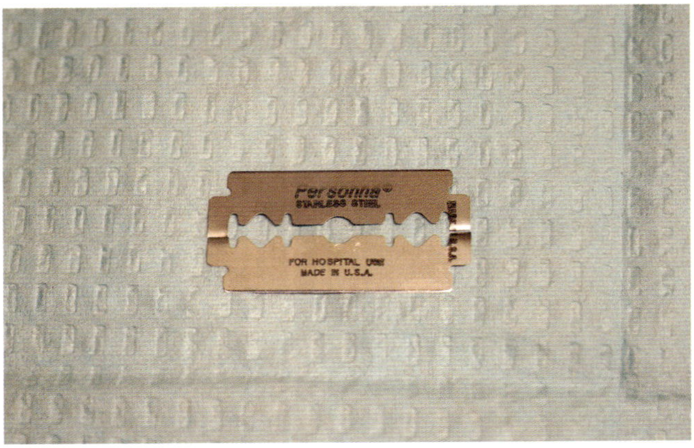

Figure 7.2 Double-edged blade.

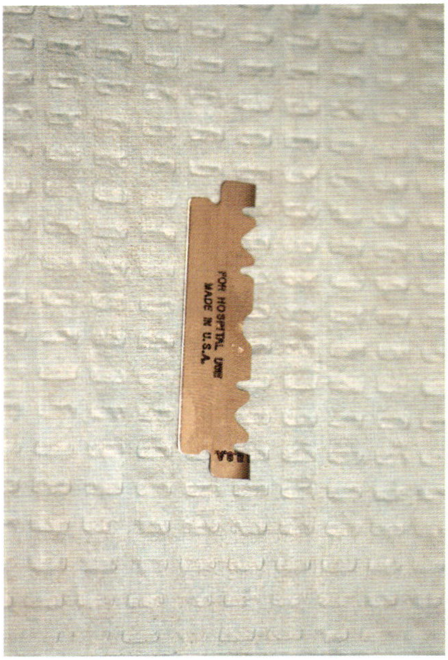

Figure 7.3 Half of a double-edged blade.

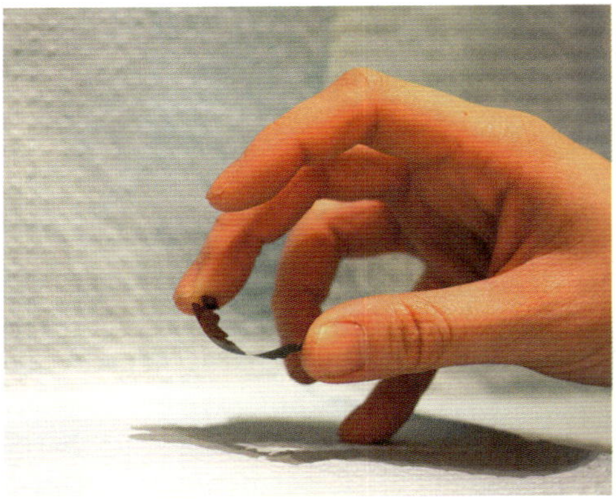

Figure 7.4 Hand positioning for a shave biopsy. The blade is held with the first and third finger, and the fifth finger provides stabilization. The second finger is free and may be used to provide traction for the specimen.

Shave biopsies can also be done with a number 15 or 10 blade on a scalpel but this technique is more challenging and suitable for small lesions that will not exceed the length of the blade. Traction is applied along the axis of lesion parallel to the direction that the blade will take. The blade is held at an angle to the skin near the edge of the lesion and an incision is created to the desired depth. The blade is then pressed horizontally under the lesion in a clean slicing motion with minimal back and forth movement and the tip end of the blade always visible to the side of the lesion. Excessive sawing motion with the blade tip sliding under the specimen will destroy the inferior surface and produce a suboptimal specimen. Sometimes if the angle is difficult to achieve, the non-dominant hand may pinch up the skin on either side of the lesion to create a more favorable angle for the blade.

Aluminum chloride 20% solution, ferric subsulfate 20% solution and electrodesiccation are all options for achieving hemostasis. Ferric subsulfate may result in discoloration

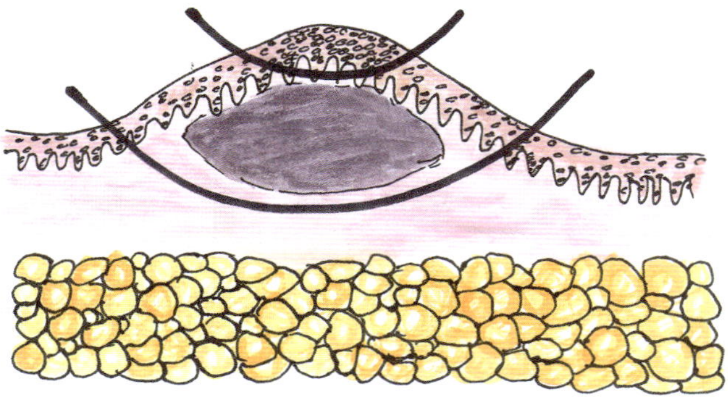

Figure 7.5 Diagram of a superficial shave biopsy of the epidermis and a deep saucerization shave biopsy into the dermis.

of the treated area and excessive electrocoagulation may inhibit wound healing and leave a more prominent scar.

7.4 Scissors Biopsy

Also referred to as a "snip biopsy," this is the preferred technique for pedunculated lesions with a very thin base such as acrochordons, certain verruca, dermatosis papulosa nigra, etc. In the case of very small lesions or in needle-phobic patients sometimes local anesthesia is not necessary.

Supplies: A pair of forceps and a pair of iris scissors are required.

Procedure: Using the forceps, the pedunculated lesion is raised perpendicularly from the skin and slight traction applied, the scissor is placed flush with the skin and the lesion is snipped off. If local anesthesia was deferred, take care when grasping the lesion gently with the forceps to avoid causing unnecessary pain.

Specialized areas: lips, tongue, genitals, scalp, dorsal hands/feet, fingers/toes

7.4.1 Lips

The mucosal lip is soft, moist, friable and has an exuberant vascular supply making a biopsy difficult. A chalazion clamp helps with traction, hemostasis and a secure grip (Figures 7.6 and 7.7). Once the area to be biopsied is anesthetized, the chalazion clamp can be fitted on either side of the lip with the ring looping over the proposed biopsy site and gently tightened to apply enough pressure to prevent bleeding during the biopsy. The clamp can be slightly relaxed and retightened as needed while obtaining hemostasis with electrocoagulation and ferric subsulfate. Punch and excisional biopsies are best suited for this site and require closure with a dissolvable soft braided or gut suture to minimize discomfort. For large lesions requiring an excisional biopsy, pressure may be obtained with an assistant firmly compressing the labial artery on either side of the biopsy site. Care should be taken to orient the long axis of the excision for the best cosmetic effect. Scars oriented horizontally can be hidden inside the lip. However, if the scar is very long, it can often shorten the depth of the lip. Vertical orientation can also be acceptable if the scar does not extend across the vermilion border. These same principles apply to biopsies of the buccal mucosa as well.

7.4.2 Tongue

The tongue is a strong muscular organ and a biopsy without sedation would require a cooperative patient. The tongue is first stabilized with a firm grip using a dry piece of gauze by an assistant. A punch, excisional or

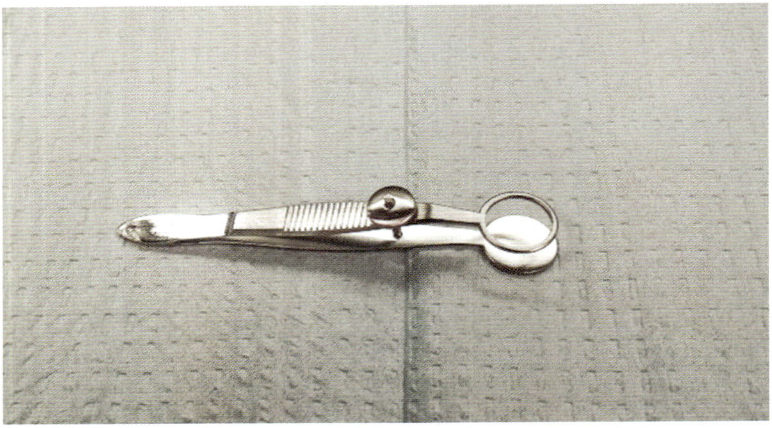

Figure 7.6 Chalazion clamp.

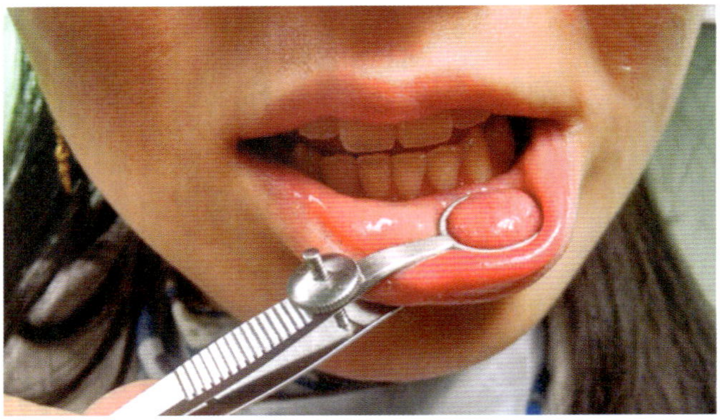

Figure 7.7 Demonstration of a chalazion clamp on the lip.

incisional biopsy may then be performed with anesthesia. If an incisional or excisional biopsy is performed, suction would be advisable to keep the field clear of blood and facilitate suture placement. A soft braided suture such as silk is preferable for patient comfort.

7.4.3 Genitalia

The genitals present a challenge as the skin is very thin and the underlying tissue pliable and loose. Superficial infiltration of the anesthesia forming a firm wheal will provide a more stable base for the biopsy, nevertheless, shave biopsies will still be difficult and the non-dominant hand may need to assist with pinching up and maneuvering the skin. Shallow punch and incisional biopsies are preferable for these areas and should be closed with a soft braided suture for comfort. In the past, it was thought that lidocaine supplemented with epinephrine should be avoided in the fingers, toes, penis, nasal tip and ear owing to a risk of necrosis. However, there have been numerous reviews in the last 20 years that have consistently disproved this theory [2–4]. It is still recommended to inject the minimum amount of lidocaine and epinephrine needed to achieve anesthesia to prevent tamponade of the draining veins of the penis.

7.4.4 Fingers and Toes

As there is similar concern for tamponade of the digits, care should be taken to use the minimum amount of lidocaine needed to achieve anesthesia. There is no need to avoid epinephrine as discussed above. A digital nerve block at the base of the digit to anesthetize the entire digit may be used in conjunction with local infiltration at the biopsy site (see Chapters 6 and 13 for the specifics for performing nerve blocks). After the biopsy a pressure dressing should be applied in a fashion that allows visualization of the tip of the digit so the patient or parent can ensure adequate perfusion of the digit. If the digit becomes dusky or purple in color, the dressing should be loosened (see Chapter 12 for more details on dressings).

7.4.5 Dorsal Hands and Feet

The dorsal hands and feet tend to have thinner skin with important underlying structures. Creating a superficial wheal while placing anesthesia will lift the skin and create a more stable base for the biopsy. Depending on whether the particular biopsy site is convex or concave one can choose to do a shave or a superficial punch as described above. The key is to raise the skin with the local anesthesia and keep the biopsy superficial to avoid injury to underlying vessels and tendons.

7.4.6 Scalp

In contrast to the dorsal hands and feet, the scalp has a much thicker dermal layer and the challenge is concerning hemostasis. In ideal conditions, the lidocaine with epinephrine 1:100000 would be placed for at least 10–20 minutes prior to performing the biopsy to allow adequate vasoconstriction to occur. Raised epidermal lesions can be sampled via shave biopsy with electrodesiccation, aluminum chloride 20% or ferric subsulfate 20%. When the biopsy is performed for hair loss disorders, two punch biopsies should be submitted, with one to be sectioned vertically (standard) and one to be sectioned horizontally. This intent should be indicated clearly on the pathology form and submitted with the specimens. Punch biopsies should be closed with non-absorbable sutures. Choosing a suture that contrasts with the hair color allows for easier location and suture removal later.

7.5 Incisional Biopsy

An incisional biopsy, by definition, does not attempt to remove the entire lesion in question but samples a portion for determining the diagnosis. Usually, it is implied that the biopsy must reach the subcutaneous fat, and thus superficial shave and snip biopsies would not fall in this category. A punch biopsy, deep punch, and elliptical incisional biopsy are good choices for an incisional biopsy. However, technically a deep shave can be done on a portion of the lesion in question and still qualify as an incisional biopsy if an attempt is made to remove a large portion of the lesion. This technique is often used to sample a large tumor or to obtain a wedge of subcutaneous tissue for inflammatory or infectious processes. A 15 or 10 blade can be used on a scalp to create an ellipse to the subcutaneous fat and closed in a layered fashion (see Chapter 8 for the basic excision).

7.6 Excisional Biopsy

An excisional biopsy, by definition, is a biopsy that intends to remove the entire lesion in toto. Depending on the size of the lesion this can be done with a punch biopsy tool or a scalpel. Deep saucerization shave biopsies can also fall in this category if the intent is to remove the lesion entirely, although these are usually simply called "deep saucerizations" while "excisional biopsy" often implies a complete elliptical excision (see Chapter 8 for basic excision technique).

7.7 Complications

Skin biopsies are generally small in nature and hemostasis is usually achieved easily with electrocoagulation, aluminum chloride

20%, ferric subsulfate 20% or silver nitrate. These hemostatic agents may be used in combination, but care should be taken to avoid electrodesiccation following aluminum chloride, which is extremely flammable. On the scalp, placing simple interrupted stitches can tamponade and stop excessive bleeding. Firm pressure for 10–15 minutes to any other area on the body is usually very effective to control bleeding. However, assisting staff must be trained to do this properly. Another method of hemostasis is to apply a pressure dressing, in which one or two pieces of gauze are firmly pressed against the bleeding area of tissue with firm backing from bony structure beneath. If the tissue at the biopsy site is loose and soft (i.e. lip, genitalia, cheek, nose) then a pinching hold should be employed instead. Again, a pressure dressing applied after the bleeding has stopped may also provide sustained benefit.

Another common complication for children is a biopsy site infection. Clean technique while performing the biopsy and good wound care afterward will prevent infection. Individuals may erroneously assume that the formation of a crust or "scab" will lead to more rapid wound healing, although research contends that a dry wound bed delays wound healing. Thus maintenance of a moist environment must be specifically explained and emphasized to families. The patient/parent should be provided with written instructions to wash the area daily, apply petrolatum and keep the site covered and clean until healed. Biopsies done in intertriginous and flexural areas are more prone to develop infections, and meticulous hygiene should be encouraged. Immunosuppression, diabetes and *Staphylococcus aureus* colonization are predisposing conditions for infection as well [5]. However, as a general guiding principal, topical antibiotics should not be routinely prescribed or recommended owing to the risk of contact allergy sensitization and lack of proven superiority over plain petrolatum/paraffin [6, 7].

7.8 Conclusion

All the traditional biopsy techniques used in adults apply to the pediatric population in terms of surgical technique. However, the difference lies in execution, as children of different developmental stages are often anxious, unwilling or unable to fully cooperate with the procedure. Speed, precision, and composure are all skills that can be fostered with practice. Safety for the patient, the staff and yourself are utmost in importance and good judgment will dictate if a biopsy can be safely performed. If it is not possible for the child to be gently restrained, sedation will be required to safely obtain a specimen in a non-traumatic way for the child.

References

1 Mendese, G., Maloney, M., and Bordeaux, J. (2014). To scoop or not to scoop: the diagnostic and therapeutic utility of the scoop-shave biopsy for pigmented lesions. *Dermatol. Surg.* 40 (10): 1077–1083.

2 Häfner, H.M., Röcken, M., and Breuninger, H. (2005). Epinephrine-supplemented local anesthetics for ear and nose surgery: clinical use without complications in more than 10,000 surgical procedures. *J. Dtsch. Dermatol. Ges.* 3 (3): 195–199.

3 Krunic, A.L., Wang, L.C., Soltani, K. et al. (2004). Digital anesthesia with epinephrine: an old myth revisited. *J. Am. Acad. Dermatol.* 51: 755–759.

4 Thompson, C.J., Lalonde, D.H., Denkler, K.A. et al. (2007). A critical look at the evidence for and against elective epinephrine use in

the finger. *Plast. Reconstr. Surg.* 119: 260–266.

5 Tai, Y.J., Borchard, K.L., Gunson, T.H. et al. (2013). Nasal carriage of Staphylococcus aureus in patients undergoing Mohs micrographic surgery is an important risk factor for postoperative surgical site infection: a prospective randomised study. *Australas. J. Dermatol.* 54 (2): 109–114.

6 Levender, M.M., Davis, S.A., Kwatra, S.G. et al. (2012). Use of topical antibiotics as prophylaxis in clean dermatologic procedures. *J. Am. Acad. Dermatol.* 66 (3): 445–451.

7 Nijhawan, R.I., Smith, L.A., and Mariwalla, K. (2013). Mohs surgeons' use of topical emollients in postoperative wound care. *Dermatol. Surg.* 39 (8): 1260–1263.

8

Common Pediatric Dermatologic Surgery Procedures

Meagan Barrett[1], Nicole Harter[1], and Ashley Wysong[2]

[1] The Keck School of Medicine of USC and LAC + USC Medical Center, Los Angeles, CA, USA
[2] Department of Dermatology, University of Nebraska Medical Center (UNMC) College of Medicine, Nebraska Medical Center, Omaha, NE, USA

8.1 Introduction

Pediatric dermatologic surgery requires several special considerations. In each stage of a child's development there are different challenges to performing procedures that should be anticipated [1]. The patient's age, cognitive development and awareness, past experiences with the health care system, and overall disposition will influence the child's understanding, level of participation, ability to cooperate, tolerance, and reaction to the procedure. This is why the appropriate approach and timing of surgery is key to a successful outcome.

8.2 Cryosurgery

8.2.1 Introduction

Cryosurgery is based on the principle that tissue destruction occurs when tissue temperatures are reduced to subzero [2]. Freezing causes direct and indirect cellular injury. The initial direct injury is through crystal formation, which produces intracellular shearing and water imbalance. Rapid cooling enhances the formation of intracellular ice, augmenting cellular death. The indirect secondary injury is via microcirculatory failure during the thawing period in which vascular stasis leads to ischemic necrosis [3]. Slow thawing is the primary mechanism of cell death and is in fact more important than rapid cooling. Repeated freeze–thaw cycles can be used to enhance destruction. The central portion of the cryogenic lesion undergoes necrosis, which is surrounded by a peripheral zone in which only partial cell death occurs [3].

Cryosurgery is a common and effective technique to treat common benign lesions of childhood. Preparing the child before the procedure can also improve tolerance. Topical anesthesia can be considered. An application of 5% mixture of lidocaine/prilocaine cream (Eutectic Mixture of Local Anesthetics, EMLA) or 4% lidocaine cream (LMX) applied 30 minutes to one hour prior to the procedure is usually sufficient. Caution must be taken in the use of prilocaine in children younger than three months of age as they may be more susceptible to the potential side effect of methemoglobinemia. Using child-friendly terms such as "cold popsicle" versus "freezing" on the skin is effective. The child should also be rewarded for cooperation and safely shown "smoking" of the liquid nitrogen following successful treatment.

Pediatric Dermatologic Surgery, First Edition. Edited by Keyvan Nouri, Latanya Benjamin, Jasem Alshaiji, and Jan Izakovic.

8.2.2 Indications

Cryosurgery is one of the most frequently used modalities in the dermatology clinic due to its wide range of applications and convenience. Liquid nitrogen can be used to treat benign, pre-malignant, and in some rare cases malignant lesions. However, when treating the pediatric population the majority of lesions will be benign, such as for common warts.

Melanocytes are killed at a temperature of −4 to −7 °C, thus less aggressive freezing is required for lesions in which melanocytes are targeted. Keratinocytes and malignant cells are killed at tissue temperatures of −20 to −30 °C, thus this should be the minimum temperature achieved for pre-malignant or malignant lesions. All cells, including fibroblasts, die at temperatures of −50 to −60 °C. In general, a light freeze will cause separation of the epidermis at the dermal-epidermal junction and will not reach temperatures that causes damage to the collagen network. In turn, this leaves intact the cells that will be responsible for wound healing. The target temperature depends upon the lesion being treated, see Table 8.1 for a list of indications and recommended freeze times.

Table 8.1 Cryosurgery – Indications and recommended freezing times [4–11].

Indication	Freeze time; seconds (s)	Notes
Acne cyst	5–15 s	
Acne scar	Face 5 s Back 5–15 s	Laser generally preferred
Acrochordon	5–10 s	
Angiofibroma	5–20 s	
Calcinosis cutis		
Capillary hemangioma		Need to treat early
Condyloma accuminata		
Dermatofibroma	30–45 s	Usually 1–3 sessions
Elastosis perforans Serpiginosa		Recurrences are common
Granuloma annulare		
Keloid	30 s	Better results with combination therapy
Milia		
Molluscum contagiosum	5–10 s	
Mucocele		
Persistent cutaneous pseudolymphoma		
Prepubertal bowenoid papulosis		Consider child abuse
Pyogenic granuloma		
Seborrheic keratosis	5–30 s	Duration based on amount of hyperkeratosis
Steatocytoma multiplex		Poor response, can see scarring
Syringoma		Good response after 2–3 sessions
Verruca plana	2–5 s	
Verruca vulgaris	10–15 s	10s sustained freeze more effective but more painful
Xanthelasma	5 s	

8.2.3 Contraindications

There are very few true contraindications to cryotherapy. A patient with a history of cold anaphylaxis or cold urticaria would not be a candidate for cryosurgery. Alternative therapies should be considered in patients with diseases that are aggravated by cold, including cryoglobulinemia or cryofibrinogenemia. Cryosurgery should not be performed on lesions where histology is important for diagnosis. Patients with darker skin types are at increased risk for post-inflammatory hyper- or hypopigmentation.

8.2.4 Techniques

There are multiple methods of application of the cryogen. Each technique influences the depth of freeze, lateral spread, and temperature achieved. Paring of hyperkeratotic lesions prior to application can enhance the effect by facilitating penetration of the cryogen into the target tissue.

The most common modality used in dermatology is the open spray method, in which a handheld canister containing evaporated liquid nitrogen is applied to the lesional skin with a pressurized spray (Figure 8.1a). Less distance between the tip of the spray canister and the target tissue results in a faster rate of tissue freezing, less lateral spread, and increased depth of freeze. An intermittent spray technique can also be used to minimize lateral spread. For more specific targeting, a neoprene cone can be added to the tip of the spray canister.

An alternative method is cotton tip application, which is more commonly used in pediatrics, as it is less intimidating and usually less painful. Cotton tip applicators penetrate more superficially, usually 2–3 mm, thus there is less destruction and fewer adverse effects. Since the lesions being treated in pediatrics are usually benign, the cotton tip method is acceptable and usually sufficient, though it may require an increased number of treatments (Figure 8.1b).

The cold instrument technique is ideal for treating exophytic or pedunculated lesions (Figure 8.1c). This is usually accomplished by dipping a metal pickup in liquid nitrogen until it is able to transfer the cold to the target lesion. The technique should be repeated until an ice frost extends to the base of the lesion. This technique allows for more accurate application to the identified lesion. It also allows the clinician to control the depth of the destruction and to presumably limit adverse effects.

There are other techniques that are less commonly used in dermatology, including the probe and spray method. A cryoprobe, a metal conductor, is connected to the liquid nitrogen unit forming a closed system. This method allows for greater destruction but also has an increased risk for adverse effects and is generally not recommended in the pediatric population.

8.2.5 Complications/Adverse Effects

A stinging, burning sensation should be expected during the freezing of the lesion, while a throbbing pain occurs during the thawing period and after. An erythematous lesion or blister can form at the dermoepidermal junction within three to six hours after treatment. The lesion will then flatten in two to three days, followed by desquamation in two to four weeks. It is important to counsel the patient and family that this is the intended effect, and allows for destruction of the lesion. The degree of erythema, edema, and pain will depend upon the depth and lateral spread of the freeze.

Dyspigmentation is another common adverse effect seen with cryosurgery. The sensitivity of melanocytes to cold injury causes this loss of pigment. Darker skin types are at higher risk for post-inflammatory hyper- and/or hypo-pigmentation. Repigmentation occurs from the margins inward and can take from months to years. This discussion should be had with the patient prior to treatment.

Treatment for less than 30 seconds usually does not cause damage to fibroblasts or

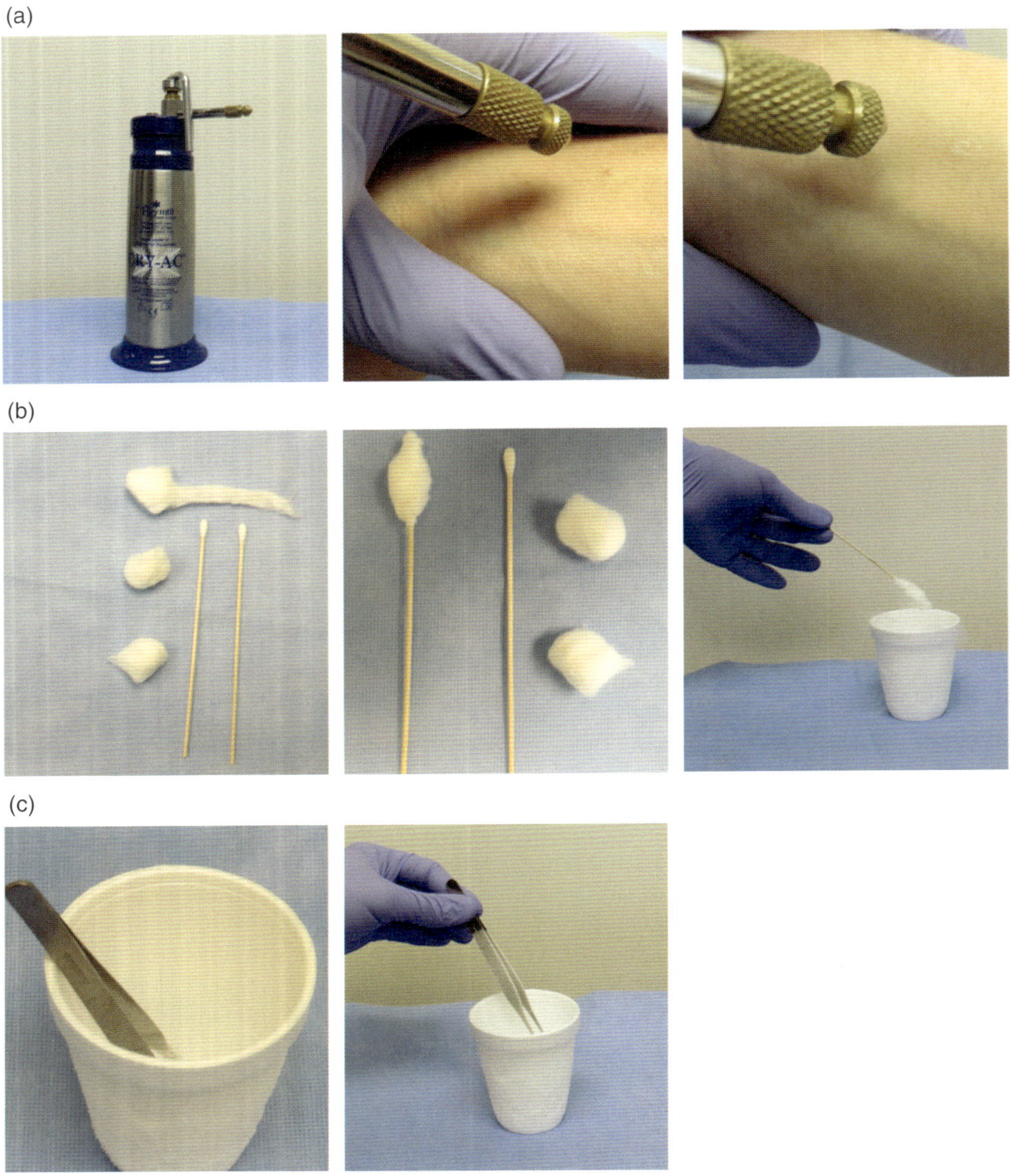

Figure 8.1 (a) Open Spray application of liquid nitrogen to lesional skin. (b) Cotton tip applicator method. (c) Forceps applicator method.

collagen. Therefore the foundation for wound healing is still present and scarring does not occur. However, with a deeper, longer freeze the risk of inducing scarring increases. In predisposed patients, hypertrophic scars or keloids may develop. Wound contraction may occur with scarring, therefore free margins on the face should be treated with extra precaution. Permanent nail dystrophy can occur if the nail plate or matrix is damaged during treatment. Alopecia may also develop when treating hair-bearing skin, due to destruction of the follicle.

Less common adverse effects include bacterial superinfection, sensory nerve damage, hemorrhage, and subcutaneous emphysema. Superinfection is rare and usually due to poor wound care. Destruction of a superficial nerve can result in paresthesias. However, the resistance of the nerve sheath to damage makes permanent loss of sensation unlikely. Delayed hemorrhage is extremely rare but may occur up to 10–14 days following treatment. Subcutaneous emphysema can occur when treating an ulcerated or open lesion if there is insufflation of the underlying tissue.

8.2.6 Conclusion

Cryosurgery is a valuable treatment for the dermatologist given its ease of use, wide range of applications, and limited adverse effects. Given that the majority of lesions in pediatric patients are benign and tolerance may be an issue, the practitioner may want to consider a shorter, lighter freeze or cotton tip application, anticipating that more treatment sessions may be required.

8.3 Curettage

8.3.1 Introduction

Curettage is defined as the superficial scraping of tissue by means of a curette for the removal of the target lesion. A curette is a cutting instrument with a circular or oval, loop-shaped cutting edge with a handle, available in varying sizes from 1 to 10 mm in diameter (Figure 8.2). Curettes are available as disposable or reusable instruments. In many instances curettage is followed by electrodesiccation to control bleeding and destroy any remaining involved tissue (see section on electrosurgery for details).

8.3.2 Indications

Curettage is commonly used in the treatment of benign or low-grade malignant tumors, or as an adjuvant modality when debulking large or exophytic neoplasms. Two of the most common indications in pediatric dermatology are milia and molluscum contagiosum [12].

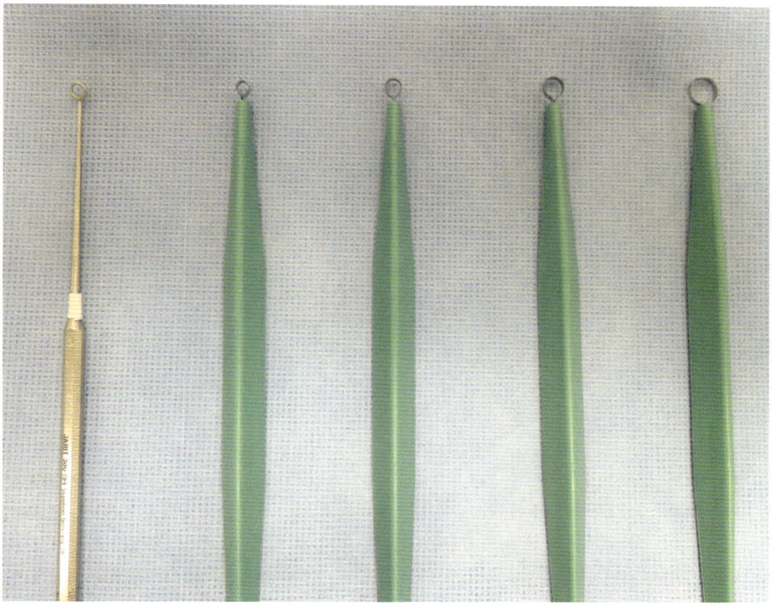

Figure 8.2 Curettes ranging from left to right: sterile reusable, 3mm, disposable, 4mm disposable, 5mm disposable, 7mm disposable.

Often these lesions can be fully removed with curettage, in contrast to multiple office visits or prolonged treatment courses with topical therapy or cryosurgery. However, in this patient population local anesthesia (such as topical and/or intralesional lidocaine) is generally required.

Curettage is also indicated for the treatment of epidermal nevi, keratoses, verruca, abscesses, soft tissue infections, and pyogenic granulomas. Treatment of pyogenic granulomas with curettage, in comparison to cryosurgery, has better cosmetic results and requires fewer treatment sessions [13]. Although providers may be concerned about post-procedural scarring there is evidence that curettage can provide smaller scars and less post-inflammatory pigmentary alteration.

Curettage has been described as a valuable treatment modality in less common pediatric diseases, such as Epidermodysplasia verruciformis (EDV)and giant congenital melanocytic nevi (GCMN) [14, 15]. EDV is a rare genodermatosis, characterized by increased susceptibility to HPV infections and development of polymorphic cutaneous lesions that clinically resemble flat warts and/or tinea versicolor. In this setting curettage allows for the treatment of multiple lesions simultaneously with a satisfactory cosmetic result, low-cost, and low rate of recurrence. Following removal of the lesion(s) the application of 35% trichloroacetic acid (TCA) can be used for hemostasis and to further reduce the risk of recurrence. Importantly, given that EDV patients are at increased risk for actinic keratosis and SCC, this technique should not be used when malignancy is suspected because it can alter the histopathologic evaluation.

Giant congenital melanocytic nevus (GCMN) is defined as a nevus present at birth that is greater than 20 cm in diameter, and is differentiated from other congenital nevi given their increased risk for developing malignant melanoma. Curettage is a unique treatment that may be applied to GCMN early in life [16]. In the first few weeks of life there is a cleavage between the upper dermis (which contains most of the pigmented cells) and deep dermis, creating a natural plane in which curettage can be applied. This technique is ideally performed within the first two weeks of life, but can be implemented up to eight weeks, and patients should be placed under general anesthesia. Compared with staged excisions for removal of GCMN, curettage is a one-stage technique, is less traumatic than excision, results in less blood loss, less post-operative pain, and less scarring with more favorable cosmetic results [17]. There is no literature to date examining the effects of curettage on the subsequent monitoring and development of malignant melanoma.

8.3.3 Contraindications

There are no true contraindications to curettage. Standard surgical precautions including risk of bleeding, wound-site infection, poor healing, and risk of scarring should be considered. Curettage can alter the histopathologic evaluation of tissue, thus should not be used to treat potentially malignant lesions without a prior definitive diagnosis.

8.3.4 Technique

Curettage technique may be guided by the type of lesion and goal of therapy [18]. Generally, smaller curette sizes are used for finer procedures, while larger curettes assist in de-bulking or removal of masses more quickly.

Anesthesia is not always necessary, but may be considered based on the clinical scenario. Tissue distortion that occurs with infiltration of local anesthetic can make curettage technically difficult, and may require lag time after infiltration. In the pediatric population, pretreatment with EMLA or LMX is typically helpful.

Prior to treatment the area should be cleansed with alcohol. The curette should be grasped like a pencil and directed toward the surgeon with the sharp side of the instrument in contact with the lesion. The instrument should be applied firmly, with downward pressure in a continuous, smooth, sweeping movement. In general pathologic tissue is more friable than unaffected skin. After the lesion is fully removed the surgeon should come in contact with normal dermis, which is firm and tough, and the operator should feel greater resistance. At this point it is recommended to scrape the base and margin of the lesion with the goal of removing any residual pathologic tissue or debris. Use of a semi-sharp curette may exaggerate the transition between abnormal and normal tissue while minimizing damage to normal skin.

A helpful pediatric pearl is the following technique. Liquid nitrogen or other cryogens may be applied to the lesion prior to curettage. This transforms malleable lesions, such as epidermal nevi and warts, to firm and brittle tissue, which is easier to curette.

Electrodesiccation is frequently used in conjunction with curettage, specifically in the treatment of non-melanoma skin cancer (NMSC). In this setting curettage and electrodesiccation are performed in alternating sequence. This method is conventionally termed electrodesiccation and curettage or ED&C. Importantly, if ED&C is planned, local anesthesia will be required prior to treatment. ED&C as the definitive treatment of NMSC may lead to an increased rate of recurrence. However, it is lower risk, less time-consuming, and utilizes fewer resources when compared with surgical alternatives.

Hemostasis following curettage may be achieved with a variety of measures, including pressure, hemostatic agent such as ferric subsulfate (Monsel's solution) or 20% aluminum chloride in ethyl alcohol (Drysol), or electrodesiccation. Healing after curettage is via second intent. Daily application of petrolatum facilitates wound healing.

8.3.5 Complications/Adverse Events

Significant complications with curettage are very rare. Patients may expect mild to moderate discomfort and minimal bleeding. The risk of scarring increases with deeper curettage, the risk of infection is negligible, and excessive bleeding is an exceedingly rare complication but must be considered in those patients who require systemic anti-coagulation or have an underlying bleeding diatheses.

8.3.6 Conclusion

Curettage is a minimally invasive, quick, low-risk technique that may be applied to a variety of cutaneous neoplasms in children. Curettage is likely underutilized and should be considered in the pediatric population, often as an alternative to cryotherapy or standard simple excision. The procedure itself is not technically difficult, can be easily mastered, and provides another treatment modality that is generally well tolerated by children.

8.4 Chemosurgery

8.4.1 Introduction

Chemosurgery, also known as Mohs chemosurgery or Mohs micrographic surgery (MMS), was developed in the 1930s by Frederic Mohs for margin control during the excision of skin cancer. In the fresh-frozen method tumor margins are evaluated by histopathologic examination in real-time, allowing for complete removal with margin control and maximal tissue conservation. This results in the highest cure rate for skin cancers, minimization of functional deficit, and best cosmetic outcome through maximal tissue preservation.

The pediatric population is uniquely suited to benefit from MMS, which maximizes tissue preservation and disease-free survival through heightened margin control [19]. This is particularly important in the setting of the genodermatoses, in which the need for multiple cutaneous surgeries can be anticipated over the lifetime.

8.4.2 Indications

Dermatofibroma sarcoma protuberans (DFSP) is a low-grade cutaneous sarcoma that usually affects young to middle-aged adults, though there are rare reports of development in childhood. The diagnosis is often delayed due to variable clinical presentations, and the tumor is often deeply infiltrative with up to 50% local recurrence rates [20]. This can be reduced to 20% with wide local excision with 3 cm margins [21]. However, this can lead to significant disfigurement. When analyzing the literature to date Paradisi et al. report recurrence rates after wide local excision at 13.2%, versus recurrence rate of 1.3% after MMS with margins averaging 1.7 cm [22].

An increased risk of basal cell carcinoma (BCC) is seen in several genodermatoses, including basal cell nevus syndrome (BCNS), xeroderma pigmentosum (XP), erythrodysplasia verruciformis (EDV), Basex syndrome, and Rombo syndrome. MMS provides a 99% cure rate for BCC, and 95% cure for recurrent BCC.

XP also predisposes patients to the early development of multiple squamous cell carcinomas (SCC), which also may develop in the scars of dystrophic epidermolysis bullosa (DEB) and in those children who are immunocompromised secondary to organ transplantation, immunosuppression, or other genetic syndromes. MMS is curative in 92–99% of primary and 90% of locally recurrent SCCs. Common to all indications, seen in Table 8.2, is the need for precise margin control and tissue preservation.

The role of MMS in melanocytic lesions in which only frozen sections are utilized continues to be controversial, due to disagreement regarding the reliability of detecting atypical melanocytes in frozen sections. The use of special stains during MMS may increase histologic sensitivity. However, some advocate also examining formalin-fixed margins to confirm final MMS margins are negative. This technique has been termed "slow Mohs" or "Mohs permanents." In this setting MMS layers are taken in the standard way, inked, and mapped in the Mohs fashion, however they are processed in formalin overnight and read as permanent sections [23]. In the adult population MMS has been used to treat melanoma in situ (MIS) with a 98% cure rate.

Table 8.2 Indications for Mohs micrographic surgery (MMS) in pediatric tumors [20–26].

Pediatric Cutaneous Tumors	Special Circumstances
• DFSP	• Prevention of local recurrence
• BCC	• Genodermatoses • Arising within a nevus sebaceus
• SCC	• Genodermatoses
• Retiform hemangioendothelioma	Recurrent
• Atypical fibroxanthoma	
• Microcystic adnexal carcinoma	
• Merkel cell carcinoma	
• Granular cell tumor	
• Infantile digital fibroma	
• MIS/Melanoma	Controversial

8.4.3 Contraindications

There are no absolute contraindications to MMS in the pediatric population. The age and cooperation of the child are of utmost importance, as this may preclude the ability of the surgeon to perform a prolonged, multiple-stage procedure. One study utilized vacuum-assisted closure with continuous pressure of 75 to 125 mmHg, which allowed the children to be mobile between layers [23].

A special consideration with regards to MMS includes its use in discontiguous tumors, which can create false-negative margins.

8.4.4 Mode of Action

MMS is performed in a precise, regimented, step-wise fashion. Serial tumor excisions are performed in stages, and 100% of the microscopic tissue margin is examined by the Mohs surgeon. This sensitive margin control allows for maximal preservation of normal tissue, thus minimizing cosmetic disfigurement.

8.4.5 Adverse Events/Complications

Complications in MMS are rare, and are those that are common to all cutaneous surgeries [27]. A recent large, multicenter, prospective study evaluated the rates of adverse events in MMS in the adult population, and found the most common complications included infections, bleeding, hematoma formation, and impaired wound healing, though the overall complication rate was 0.72% [28]. Notably, 95% of patients who experienced bleeding complications were being treated with anticoagulants. However, most patients taking anticoagulants did not have bleeding complications. In this study the use of sterile gloves, pre-operative chlorhexidine, and perioperative oral or topical antibiotics were associated with decreased risk of infection.

To some degree, sensory nerve injury is likely to occur in all cutaneous surgery and must be discussed as part of the pre-operative consent, especially when operating in high-risk anatomic sites. Motor nerve injury may be required if the tumor is deeply invasive, which is again true for all methods of surgical excision.

As patients are conscious during these long procedures anxiety or fear may be more pronounced and must be managed by the surgeon with empathy for the patient and/or parent experience.

8.4.6 Conclusion

Although Mohs surgery is classically used to treat high-risk cutaneous malignancies in the adult population, there is evidence to support the appropriate utilization of this precise surgical modality in pediatric dermatologic surgery. It is imperative to highlight the importance of tissue preservation in children given the reduction in available tissue due to smaller patient size, as well as the intensified psychosocial implication of cutaneous surgery in the pediatric population. In those with genetic predisposition to skin cancer it is important to consider use of MMS given the likelihood of need for multiple surgeries throughout the lifetime.

8.5 Electrosurgery

8.5.1 Introduction

Electrosurgery is the application of heat and/or electrical current to tissue to produce coagulation with or without cutting. It is primarily used to destroy benign and superficial lesions, to achieve hemostasis, in the ablation of vascular growths, and in the destruction of some malignant tumors of the skin. The basic principle is that an electrical current is applied to the tissue, which is a poor conductor of electricity, and thus creates resistance. This resistance leads to conversion of electrical current to heat energy and results in either coagulation or cutting.

Depending on the device used, electrosurgery has three major capabilities, with indications summarized in Table 8.3. The first is superficial tissue destruction, which includes electrodesiccation and electrofulguration; the second is deep tissue destruction, which employs electrocoagulation; and the third is cutting, which utilizes electrosection.

8.5.2 Electrosurgical Modalities

The forms of electrosurgery, which include electrodesiccation, electrofulguration, electrocoagulation, electrolysis, and electrosection are summarized in Table 8.4 [29]. The fundamental differences in electrosurgical forms are based on their interactions between current, waveform, and voltage.

Electrocautery, which is most commonly used in the pediatric dermatology clinic for hemostasis, is not a true form of electrosurgery as it does not directly apply electrical current to the patient. Instead it uses a low-voltage,

Table 8.3 Indications for the various forms of electrosurgery.

Electrosurgical Modality	Indications
Electrofulguration/ desiccation • superficial skin ablation	Acrochordon, actinic keratosis, small angioma, BCC (superficial and nodular), Bowen's disease (SCC-in situ), epidermal nevus, hemostasis (capillary bleeding), lentigo, seborrheic keratosis, verruca vulgaris
Electrocoagulation • deep skin ablation	Angiofibroma, large angioma, BCC, Bowen's (SCC in situ), hemostasis (arterial bleeding), hirsutism, ingrown toenail, matrixectomy, banal melanocytic nevi, sebaceous hyperplasia, SCC, syringoma, telangiectasia, tricho-epithelioma, verruca vulgaris
Electrosection • skin incision/excision	Acne keloidalis nuchae, blepharoplasty, debulking procedures, scar revision, shave removal of benign lesions, skin flap incisions and undermining, surgical excision of benign or malignant skin lesions

Table 8.4 Major modalities of electrosurgery.

Electrosurgical Form	Terminal and Current	Use	Mechanism
Electrofulguration	• AC • Monoterminal • Monopolar • - High voltage, low amperage	A single treatment electrode that produces a spark without touching the tissue (reticular dermis usually not affected)	• High voltage can be used because the patient is not part of the circuit. With low amperage this produces less heat and less tissue destruction and functions by dehydrating cells
Electrodesiccation	• AC • Monoterminal • Monopolar • - High voltage, low amperage	• Same as electrofulguration except electrode is in contact with tissue and thus no spark is produced	• Same as electrofulguration
Electrocoagulation	• AC • Biterminal • Monopolar or bipolar • Low voltage, high amperage	• Large tumors requiring more extensive destruction • Highly vascular tumors • Causes wider/deeper destruction & improved hemostasis, though greater scarring	• Penetrates more deeply than electrodesiccation • Coagulation is *not* specific to this form (despite the name). However, it does cause tissue coagulation • Contrary to the name ED&C, electrocoagulation may be the preferred waveform for all but the most superficial tissue destruction
Electrosection	• AC • Biterminal • Low voltage, high amperage	• Ability to cut while achieving hemostasis • Bovie: blended damped and undamped wave (coagulation and cutting)	• Cuts like a scalpel • Less bleeding

high-amperage direct current (DC) to generate thermal energy, which heats a metal element which is directly applied to tissue causing superficial destruction or hemostasis. Due to the absence of electrical current these devices may be handheld, battery-operated, low-cost, and readily portable. The absence of electrical current is advantageous in patients with pacemakers and implantable cardiac devices (ICDs) (see below). However, in this setting the mechanism of direct transfer of heat could produce a burn which may impair wound healing or impact cosmesis.

Electrolysis utilizes a low-voltage, low-amperage direct electrical current used primary for hair removal. The negative electrode is inserted into the hair follicle, the positive electrode is held in the patient's hand, and the current generated causes liquefaction of the hair follicle.

8.5.3 Electrofulguration, Electrodesiccation, Electrocoagulation, and Electrosection

In contrast, electrosurgical modalities including electrofulguration, electrodesiccation, electrocoagulation, and electrosection employ an alternating current (AC). This produces two types of waveforms or current flow, termed damped and undamped. Damped current has a strong initial electrical burst followed by waves of decreasing amplitude, while undamped current is a series of sinusoidal waves, all with the same amplitude. Practically speaking, the amount of hemostasis achieved with a device is directly proportional to the degree of current damping (more damping = more hemostasis). All electrosurgical methods using AC have a damped waveform. Additionally, electrosection also utilizes an undamped current and cuts tissue without hemostasis. The method used must be tailored to the specific indication and goal of treatment. Because damped current coagulates tissue, it causes more tissue damage. Combination methods use blended waves of damped and undamped current, so both coagulation and cutting options are available.

Electrosurgical terminology is often confusing and applied incorrectly. The number of poles (monopolar vs. bipolar) denotes the number of tissue-contacting tips at the end of the electrosurgical unit, whereas the number of terminals (monoterminal vs. biterminal) indicates the number of treatment electrodes applied to the patient. A monopolar device employs a single tip, and current flows from this single treatment electrode to the patient. A bipolar device utilizes two tips, and current flows between the two prongs of the forceps. A monoterminal device (i.e. electrodesiccation, electrofulguration) utilizes a single electrode, which transfers electricity to the patient, and then disperses to the environment. A biterminal device (i.e. electrocoagulation) employs a grounding plate, which is attached to the patient's skin at an area distant from the treatment site. Current flows between the treatment electrode and the grounding plate, completing an electrical circuit. Whether an electrosurgical unit is monoterminal or biterminal will determine the spread of the electrical current through the patient. Monopolar or bipolar devices may each operate in monoterminal or biterminal configuration.

Electrodesiccation and electrofulguration are both monoterminal, high-voltage, low-amperage devices used for superficial destruction. Electrodesiccation can also be used for capillary hemostasis. In electrodesiccation the current should be applied directly onto the tissue, while in electrofulguration the device is held 1–2 mm from the tissue, which damages tissue with a bridging current. When performing electrofulguration or electrodesiccation of these epidermal lesions the tip of a fine epilating needle can be inserted into the tumor followed by application of low current until surface bubbling occurs, which signifies separation of epidermis from dermis. Precision may also be obtained via inserting a 30-gauge needle attached to a syringe directly into the lesion, and then touching the active electrode to the needle shaft. It is best practice to avoid large sparks as this chars tissue and increases destruction.

Electrosection is a biterminal, low-voltage, high-amperage current used for tissue cutting. It provides an advantage over classic scalpel surgery by reduction in incisional time and blood loss. To minimize tissue damage a pure cutting setting can be used as it causes the least amount of lateral heat spread. This can be followed by spot electrocoagulation. The benefit of a blended cutting/coagulation current is hemostasis at the time of incision, which is ideal for obtaining a bloodless field. A drawback when using electrosection is the smoke plume generated by tissue vaporization. This not only obscures the surgeon's vision, but also may create a vector of disease transmission (see below).

Anesthesia is nearly always required in electrosurgery, except for the most superficial destruction. Small, superficial lesions such as verruca and acrochordons may be treated with low energies, and topical anesthetics can be used to decrease discomfort. However, the patient will still feel a stinging or burning sensation. Children should be allowed to feel the tip of the instrument on the skin before electricity is applied, as well as hear the sound of the electrosurgical machine to minimize jerking or retraction upon initial application of the device.

If the lesional tissue will be evaluated histologically the method of removal should preserve tissue architecture prior to application of electrosurgery. Tissue must be as dry as possible when performing electrosurgery as blood decreases resistance and prevents adequate heat from being generated.

8.5.4 Burn Prevention

Electrical burns are a concerning risk in electrosurgery. Risk factors include the use of flammable materials, cleansers with alcohol, or the presence of oxygen in the area. A nonflammable cleanser such as chlorhexidine or povidone-iodine should be used, and alcohol should be avoided. Flowing oxygen should be avoided near the treatment site. If using a biterminal device (i.e. with grounding pads) the indifferent electrode must have complete contact with skin, and avoid placement over bone, scar, or implanted metal. The electrode should be placed away from vital structures to decrease the risk of current channeling into a substance more conductive than skin, such as a nerve or vessel. One must ensure the patient is not touching any grounded metal objects, such as the operating table. If the patient is accidentally grounded a burn and/or electric shock at the contact point can occur. Importantly, this can happen with electrofulguration/desiccation as a dispersive electrode is not used.

8.5.5 Adverse Events/Complications

Overall, complications in electrosurgery are extremely rare [30]. However, given that electrical energy is used the question arises regarding electromechanical interference (EMI) with patients' ICD and cardiac pacemakers, which could result in inhibition or triggering of pacemakers, conversion to asynchronous pacing, bradycardia, asystole, or firing of an ICD. The risk of this complication has been reported as 0.8/100 years of surgical practice, and is greatest with electrosection due to the higher energy output. To date there have been no reported cases of EMI with a pacemaker or ICD in the dermatologic setting.

Despite this, controversy remains regarding the risk of interference with these devices, and there are no clear guidelines outlining the use of electrosurgery in this setting, but there are general recommendations to minimize the risk of EMI. Bipolar forceps are beneficial as the electrical current is contained between the forceps and minimizes spread to the patient. Electrocautery is also very useful in this setting as no current is transferred. Short, <5 second bursts with minimum power, the application of the dispersive electrode away from the cardiac device, and avoidance of electrosurgery within 10 in. of the device itself further minimize risk. Channeling occurs when electrical current is conducted along neurovascular bundles and usually occurs when operating near a nerve, resulting in pain and tissue damage at sites distal to the treatment area. This may be prevented with the use of bipolar forceps or electrocautery, and the lowest possible energy settings.

The risk of electrical burn can be minimized with the techniques outlined above. Electric shock is prevented by using a grounded, three-pronged outlet, which is not installed in the treatment table. Do not make or break contact with the patient during delivery of the electrical current.

8.5.6 Transmission of Infection

A smoke plume may be generated during electrosurgery, most commonly during electrosection, due to thermal destruction of tissue, which may contain toxic gases, blood fragments, and viruses, and potentially transmit infectious disease. Human papilloma virus (HPV) and herpes simplex virus (HSV) have been detected in this smoke plume. However, neither Hepatitis B virus nor HIV have been shown to be transmitted by this route. A smoke evacuator should be held 2–6 cm from the operative site while a plume is produced, and surgeons should adhere to standard surgical precautions, including use of a mask and protective eyewear.

8.5.7 Tissue Destruction/Scarring

Inherent in electrosurgery is the destruction of tissue. However, avoidance of excessive destruction or scarring is important for wound healing and a favorable cosmetic outcome. The most common adverse outcome is hypopigmentation. Excessive charcoal formation or treatment of wound edges should be avoided, with use of minimum power settings. Generally treatment near the eye should be avoided, though if working near this area the patient should be provided with corneal shields to prevent injury.

8.5.8 Conclusion

Once a surgeon has become familiar with the principles of electrosurgery its methods can be widely applied to a myriad of pediatric dermatologic procedures. The use of electrosurgery can optimize and facilitate other procedures, such as with curettage in ED&C, and is vital for basic surgery such as with hemostasis during excision. Careful attention to detail when gathering the patient's history, medical examination and the appropriate choice of electrosurgical modality for the target tissue and treatment goal can further reduce the already low risk of complications.

8.6 Techniques for Intra-Lesional Injection

Intralesional injections in children can be highly anxiety-provoking, thus there are multiple strategies to reduce the pain and fear associated with injections. Application of ice to the area prior to injection or pinching of the skin are simple methods that may blunt discomfort. The injection site itself can be pinched prior to injection to de-sensitize local nerve endings, or adjacent skin can be pinched during infiltration as a distractor. Topical anesthetics are typically efficacious in this setting, with application of EMLA (5% mixture of 2.5% lidocaine and 2.5% prilocaine) or ELA-Max (4% lidocaine cream) 30 minutes to one hour prior to procedure. If multiple treatments are anticipated minimizing the trauma of the initial procedure will likely aide in patient compliance and tolerance at future visits. To facilitate the use of topical anesthetics in the outpatient surgical setting prescriptions may be provided to parents prior to the scheduled procedure, with instruction for application and occlusion at home one hour prior to appointment time. It is important to ensure parental understanding of correct application to prevent potentially rare but serious consequences of systemic toxicity.

Intralesional steroids are one of the most commonly used intralesional agents in the pediatric dermatologic practice. Intralesional triamcinolone (IL-TAC) is an effective local anti-inflammatory medication. Local infiltration of IL-TAC allows for high concentration in the affected area without concern for significant systemic absorption. IL-TAC is indicated in the treatment of multiple common pediatric dermatologic conditions, including acne cysts, psoriatic plaques, keloids, alopecia areata, and nail disorders, to name a few [31]. IL-TAC (Kenalog®) is used in varying concentrations, and comes in 10 mg/cc or 40 mg/cc injectable suspensions, which can be diluted with 0.9% normal saline to the desired concentration.

Injection is best performed with a 1 ml tuberculin syringe using a 30-gauge needle. However, increasing concentrations of IL-TAC have greater viscosity and may be difficult to inject. Fibrotic or firm lesions may result in increased resistance to injection, thus requiring a lower-gauge needle for infiltration. Frequently a lower concentration is initially tried and assessed in follow-up. At the subsequent visit dosage may be titrated up based on response.

8.7 Indications for Intralesional Injections

8.7.1 Intralesional Steroids for Alopecia Areata of Brows and Scalp

Alopecia areata (AA) is a non-scarring, T-cell mediated autoimmune alopecia, the majority of which presents with well-demarcated patches of alopecia. IL-TAC is a first-line treatment for patchy, localized disease [32]. There are variable response rates between individual patients.

Treatment typically requires multiple injections into the affected areas to target the inflammatory infiltrate [33]. A major consideration in treatment with IL-TAC is the pain associated with injection, which is a significant factor when discussing this option in the pediatric population. Topical anesthetic may be applied to reduce discomfort and increase treatment tolerance. IL-TAC 2.5-5 mg/ml is recommended for areas on the face, and up to 10 mg/ml on the scalp, with a maximum total dose of 20 mg TAC per treatment session. Injections should be administered superficially at the level of the hair bulb to avoid dermal atrophy. Approximately 0.1 ml spaced 0.5–1 cm apart should be instilled around the circumference and within the center of the alopecic patch, with gentle messaging of the area to evenly distribute the IL-TAC. When treating the eyebrows and face 2.5 mg/ml with a maximum total volume of 0.5 ml to each eyebrow may be used as a general treatment guideline. Treatments should be repeated every 4–6 weeks, and discontinued if no effect is seen after three to six months. The first signs of regrowth may be seen four to six weeks following treatment. It is important to note that spontaneous regrowth may also occur during this interval. Up to 33% of patients will have treatment failure, which may be more likely in rapidly expanding patches or areas of long-standing hair loss.

Close monitoring for steroid side-effects including atrophy, telangiectasia, hypopigmentaton, and striae should be performed at each visit prior to repeat injection. The most common adverse effect is local skin atrophy, which is a dose-dependent response. This can be prevented with careful selection of IL-TAC concentrations and volumes, placement and close monitoring for early clinical evidence of steroid atrophy. The clinician should avoid deep injections and excessive treatment sessions to further reduce this risk.

8.7.2 Intralesional Steroids for Scars and Keloids

Hypertrophic scars (HTS) are elevated and thicker than expected, though confined to the area of initial injury. Keloids are pink-brown, firm, rubbery, raised plaques that grow uncontrollably, extending beyond the original site of injury. Patients may complain of pain, burning, or pruritus within keloids, which is generally a sign of active fibroblast proliferation.

The goal is prevention of HTS/keloid development in the surgical and early postoperative phase. This can be achieved by avoidance of tension on the wound, minimization of electrosurgery, chemosurgery, and early implementation of preventative treatments (i.e. IL-TAC, pressure earrings/bandages, Cordran tape, silicone sheeting). Cutaneous surgery should not be performed if a pediatric patient has been taking isotretinoin in past 6–12 months as this puts them at increased risk for the development of HTS and keloid formation.

HTS/keloid generally speaking responds well to corticosteroid therapy. For this reason IL-TAC is the first-line treatment for keloids. Glucocorticoids target the uncontrolled proliferation seen in keloidal tissue by decreasing collagen synthesis and enhancing its breakdown.

Concentration of IL-TAC is dependent upon the site of the keloid, as well as size, degree of elevation, and amount of induration. In general, higher concentrations are used than in the treatment of other dermatologic disorders as the goal of treatment is atrophy of keloidal tissue, which is the dose-limiting factor in other conditions. Concentrations ranging from 20 to 40 mg/ml are usually required for therapeutic benefit, with repeat injections at four to six week intervals. As treatment response is seen, the concentration should be decreased to prevent adverse effects in surrounding or underlying normal tissue. Lower-gauge needles are often needed to instill IL-TAC into firm keloidal tissue. In another technique, liquid nitrogen is applied to the keloid prior to the injection. This causes edema and makes the lesion less dense, facilitating fluid injections into the scar. Cryotherapy alone is also known to have a therapeutic effect. Treatment with Pulsed-dye laser is another option that has also been shown to have a similar benefit.

Given the refractory nature of keloids there have been reports of combination intralesional therapies. A mixture of 5-fluorouracil (5-FU) 5 mg/ml with TAC 10 mg/ml (obtained via 9:1 dilution of 50 mg/ml 5-FU to 10 mg/ml TAC) has been used one to two times per week, followed by monthly injections. In one study outcomes were superior to IL-TAC alone with reduction in side-effects. Combination treatment was noted to be less painful. Alternatively, topical bleomycin can be used to treat keloids with a 25-gauge needle, inserted to transfer the solution into the dermis.

8.7.3 Intralesional Steroids for Hemangiomas of Infancy

Infantile hemangiomas (IH) are benign vascular growths and are the most common benign tumors of infancy, affecting up to 10% of children. Since these lesions almost always involute spontaneously, the first-line treatment is clinical monitoring and reassurance. However, it is important to note that telangiectasias, anatomic distortions, fibrofatty residuae, or scar may persist following involution, which can lead to permanent cosmetic disfigurement. Ulceration, uncontrolled bleeding of the lesion, infection, current compromise of internal organs or airway or future risk for functional impairment or disfigurement are the primary indications for treatment. If continued growth will lead to or worsen any of the above outcomes then treatment should be initiated. Currently topical or systemic beta-blockers are the mainstay of therapy.

Intralesional steroids are thus less commonly indicated. However, they can be an effective first-line treatment modality in small, localized lesions.

Triamcinolone 3–5 mg/ml can be administered intralesionally in an attempt to halt further growth and may lead to a reduction in tumor size. In many cases, multiple treatments may be necessary in order to optimize the effects. Children less than one year of age with the superficial subtype during the proliferative phase are the most likely to have a robust response. Since intralesional treatments are administered in an office setting this may be an ideal treatment for a pediatric patient with or without the use of a topical anesthetic.

The risk of atrophy, the most common side effect, can be reduced by injecting into the center of the lesion. Although intralesional injections are generally safe there are a few severe adverse effects reported in conjunction with the treatment of IH. Injection of peri-ocular lesions has led to central retinal artery occlusion through retrograde embolization of the injected drug which can lead to permanent loss of vision. Ophthalmologists recommend injecting perpendicular to the vasculature of the orbit or in the direction of anterograde flow to try to further reduce this risk. There have been reports of systemic symptoms such as Cushing's syndrome following local injection, which may be due to the vascular nature of the lesion being treated and enhanced absorption. Since there have been more notable side effects with IL-TAC this is being replaced by the non-painful approach using topical or systemic beta-blockers in children.

8.7.4 Intralesional Steroids for Acne and Inflamed Cysts

Administration of intralesional corticosteroid into an inflamed acne lesion can rapidly improve its appearance and tenderness. Treatment of inflamed acne cysts may also reduce the risk of scarring which can be permanently disfiguring. In general the recommended concentration is 2.5 mg/ml. However, up to 5 mg/ml can be used for larger deep-seated lesions. The IL-TAC should be administered until the cyst is just slightly distended, the volume utilized may range from 0.025 ml up to a maximum of 0.1 ml per lesion. Since acne lesions are self-resolving the risk of injection, although small, must be weighed before injecting a lesion. The most common adverse effects include pain with injection, hypopigmentation, especially in darker skin types, atrophy, telangiectasias, and needle track scarring. Within 48 hours of injection, most lesions will flatten and then resolve.

8.7.5 Botox for Localized Hyperhidrosis

Hyperhidrosis is a disorder of excessive sweating, beyond what is needed to maintain thermoregulation. Localized hyperhidrosis often involves the axilla, palms, and soles. Treatment of hyperhidrosis can be difficult, with topical aluminum chloride often used as first-line treatment. Botulinum toxin A has been shown to be an effective treatment for localized disease [34]. Alternatively, inotophoresis, systemic agents, and surgical sympathectomy are also used in more generalized or refractory cases.

Botulinum toxin is a neurotoxin produced by the gram-negative, spore forming bacillus Clostridium botulinum. The toxin inhibits the release of acetylcholine in cholinergic nerves, which chemically denervates eccrine sweat glands, thus producing anhidrosis. In 2004 botulinum toxin A (Botox cosmetic) was approved by the FDA for the treatment of axillary hyperhidrosis, though it is also used to treat the palmoplantar variant.

The minor's starch iodine test can be performed to determine the location and severity of excess sweating. Iodine solution is applied to clean, shaven skin, allowed to dry, and cornstarch powder is then brushed over the area. A blue-black pigmentation appears in areas of sweating, which can be used to map areas prior to treatment with botulinum toxin.

The greatest drawback in the use of botulinum toxin is pain with injection. Topical anesthetics and ice packs may be used but are not 100% effective. For palmoplantar hyperhidrosis median and ulnar nerve blocks are safe and effective, though may cause temporary hand paralysis for one to two hours after treatment and have a more limited role in the pediatric population. There are reports of some success with the use of refrigerant sprays containing dichlorotetrafluoroethane.

Each axilla is treated with 50 units of botulinum toxin, injected intradermally, 1 cm apart in a grid pattern over the affected area. In approximately one week sweating is reduced or absent, with the effect lasting three to six months, and in some reports up to one year.

In treatment of palmar hyperhidrosis 100–150 units per palm are used due to the greater surface area and limited diffusion into acral skin. Given the extreme sensitivity of volar skin pain is significantly more intense in this location. Superficial injection of the toxin can decrease the risk of post-procedural muscle weakness of the hands (discussed below). Injections are repeated at three to six month intervals.

The most common complication is pain with injection, which can be minimized with the above techniques. After treatment of the palms patients may have a slight weakness in the hands with a decrease in fine motor skills. This usually self-resolves over two to five weeks, and thus it is recommended to perform treatments on one hand at a time if this is the case. With axillary treatment there have been rare reports of increased sweating at distant sites, termed compensatory hyperhidrosis. Xerotic skin may be an unpredicatable complication, though it is also a treatment goal. Small hematomas may develop at injection sites. Patients should be counseled to avoid aspirin and non-steroidal anti-inflammatory medications for 10 days prior to treatment to reduce post-procedural bruising. Injections should never be performed over an active infection.

Studies on the use botulinum toxin for the treatment of hyperhidrosis have primarily been performed in the adult population. However, there have been several reports of use in adolescents with positive result and no significant adverse events. Intramuscular (IM) botulinum toxin A has been successfully used in the pediatric population in treatment of neuromuscular disease. Adverse events (stumbling, leg cramps, leg weakness, calf atrophy) in these studies were seen with doses that greatly exceed those used in the treatment of hyperhidrosis, and these local effects may occur due to IM instillation of botulinum toxin, and therefore are not easily extrapolated to the treatment of hyperhidrosis.

References

1 Metz, B.J. (2013). Procedural pediatric dermatology. *Dermatol. Clin.* 31 (2): 337–346.

2 Nouri, K. *Complications in Dermatologic Surgery*, vol. 7, 119–135.

3 Baust, J.G. and Gage, A.A. (2005). The molecular basis of cryosurgery. *BJU Int.* 95 (9): 1187–1191.

4 Connolly, M., Bazmi, K., O'Connell, M. et al. (2001). Cryotherapy of viral warts: a sustained 10-s freeze is more effective than the traditional method. *Br. J. Dermatol.* 145 (4): 554–557.

5 Boull, C. and Groth, D. (2011). Update: treatment of cutaneous viral warts in children. *Pediatr. Dermatol.* 28 (3): 217–229.

6 Boyd, A.S. (1990). Condylomata acuminata in the pediatric population. *Am. J. Dis. Child.* 144 (7): 817–824.

7 Gamble, R.G., Echols, K.F., and Dellavalle, R.P. (2012). Imiquimod vs cryotherapy for molluscum contagiosum a randomized controlled trial. *Arch. Dermatol.* 148 (1): 109–112.

8 Drake, L.A., Ceilley, R.I., Cornelison, R.L. et al. (1994). Guidelines of care for cryosurgery. *J. Am. Acad. Dermatol.* 31: 648–653.

9 Reischle, S. and Schuller-Petrovic, S. (2000). Treatment of capillary hemangiomas of early childhood with a new method of cryosurgery. *J. Am. Acad. Dermatol.* 42 (5 Pt 1): 809–813.

10 Trost, L.B. and Bailin, P.L. (2009). Cryosurgery. In: *Dermatologic Surgery* (ed. A.T. Vidimos, C.T. Ammirati and C. Poblete-Lopez), 107–115. Edinburgh: Saunders Elsevier.
11 Thai, K.E. and Sinclair, R. (1999). Cryosurgery of benign skin lesions. *Australas. J. Dermatol.* 40: 175–186.
12 Smolinski, K.N. and Yan, A.C. (2005). How and when to treat molluscum contagiosum and warts in children. *Pediatr. Ann.* 34 (3): 211–221.
13 Ghodsi, S.Z., Raziei, M., Taheri, A. et al. (2006). Comparison of cryotherapy and curettage for the treatment of pyogenic granuloma: a randomized trial. *Br. J. Dermatol.* 154 (4): 671–675.
14 De Raeve, L.E. and Roseeuw, D.I. (2002). Curettage of Giant congenital melanocytic nevi in neonates: a decade later. *Arch. Dermatol.* 138 (7): 943–947.
15 Hoffner, M.V. and Camacho, F.M. (2010). Surgical treatment of epidermodysplasia verruciformis. *Dermatol. Surg.* 36 (3): 363–367.
16 De Raeve, L.E., De Coninck, A.L., and Dierickx, P.R. (1996). Neonatal curettage of giant congenital melanocytic nevi. *Arch. Dermatol.* 132 (1): 20–22.
17 De Raeve, L.E. and Roseeuw, D.I. (2002). Curettage of giant congenital melanocytic nevi in neonates: a decade later. *Arch. Dermatol.* 138 (7): 943–947.
18 Adam, J.E. (1986). The technic of curettage surgery. *J. Am. Acad. Dermatol.* 15 (4 Pt 1): 697–702.
19 Mann, J.A. (2014). Update on pediatric dermatologic surgery from tots to teens. *Curr. Opin. Pediatr.* 26 (4): 452–459. https://doi.org/10.1097/MOP.0000000000000123.
20 Roh, M.R., Bae, B., and Chung, K.Y. (2010). Mohs' micrographic surgery for dermatofibrosarcoma protuberans. *Clin. Exp. Dermatol.* 35 (8): 849–852.
21 Abeni, D., Rusciani, A. et al. (2008). Dermatofibrosarcoma protuberans: wide local excision vs. Mohs micrographic surgery. *Cancer Treat. Rev.* 34: 728–736.
22 Paradisi, A., Abeni, D., Rusciani, A. et al. (2008). Dermatofibrosarcoma protuberans: wide local excision vs. Mohs micrographic surgery. *Cancer Treat. Rev.* 34: 728–736.
23 Barysch, M.J., Weibel, L., Neuhaus, K. et al. (2013). Dermatofibrosarcoma protuberans in childhood treated with slow Mohs micrographic surgery. *Pediatr. Dermatol.* 30 (4): 462–468.
24 Abraham, T., Jackson, B., Davis, L. et al. (2007). Mohs surgical treatment of a granular cell tumor on the toe of a child. *Pediatr. Dermatol.* 24 (3): 235–237.
25 Keiler, S.A., Honda, K., and Bordeaux, J.S. (2011). Retiform hemangioendothelioma treated with Mohs micrographic surgery. *J. Am. Acad. Dermatol.* 65 (1): 233–235.
26 Taher, M., Feibleman, C., and Bennett, R. (2010). Squamous cell carcinoma arising in a nevus sebaceous of Jadassohn in a 9-year-old girl: treatment using Mohs micrographic surgery with literature review. *Dermatol. Surg.* 36 (7): 1203–1208.
27 Elliott, T.G., Thom, G.A., and Litterick, K.A. (2012). Office based dermatological surgery and Mohs surgery: a prospective audit of surgical procedures and complications in a procedural dermatology practice. *Australas. J. Dermatol.* 53 (4): 264–271.
28 Alam, M., Ibrahim, O., Nodzenski, M. et al. (2013). Adverse events associated with Mohs micrographic surgery, multicenter prospective cohort study of 20,821 cases at 23 centers. *JAMA Dermatol.* 149 (12): 1378–1385.
29 Vidimos, A.T., Ammirati, C.T., and Poblete-Lopez, C. Electrosurgery. In: *Dermatologic Surgery,* 101–105. 1e, 2009. Elsevier, New York.
30 Nouri, K. Complications. In: Complications in *Dermatologic Surgery,* 5e, 91–100. 2008. Elsevier Heath Sciences.
31 Arndt, K.A. and Hsu, J.T.S. (2002). Topical and intralesional corticosteroids – acne, hemangiomas, alopecia areata. In: *Manual of Dermatologic Therapeutics,* 6e.

Philadelphia, PA: Lippincott, Williams & Wilkins.

32 Shapiro, J. (2013). Current treatment of alopecia areata. *J. Investig. Dermatol. Symp. Proc.* 16 (1): S42–S44. https://doi.org/10.1038/jidsymp.2013.14.

33 Alkhalifah, A., Alsantali, A., Wang, E. et al. (2010). Alopecia areata update: part II. Treatment. *J. Am. Acad. Dermatol.* 62 (2): 191–202, quiz 203–4. doi: https://doi.org/10.1016/j.jaad.2009.10.031.

34 Gelbard, C.M., Epstein, H., and Hebert, A. (2008). Primary pediatric hyperhidrosis: a review of current treatment options. *Pediatr. Dermatol.* 25 (6): 591–598. https://doi.org/10.1111/j.1525-1470.2008.00782.x.

9

Suturing Techniques

Israel D. Andrews[1,2,3], *Jennifer J. Schoch*[4], *and Kathryn Ann Potter*[5]

[1] Department of Dermatology, Phoenix Children's Hospital, Phoenix, AZ, USA
[2] Department of Pediatrics, Mayo College of Medicine, Rochester, MN, USA
[3] Department of Child Health, University of Arizona – College of Medicine, Tucson, AZ, USA
[4] Department of Dermatology, University of Florida, Gainesville, FL, USA
[5] Division of Dermatology, University of Vermont Medical Center, Burlington, VT, USA

9.1 Introduction

Suture technique is essential to optimize both surgical and cosmetic outcomes. In pediatric patients, suture placement is particularly important due to unique factors, including poor wound care compliance and increased physical activity. One must also consider candidate selection and timing of the procedure. A thorough history, including involvement in extracurricular activities, may help to plan the procedure at a time when activity restriction would be minimally disruptive for the child [1, 2].

Suture material and needle selection are contingent upon the type of procedure, location of the defect, and activity level of the patient. Suture properties such as tensile strength, tissue reactivity, and knot security should be considered in light of the unique challenges presented by pediatric patients (see Chapter 11) [3, 4]. While non-absorbable nylon sutures have great tensile strength and are a reasonable selection for superficial sutures, multifilament or braided nylon has fair knot security and a moderate amount of tissue capillarity, and may not be best suited for potentially unclean locations such as the extremities, buttocks, or neck in children [4, 5]. Suture techniques may dictate suture selection in order to maximize both closure and cosmesis. For example, polypropylene monofilament is an ideal selection for a running subcuticular suture on the face, as it leaves no track marks and has low tissue reactivity; however, its moderate tensile strength makes this suture material and suture technique less applicable in areas where there is high wound tension and greater risk of tissue strangulation [2, 5–6].

Prior to suture placement, it is also important to ensure that the wound edges, wound bed, and surrounding tissue are appropriately prepared for closure. This includes removing de-vitalized tissue, achieving adequate hemostasis, sufficient undermining, and perpendicularly aligned wound edges [2, 3, 7]. Care must be taken not to compromise the dermal vasculature with excessive cauterization or pressure with forceps, which may decrease the tensile strength of the dermis [2, 8]. Undermining, to achieve sufficient release of surrounding tissue tension, increases the likelihood of precise approximation of the free wound edges during suture placement [7]. Excision techniques that achieve these factors facilitate optimal suture placement and optimal surgical outcomes.

Pediatric Dermatologic Surgery, First Edition. Edited by Keyvan Nouri, Latanya Benjamin, Jasem Alshaiji, and Jan Izakovic.

Numerous wound closure techniques exist and are utilized in the management of adult and pediatric dermatologic surgery, with the common goal of tissue approximation and wound eversion. The following sections will describe suture techniques employed most often during the surgical care of our pediatric patients.

9.2 Principles of Suturing

9.2.1 Preparing to Close

Prior to closure, the physician performing the procedure should be familiar with the available sutures and instruments. Ease and comfort with the chosen needle driver, forceps and suture scissors is key to ensuring an efficient and safe procedure.

The instrument tray should be in close proximity to the physician performing the procedure to optimize efficiency, safety and decrease potential instrument contamination. The patient shall be positioned to minimize ergonomic injuries. Most importantly, everyone involved in the procedure should maintain awareness of all sharp instruments utilized throughout the procedure. Sutures should not be loaded into needle drivers prior to suture placement in an effort to prevent needle-stick injuries. Magnetic suture holders may be used to organize sharps and sutures during a procedure. Needle-stick or other sharps injuries serve as an increased risk factor for transmission of blood-borne pathogens, and every precaution when handling sutures or other sharp instruments should be taken [4–5, 9].

9.2.2 Loading the Suture

Sutures are divided into two main components, the thread and the suture needle. The suture needle is further sub-divided into the point (or tip), the body, and the shank. The shank is the most proximal part of the suture needle. Its diameter is the largest and determines the final gauge of the needle. It also is the area of greatest weakness and is not an optimal location for placement of the needle driver. Suture needles are hollow in order to create a seamless transition between the thread and the suture needle. The suture needle is adhered to the thread by applying mechanical pressure to the shank after the thread has been fed into the hollow portion of the suture needle. This process gives the shank its characteristic weakness.

The body of the suture needle has the greatest strength and occupies the area between the tip and the shank. It is the ideal area of handling during suture placement. The tip of the suture needle extends to the aspect of the body at which there is the largest cross-sectional diameter [4, 5, 9–11].

Needle drivers (holders) are scissor-like instruments with similar appearing handles, but they have ratchets that allow for locking the suture in place. Needle drivers are divided into three parts: the handle, the joint, and the jaws. The surface of the jaws can be smooth or serrated, and selection will depend on the procedure and surgeon preference. Smooth-edged jaws offer greater protection to fine suture needles and are excellent for use in delicate procedures, but increase the risk of the suture needle slipping. Drivers with teeth or larger serrations offer a diminished risk of needle slip and greater handling capability, but also increase the risk of damage to the suture needle. The size of needle drivers can vary greatly; however, typically needle drivers are chosen proportional to needle size [9].

Needle driver technique varies from surgeon to surgeon. While some prefer to use needle driver rings by inserting the thumb and fourth finger during suture placement, others will grasp the rings of the driver in the palm of the dominant hand, which allows for more wrist rotation [3]. Either technique is acceptable.

Loading the suture requires placement of the suture needle into the jaws of the needle driver. Proper placement can prevent bending and breakage of the suture needle. The needle driver should grasp the body of the suture needle so that there are two-thirds of the suture needle distally to the tip, and one-third proximally to the thread. This avoids placement of the jaws of the needle driver on the shank, the most proximal component of the suture needle, where the risk of needle deformity during suture placement is greatest [11]. Sutures should be loaded into needle drivers while holding the suture needle with a forceps. Manual loading without holding the needle with an instrument increases the risk of needle-stick injury.

Once the suture needle is firmly in place within the needle driver, the next step is to stabilize the tissue in preparation for the suturing process.

9.2.3 Suture Placement

Tissue stabilization is achieved by everting the free margin of the wound edge for adequate visualization and planning of suture placement. It is often utilized during deep suture placement to ensure symmetry, as uneven placement of sutures can contribute to poor outcomes such as step-off deformity. Tissue stabilization and good suture technique will create optimal outcomes.

Forceps and skin hooks are most often utilized to create counter-traction of the free wound edge, thus allowing visualization of the planned suture trajectory. Care must be taken when using skin hooks or forceps, as excess pressure or trauma to the superficial papillary dermis can compromise the vascular supply of the surrounding skin. This increases the risk of skin necrosis and may lead to increased risk of the suture tearing through the skin. Preference of skin hooks over tissue forceps is operator independent, but in general, skin hooks are less traumatic to the epidermis and allow excellent retraction. The trade-off is that skin hooks may increase the risk of sharps injury to the surgeon or assistant. Alternatively, toothed forceps can be used for wound edge eversion, but there is greater risk of tissue damage secondary to pressure ischemia. Using only one arm of a toothed forceps to retract and evert a free wound edge may avoid this risk [2, 3–5, 8].

Excessive counter-traction of a free wound edge can limit the size of the target trajectory for suture. The superficial papillary dermis should be the target for tissue eversion [3].

Once tissue stabilization is achieved with adequate counter-traction, suture placement can ensue and culminates in the instrument tie. Suture technique is chosen based on the objective of the suture and the anatomic location. Specific suture techniques will be reviewed in subsequent sections in this chapter.

9.2.4 The Instrument Tie

The goal of the instrument tie is to support free wound edge approximation with tension evenly distributed across the wound. Excess tension across the wound edge increases the risk of wound dehiscence and a less cosmetically favorable scar.

The square knot (also known as the surgeon's or reef knot) is the basic surgical knot and is most commonly used during dermatologic procedures. It has wide application and is utilized in tying both deep and superficial sutures. For descriptive purposes, the free end of the suture will refer to the end of the suture thread, while the running end of the suture will refer to the suture needle. Once the suture has passed through the intended tissue trajectory, a small amount of the free end should remain where the suture entered the tissue [5, 13].

A V-configuration of the suture legs should exist following entering and exiting of the wound. The suture tail should be pulled through the wound up to about a few millimeters, far enough to allow for the suture tie, but not so little as to waste suture. Too little free end may compromise tying and knot stability.

Following establishment of the V-configuration, the running edge can be held in between the thumb and index finger of the non-dominant hand, and looped around the tips of the closed needle driver being held in the dominant hand. It is important that the needle driver remain in the center of the V-configuration at all times at the start of each tie. With the non-dominant hand holding the suture end, while at all times maintaining awareness of the location of the suture needle, the thread is wrapped around the needle driver twice. A double-throw is recommended for the initial knot to prevent knot slippage and provide knot security while subsequent knots are being tied. Once the double loops (also known as throws) have been placed around the tips of the needle driver, the free end of the suture is grasped between the jaws of the needle driver and pulled through the loops gently. The resulting knot should lie on top of the wound perpendicular to its long axis, but this orientation may vary depending on suture technique utilized. For example, the initial knot in a simple interrupted suture lies perpendicular to the wound axis, but a buried vertical mattress has its initial knot in parallel to the wound axis.

The initial knot should not be tied too tight. Since the first knot has most approximation with the tissue, excessive force used to tie this knot can create tissue strangulation. Instead, the initial knot should be placed gently, while subsequent knots can be utilized to tighten down the knot. This is particularly true for single filament sutures. In many superficial sutures, such as simple interrupted sutures, if knots are not tied tightly enough, a failure to achieve wound approximation and eversion can result.

After the initial knot is placed, the free end of the suture should now remain on the opposite end of the wound axis from its initial position. A similar technique to the first knot is used to grasp the free end; however, it is essential to reverse the directionality of the loops around the tips of the needle driver in order to maintain the square knot. Each throw is thus opposite to the prior knot. For example, if a counter-clockwise motion was used initially to double-loop the suture end around the needle driver, the subsequent knot will utilize a clockwise direction of looping the suture end around the tips of the needle driver.

Additional knot placement will depend on the suture technique utilized, the location of the suture that is being placed (buried vs. superficial), and the anatomic location of the procedure. More knots improve outcomes when utilized on the extremities and trunk, while fewer are needed on the face or dorsum of the hands. Once the appropriate number of knots is placed, suture scissors are used to free the running end of the suture from the knot. Length should be determined by the performing surgeon; long suture ends may create discomfort, while short suture ends make suture removal difficult and compromise knot security. This is an important consideration, especially in the pediatric population.

Following the instrument tie, depending on suture type and technique, effort should be made to assess for suture stability. If buried sutures are placed, a "pull test" or counter-traction away from the wound edge margin can be employed to determine if there are gaps in the dermal components of the free wound edge. If superficial sutures are placed asymmetrically, wound edges may be visible, indicating improper dermal-epidermal alignment.

The remaining sections of this chapter will delve into the various suture techniques employed in pediatric dermatologic surgery [2, 3–5, 7–8, 11–12].

9.2.5 Suture Techniques

Various suture techniques are used during dermatologic surgical procedures. Sutures can be buried, without exposure to or penetration of the epidermis, or superficial, meaning that their primary point of entrance and exit is through the epidermis. They can also be interrupted, meaning that a single suture is placed, the knot is tied, and the remaining running end is cut free. Sutures may also be "running" in that there is a continuous threading of the suture through the entire defect of the tissue before being tied off in a solitary knot. Modifications exist for each suture type, and familiarity with the basic suture techniques will enable appropriate decision-making when planning a closure.

Proper closure of a full-thickness defect (a defect extending down to the subcutaneous fat and tissue) requires two independent layers of sutures: a deep layer and a superficial layer. In the next section we will cover suture techniques to close the deep dermis and subcutaneous tissue, while the subsequent section will address techniques utilized to close surgical wounds superficially.

9.2.6 Deep Sutures

The most commonly employed suture technique to achieve wound closure of the deep dermis and subcutaneous tissue is the buried vertical mattress suture [2–5]. It provides excellent cosmetic outcomes, and in conjunction with absorbable sutures, decreases the amount of post-operative care [4, 13–14].

A mattress suture is any suture that uses a double stitch to form a loop around the free wound edge on both sides of a wound, resulting in eversion. A vertical mattress aligns the suture loop perpendicular to the skin such that the apex of the loop lies more superficially, closer to the epidermis, and the base of the loop lies deep, closer to the subcutaneous fat. A horizontal mattress is oriented in the same plane of the skin, and will be discussed later.

9.2.7 The Buried Vertical Mattress

The buried vertical mattress is an interrupted mattress suture, oriented vertically, that does not run through the epidermis as it passes from one side of the wound edge to the other. This is not to be confused with a vertical mattress or half-buried vertical mattress during which the suture is passed through the epidermis of the wound with the final knot tie lying on top of the epidermis. In contrast, the knot of the buried (inverted) vertical mattress remains at the deepest point of the mattress loop.

The buried vertical mattress has excellent utility and can be used in most dermatologic surgical procedures where there is little potential for impact on delicate cosmetic subunits, such as the eyelid or vermilion lip margin. Like most deep sutures, it eliminates dead space by approximating the free wound edges of the subcutaneous fat, dermis, and epidermis. It is of great value in wounds under tension and provides strength to maturing wounds [3, 13]. Most importantly, if executed properly, the buried vertical mattress decreases wound gaps and provides outstanding eversion of the free wound edges, enabling for optimal cosmesis [3, 13].

Visualizing the wound edge is imperative during the placement of a buried surgical mattress. Counter-traction using skin hooks or forceps enables the surgeon to visualize the entry and exit point of the suture needle on each side of the free wound edge, increasing the potential for a symmetric suture trajectory through the deep tissue.

Placement of the initial buried vertical mattress is dependent on preference of the surgeon and the features of the wound. Many will place the initial suture at the area of greatest tension, typically at the center of the defect where the distance between the free wound edges is greatest. This offers the advantage of better visualization and maneuverability in the area of greatest tension, but also affords the ability to place additional buried vertical mattress sutures in lower-tension areas to better approximate the high-tension area. The alternative is to place buried vertical mattress sutures in areas of low tension initially, in order to decrease excess tension on the defect at its widest diameter. This is then followed by placement of sutures in the high-tension areas, where the level of tension has been decreased by the surrounding buried vertical mattress sutures [3, 11, 13–14].

Once visualization of the dermis through counter-traction has been achieved, the surgeon will orient the suture needle with the dominant hand and retract the wound edge with the non-dominant hand. The suture enters in the deep reticular dermis at a 90° angle, followed by extension and rotation of the wrist in an upward motion in order to create the peak of the loop. At this point, the suture needle should be located immediately below the epidermis in the superficial papillary dermis.

It is important to point out the potential complication of penetrating the epidermis during this initial motion. Occasionally, if the upward rotational motion is too brisk, the running end of the suture could exit and re-enter the epidermis at the surface prior to completion of the arc. This results in a "track mark" across the epidermis. To prevent this, we recommend relaxing the counter-traction prior to completion of the arc to ensure this has not taken place. Any dimpling on inspection signifies penetration of the epidermis, and the entire suture should be removed.

Once proper position of the suture is confirmed, the wrist completes its rotation, aiming the suture toward the base of the wound, where it exits at the free wound edge superficially. This completes the first half, the deep to superficial component, of the buried vertical mattress. The upward motion of the suture following initial insertion creates the peak, and the downward and out path of the suture following peak creation creates the valley. It is imperative to achieve mirror-image symmetry in both passes of suture through the wound edge to prevent step-off deformity, which will be addressed later in this section.

The final component of the buried vertical mattress requires passing the suture needle into the dermis superficially, at the same level of where it exited the opposing wound edge. This component of the buried vertical mattress suture may require alternating the needle driver loaded with the suture to the non-dominant hand while the dominant hand provides counter-traction. Again, the needle should enter at a 90° angle, but should then be aimed toward the epidermis to establish the second peak. Additional wrist rotation then passes the suture through the deeper dermis, where it exits at the same level of the initial deep suture placement on the opposing wound edge. Producing the second arc following entrance at the 90° angle is facilitated both by the suture needle shape (preferably a 3/8 or 1/2 arc suture) as well as counter-traction of the free wound edge. At this stage, two symmetric loops on each side of the wound edge create a "heart-shaped" loop, and entrance and exit points in the deep and superficial dermis should be aligned.

Following suture placement, the knot tie creates approximation of the wound edges. There are subtle differences from the standard knot tie with all buried suture techniques. However, the principal technique remains the same. One key difference is the location of the final knot. In a buried vertical mattress the knot rests at the base of the loop. To achieve proper knot placement, the running suture end is pulled out of the tissue in the same direction of the free end, creating a "V" that lies on the wound bed and points to the center of the wound [3]. Gentle tension to the running end and the free end of the suture can be used to determine if the V is properly aligned. The instrument tie is then performed, as outlined above, with care to secure the knot parallel to the long axis of the wound defect. This step should be performed slowly as the opposing tissue is drawn together, to avoid pulling the suture through the tissue. An assistant may apply lateral pressure to the wound edges during the initial knot placement to decrease excess tension.

"Locking the knot" can be achieved by manually maintaining tension on the running end of the suture with the thumb and index finger, while simultaneously using the needle driver to orient the free end of the suture in the same direction as the running end, such that equal tension is placed on both the running and free end. Sufficient locking allows for release of the free end of the suture with the needle driver and is demonstrated by lack of tissue pull following locking. It also allows subsequent throws to be placed without collapse of the free wound edge [3, 4, 7, 10–11, 13–14].

Proper placement of a buried vertical mattress will create a slight indentation in the epidermis at the most superficial arc of the buried suture loop, immediately lateral to the epidermal wound edge. This suture technique simultaneously tents upward the medial aspect of the epidermal wound edge, thus establishing wound edge eversion. If the suture path through deep tissue proceeded symmetrically, eversion will be apparent on tissue. The value of eversion is demonstrated during wound maturity. As wounds heal and there is tension applied evenly and radially from the center of the wound, the everted skin will flatten leaving a flat and cosmetically acceptable scar [3].

Anatomic variation in the thickness of the dermis should be considered when using the buried vertical mattress in order to achieve eversion. Thicker dermis, such as the back, requires wider "bites," or a wider distance between the free wound edge and the lateral most aspect of the suture arc. These wider bites create the necessary difference between the peak of the arc and the valley, where the running end exits superficially. This enables adequate downward and medial pull during the knot tie and increases both approximation and eversion. In contrast, thinner dermis, such as the skin of the face or neck, requires smaller bites [2, 3, 11].

On completion of subsequent buried vertical mattress sutures, no gap between wound edges should exist. A skin hook or forceps should be able to gently retract the epidermal wound edge, demonstrating the dermis immediately above the buried vertical mattress, and resulting in "snap-back" upon release. While this outcome is optimal, it may not always be achievable.

9.2.8 Wound Gaps

It is vital to assess for wound gaps between wound edges prior to placement of superficial sutures. A wound gap can be identified if there is noticeable blood from the wound edges or if the wound edges are visible without manipulation. Wound gaps may result from an inadequate number of buried sutures or from lack of symmetry of the buried vertical mattress sutures. Assessing for adequacy of buried sutures can be easily accomplished by gently pulling laterally on the wound edge of each side manually. Any significant gaps discovered should signify the necessity for additional buried sutures. As the wound heals, the skin is stretched radially around the axis of the defect in all directions. If a wound gap exists, or if the wound is closed without eversion, skin at the free wound edge will invert, resulting in a poor cosmetic outcome [2–4, 8, 10–12].

Wound gaps caused by one wound edge lying superficial to the opposing wound edge, also known as the "step-off deformity", can result from asymmetric suture paths of the buried vertical mattress. If the arc on one side of the wound edge is more superficial than that of the opposing side, there is greater downward and medial tension applied to the epidermis, which is reflected by a depression of the ipsilateral wound edge. The contralateral wound edge lies superior to the depressed wound edge creating a "step-off" with visible wound gap. The buried vertical mattress could be removed and replaced in its entirety or corrected with an interrupted superficial suture. A small "bite" or arc is placed in the more elevated wound edge, and a wider bite is placed on the more depressed side. This results in depression with medial tension and alignment of the elevated side [3–4, 11].

A wound gap can exist without step-off deformity, and frequently occurs when a buried vertical mattress is placed too deep, such that the arc on either side does not reach a point superficial enough to create the necessary downward and medial tension on the wound edges. This results in wound edges that invert toward the center of the wound because of lack of support from the dermis. Excess inversion can be corrected by using a scalpel to trim the excess overhanging tissue on each side of the wound edge, followed by placement of a superficial interrupted suture with equal bites to create eversion [3].

Another common cause for wound gaps is the lack of arc creation by the suture path, resulting in a buried circular suture. A buried circular suture, when closed, pulls the free wound edges directly across the wound equilaterally without downward and medial tension. This creates an absence of eversion and possibly a wound gap. Correction of a widely splayed wound gap with superficial sutures can lead to excess tension placed on the epidermis, resulting in tissue damage. It is best to remove and replace buried circular sutures with a buried vertical mattress.

9.2.9 Other Deep Suture Techniques

Alternatives to the buried vertical mattress can be employed to achieve wound edge approximation, and some may have advantages over the buried vertical mattress in select situations.

The pulley stitch has the advantage that it can be used in areas of high tension, where there is a significant amount of rotation, for example the superior-lateral aspect of the shoulder. The suture enters the epidermis distal to the wound edge passes into the reticular dermis, across the wound bed, and then up through the contralateral wound edge through the epidermis, exiting near the wound edge. It is then re-entered into the epidermis near the wound edge on the initial side of entry, looped down into the dermis, passing again to the contralateral wound edge, where it exits the epidermis farther from the wound edge. Through multiple passes in the reticular dermis and subcutaneous fat, the pulley stitch provides great approximation of the deep tissue and decreases tension across the wound. It can either be left in place to decrease tension during the placement of subsequent deep sutures or removed following the distribution of tension across the wound bed after with additional deep sutures. Disadvantages of the pulley stitch include the superficial placement of a knot under significant tension, and the multiple passes through the epidermis leaving track marks. Many will utilize this technique to decrease significant tension across the widest portion of the wound bed, place buried vertical mattresses adjacent to the pulley stitch, and then remove it [4–5, 11].

The vertical and horizontal mattress sutures, mentioned later in this chapter, can also be utilized to close dead space, approximate wound edges and reduce tension. In certain situations, they can be used solely to close wounds, but are often utilized in conjunction with deep sutures.

9.3 Superficial Sutures

9.3.1 Simple Interrupted Sutures

Simple interrupted sutures are utilized to approximate epidermal wound edges, while also offering eversion. After dermal sutures are placed, superficial epidermal sutures may be utilized to correct the asymmetry in wound edges. The superficial suture should bear minimal tension.

The stitch is placed by passing the needle through the epidermis into the superficial dermis, through the wound, and exiting through the dermis and epidermis on the other side [10]. Both ends of the suture are then tied with a square knot, and the suture is cut. Individual sutures are placed until the wound is closed. To ensure that the suture is not under too much tension, the surgeon should be able to place a forcep under the loop without difficulty. Leaving a suture too tight can result in “railroad track mark” formation after suture removal.

The distance between needle entry into the epidermis and the wound should create eversion. If the needle enters too far from the wound edge, inversion will occur [3]. To correct a step off, the needle should pass through the dermis more superficially on the high side of the step off and deeper on the lower side.

9.3.2 Simple Running Sutures

Simple running sutures are best utilized to approximate epidermal wound edges, and are generally used in low-tension anatomic sites. Appropriate sites for this suture include the eyelids, neck, and scrotum, among others. This suture also allows for wound eversion and can be placed rapidly, which is beneficial in pediatric patients [11]. Simple running sutures also allow for the tension to be distributed evenly across the wound.

First, a simple interrupted suture is placed; however, after the square knot is tied, the free end is cut while the running end remains attached to the suture. The needle then re-enters the wound edge on the first side of the epidermis a few millimeters down the wound, and then exits the opposite side of the epidermis. This is continued for the full length until the superficial wound is closed. To tie the final knot, the last stitch is completely pulled through, and the loop that is left is used to tie the final square knot [3]. The resulting two knots at entry and exit of the running suture also enable relative ease during suture removal.

9.3.3 Running Sub-Cuticular Sutures

Running sub-cuticular sutures are best utilized for superficial wound closure, but do not provide the eversion that the simple running and interrupted sutures offer. The benefits of this suture include decreased suture marks and skin irritation. The running sub-cuticular suture can be left in place for up to two weeks (without the risk of track marks left by the epidermal sutures), which is beneficial in children that are active after surgery. The absence of sutures on the skin surface decreases the risk of manipulation by pediatric patients. The sub-cuticular stitch is the least "cosmetically deforming" suture [1–2, 15].

Following the entrance of the running end of the suture through the epidermis and dermis at the apex of an elliptical wound, a running sub-cuticular suture is placed by inserting the needle parallel to the wound at a 90° angle in the same plane of the superficial dermis and rotating the wrist so that the needle exits distally at the same level of the dermis down the wound. Then, the needle is turned and enters on the opposite side of the wound in the same way, alternating sides at the level half way down the length of the throw until the wound is closed. Increasing overlap of each pass through the dermis on contralateral sides of the wound edge enhances wound closure and decreases wound gap. Once the wound edges are adequately opposed, which can be demonstrated by gentle tension along the suture length, the running end is passed into the wound bed through the dermis at the apex and exits the epidermis. With the running end of the suture, a double-loop is placed around the tips of the needle driver and the suture lying closest to the skin is pulled through the loops to create the knot.

9.3.4 Horizontal Mattress Sutures

Horizontal mattress sutures are employed for hemostasis and eversion, particularly in highly vascular areas such as the scalp. This type of suture also is helpful in closing dead spaces. The risk of the horizontal mattress suture is potential for strangulation of dermal vasculature and subsequent necrosis of wound edges [11].

The surgeon places this type of suture by first throwing a simple interrupted suture, but instead of tying the knot, the needle is then inserted into the epidermis parallel to and on the same side as it exited, closer to the apex of the wound. The needle exits the wound edge on the first side of the wound, and a square knot is tied [5, 12, 16].

9.3.5 Vertical Mattress

The vertical mattress and half-buried vertical mattress are somewhat hybrid suture techniques in that they approximate the deep tissue, but have several passes through the epidermis, and result in a superficial knot. This leads to track marks and a compromised cosmetic result. In shallow wounds with low tension, they serve as adequate alternatives to the buried vertical mattress with some advantages. The vertical mattress may be utilized if there is considerable wound gap following closure with deep sutures, and when adequate eversion of the superficial wound edges has not been achieved [1–5, 10–12].

The vertical mattress, or the "far-far-near-near" stitch, is executed by inserting the running end of the suture into the epidermis lateral to the wound edge, then passed across the depth of the wound bed, up and out the contralateral epidermis at an equilateral distance from the wound edge. Remaining on that contralateral edge, the running end needle is reversed, entering into the epidermis near to the wound edge, passing across the wound, and exiting the contralateral epidermis near the wound edge. A square knot then completes the suture near the initial insertion point.

A variation of this, the half-buried vertical mattress, can be utilized in areas of the skin where the superficial knot can be hidden, such as the hairline or pre-auricular cheek. In this technique, one side of the suture remains buried, with the initial entry and exit point through the epidermis occurring on the same side. It provides adequate eversion and a more cosmetically acceptable result than the vertical mattress, but should not be utilized in areas of high tension [11].

9.4 Closure Material Alternatives

9.4.1 Staples

Staples allow for high tensile strength, with decreased tissue reaction and infectious complications. When placed properly, staples also allow for eversion of the wound edge and increased speed of closure. Staples are frequently placed in scalp wounds, given the increased tension and diminished concern for the cosmetic result in this location [16]. In one study, Kanegaye et al. compared staples versus suturing repair for scalp lacerations in a pediatric Emergency Room. Stapling resulted in six times shorter suture repair time; at follow-up, there were no cosmetic or infectious complications in either group [17].

9.4.2 Tissue Adhesives

Tissue adhesives are employed in the place of, or as an adjunct to, superficial epidermal sutures. Surgeons may also choose to add tissue adhesives with running sub-cuticular sutures, or if there is an area of increased wound tension following the placement of all epidermal sutures. There are multiple commercially available tissue adhesives including octyl cyanoacrylate (Dermabond), butyl cyanoacrylate (LiquiBand), and N-butyl-2-cyanoacrylate (GluSeal). In a prospective controlled trial, Maloney and colleagues showed that LiquiBand and Dermabond had no statistically significant difference in cosmesis and surgeon satisfaction at 90 days after closure, but the LiquiBand device did allow for reduced closure time [18]. The tissue adhesive can impair wound healing if it enters the wound, so it should only be placed on a well-approximated wound [19]. Additionally, there is a risk of allergic reaction with adhesives [11].

9.4.3 Skin Closure Tapes

Skin closure tapes are frequently used to repair lacerations, or after suture removal to provide increased mechanical strength. The benefit of skin closure tapes is that they hold wound edges together without causing iatrogenic trauma to the epidermis. Skin closure tapes may augment deep dermal sutures in low-tension wounds. Even when used with epidermal sutures, closure tapes can decrease the wound tension. The tapes are often used with a liquid adhesive (Mastisol) on either side of the wound, keeping the tape in place for one to two weeks [10]. Katz and colleagues found that optimal application technique is demonstrated by applying the strips in a parallel non-overlapping pattern, after coating the entire area with adhesive. The tapes can be easily removed with manipulation, a concern in the care of pediatric patients, and thus should not be used on their own for wound closure but rather as a part of a complex pressure dressing [20].

9.5 Conclusion

Within this chapter, we have introduced a multitude of techniques frequently utilized during wound closure. Without doubt, many more exist, and typically, preference of use will depend on the surgeon and the situation. Familiarity with these basic techniques will allow for elaboration and variation as the opportunity arises. Through repetition, the practicing surgeon can achieve comfort with various suture techniques to close deep and superficial wounds.

Although suture technique is paramount to achieve optimal outcomes, optimizing the wound through elimination of dead space, establishment of eversion, and decreasing wound tension is equally important. Preparing the surgical wound, and meticulous placement of both deep and superficial sutures, will lead to optimal surgical and cosmetic outcomes.

References

1 Wilson, B., Wiley, A., and Lee, K.K. (2009). Suture techniques. In: *Requisites in Dermatology: Dermatologic Surgery* (ed. A.D. Vidimos, C.T. Ammirati and C. Poblete-Lopez), 139–156. Edinburgh: Elsevier Saunders.

2 Bickel, K.D., Gibbs, N.F., and Cunningham, B.B. (1998). The subcuticular "spider" stitch: a simple solution to suture breakage and patient discomfort in long incisions. *Pediatric Dermatology* 15: 480–481.

3 Miller, C.J., Antunes, M.B., and Sobanko, J.F. (2015a). Surgical technique for optimal outcomes: part II. Repairing tissue: suturing. *Journal of the American Academy of Dermatology* 72: 389–402.

4 Zitelli, J.A. and Moy, R.L. (1989). Buried vertical mattress suture. *The Journal of Dermatologic Surgery and Oncology* 15: 17–19.

5 Wisco, O.J. and Ricks, M.R. (2009). Suture materials. In: *Requisites in Dermatology: Dermatologic Surgery* (ed. A.D. Vidimos, C.T. Ammirati and C. Poblete-Lopez), 157–162. Edinburgh: Elsevier Saunders.

6 Regula, C.G. and Yag-howard, C. (2015). Suture products and techniques: what to use, where, and why. *Dermatologic Surgery* 41 (Suppl 10): S187–S200.

7 Weitzul, S. and Taylor, R.S. (2013). Suturing techniques and other closure materials. In: *Surgery of the Skin: Procedural Dermatology*, 2e (ed. J.K. Robinson, C.W. Hanke, D.M. Siegel and A. Fratila), 189–209. Philadelphia, PA: Elsevier Mosby.

8 Bhatia, A.C. and Taneja, A. (2009). Surgical instruments. In: *Requisites in Dermatology: Dermatologic Surgery* (ed. A.D. Vidimos, C.T. Ammirati and C. Poblete-Lopez), 59–71. Edinburgh: Elsevier Saunders.

9 Fincher, E.F., Gladstone, H.B., and Moy, R.L. (2005). Layered closures, complex closures with suspension sutures and plication of SMAS. In: *Surgery of the Skin: Procedural Dermatology* (ed. J.K. Robinson, C.W. Hanke, R.D. Sengelmann, et al.), 273–290. Philadelphia, PA: Elsevier Mosby.

10 Miller, C.J., Antunes, M.B., and Sobanko, J.F. (2015b). Surgical technique for optimal outcomes: part I. Cutting tissue: incising, excising, and undermining. *Journal of the American Academy of Dermatology* 72: 377–387.

11 Olbricht, S. (2012). Biopsy techniques and basic excisions. In: *Dermatology* (ed. J. Bolognia, J.L. Jorizzo and J.V. Schaffer), 2381–2397. Philadelphia, PA: Elsevier Saunders.

12 Weitzul, S. and Taylor, R.S. (2005). Suturing techniques and other closure materials. In: *Surgery of the Skin: Procedural Dermatology* (ed. J.K. Robinson, C.W. Hanke, R.D. Sengelmann, et al.), 225–244. Philadelphia, PA: Elsevier Mosby.

13 Poblete-Lopez, C. (2009). Basic excisional surgery. In: *Requisites in Dermatology: Dermatologic Surgery* (ed. A.D. Vidimos, C.T. Ammirati and C. Poblete-Lopez), 123–137. Edinburgh: Elsevier Saunders.

14 Adams, B., Levy, R., Rademaker, A.E. et al. (2006). Frequency of use of suturing and repair techniques preferred by dermatologic surgeons. *Dermatologic Surgery* 32: 682–689.

15 Wagner, A.M. (1998). Slick suturing for impatient patients. *Pediatric Dermatology* 15: 62–64.

16 Cunningham, B. and Wagner, A.M. (2011). Surgical techniques. In: *Pediatric Dermatology* (ed. L.A. Schachner and R.C. Hansen), 162. Philadelphia, PA: Elsevier Mosby.

17 Moy, R.L., Waldman, B., and Hein, D.W. (1992). A review of sutures and suturing techniques. *The Journal of Dermatologic Surgery and Oncology* 18: 785–795.

18 Kanegaye, J.T., Vance, C.W., Chan, L., and Schonfeld, N. (1997). Comparison of skin stapling devices and standard sutures for pediatric scalp lacerations: a randomized study of cost and time benefits. *Journal of Pediatrics* 130: 808–813.

19 Maloney, J., Rogers, G.S., and Kapadia, M. (2013). Surgical corner: a prospective randomized evaluation of cyanoacrylate glue devices in the closure of surgical wounds. *Journal of Drugs in Dermatology* 12: 810–814.

20 Katz, K.H., Desciak, E.B., and Maloney, M.E. (1999). The optimal application of surgical adhesive tape strips. *Dermatologic Surgery* 25: 686–688.

10

Wound Closure Technique

Daniel Belkin[1] and Ashley Wysong[2]

[1] *The Keck School of Medicine of USC and LAC + USC Medical Center, Los Angeles, CA, USA*
[2] *Department of Dermatology, University of Nebraska Medical Center (UNMC) College of Medicine, Nebraska Medical Center, Omaha, NE, USA*

10.1 Introduction

Excision or excisional biopsy often leaves a defect that must be closed. To this end, it is important that the pediatric dermatologist understand certain basic wound closure principles and techniques. This chapter will discuss the basic types of closure, factors to consider in closure design, and techniques for optimal execution.

10.2 Common Pediatric Dermatologic Surgical Indications

Some common conditions considered for cutaneous surgical excision in pediatric dermatology are Spitz nevus, nevus sebaceus, infantile hemangioma, pilomatricoma, and large congenital melanocytic nevus. Excision for large congenital melanocytic nevus is a special case and will be discussed later in this chapter. More detail on indications for dermatologic surgery in pediatrics can be found in Chapter 16.

Excisional biopsy for a suspected Spitz nevus is indicated in any child after puberty and in a child of any age when it has atypical features [1]. Atypical clinical features in a Spitz nevus include size greater than 1 cm, asymmetry, pain, ulceration, or a history of rapid evolution [1].

Historically, most dermatologists recommended excision for nevus sebaceus. This was likely due in large part to the vast overestimation of the incidence of secondary basal cell carcinoma. Now, many pediatric dermatologists recommend excision only if the lesion is bothersome to the patient, usually because of its unattractive appearance [1]. For small lesions, it is best to wait until adolescence to avoid the use of general anesthesia. Parents can be assured that though the incidence of basal cell carcinoma remains slightly unclear, the tumor almost never arises before adulthood [1]. However, for larger lesions, such as over 1.5 cm in diameter at birth, excision in infancy is recommended, as the skin's great elasticity at this age allows for a one-stage procedure [1]. The trend to delay or decline surgery for nevus sebaceus, especially in more cosmetically sensitive sites, has also been affected by new studies showing promise of laser and other minimally invasive procedures. Promising treatments include pulse dye laser as well as fractional and non-fractional ablative lasers.

Infantile hemangioma is generally managed with watchful waiting or, if necessary, medical therapy, until after involution. Excision of infantile hemangioma should be delayed until after involution because before

Pediatric Dermatologic Surgery, First Edition. Edited by Keyvan Nouri, Latanya Benjamin, Jasem Alshaiji, and Jan Izakovic.

this time, the lesion is still evolving and it is unclear to what extent the lesion will resolve on its own. Waiting until after involution has also been shown to prevent recurrence after excision [1]. Superficial hemangiomas leave behind telangiectasias and pigment change in about three quarters of cases, while deep hemangiomas leave noticeable scarring or fibrofatty change in about a quarter of cases [1]. Surgical excision is particularly useful for the redundant fibrofatty tissue from deep hemangiomas.

Pilomatricoma is a common neoplasm in the pediatric population. It most commonly occurs on the head, neck, and upper extremities. These benign tumors are well circumscribed and will not spontaneously regress, so surgical excision is the treatment of choice [2, 3]. Excision is frequently done prior to histopathologic diagnosis due to clinical suspicion. Overlying skin can be included in the excision or spared with an incision and dissection method.

10.3 The Basics of Wound Closure

10.3.1 Primary and Secondary Intention

A surgical wound in dermatologic surgery is typically closed in one of four ways. Wounds are closed by secondary intention, by side-to-side or "primary" closure, with a flap, or with a graft. When evaluating a lesion or wound with closure in mind, the surgeon will first decide which of these four methods is most appropriate.

Secondary intention is the simplest method of closure, whereby a wound is left open to heal on its own. It is named so in contrast to primary intention in which a wound is sutured closed intraoperatively, as in the other three methods. In some cases, the surgeon may wish to leave the entire wound open, while in others, the wound is left only partially open. Though immediate reconstruction is most often the method of choice, secondary intention healing can produce excellent results on the right setting if the right wound, the right anatomic site and the right patient are selected. Specifically, it may achieve excellent cosmesis when there are small wounds in concave surfaces of the face and ears, such as in the medial canthus, alar crease, nasolabial area, temple, and fossae and concha of the ear. Full-thickness wounds of the lower eyelid have also been shown to heal exceptionally well [4].

A spontaneously healing wound undergoes wound contraction, granulation, and epithelialization. Contraction in areas of laxity or elasticity will pull in adjacent skin, which tends to have the best color and texture match to the excised skin [4]. The longer a wound is contracting, the more granulation tissue develops; by this mechanism, enough granulation may result to ultimately fill the depth of even deeper wounds [4]. Subsequently, epithelialization occurs over the granulation tissue. Parents should be informed that secondary intention is an option in appropriate cases, as they may prefer the more natural appearing scar it produces and the shorter surgical time required. Care should be taken when considering second intent healing near free margins, as wound contraction creates tension that may disrupt these structures (free margins will be discussed later). Second intent healing should also be avoided generally in wounds devoid of periosteum or perichondrium. Exposed bone and cartilage are poorly vascularized, so granulation will be weak and delayed, leading to slow healing and poor results. Wound infection is a consideration in pediatric surgery and postop care instructions with preventative strategies should be adequately discussed with the parents.

Most other wounds will be closed via primary intention. Side-to-side closure, also known as primary closure, is by far the most common closure for simple excisions. Side-to-side closure of a round defect with excision of redundant tissue in the form of two diametric cutaneous cones or "dog ears" to create a fusiform shape (i.e. elliptical excision) will in most cases create a simple and elegant linear closure. The long axis of the ellipse should be designed along relaxed skin tension lines (relaxed skin tension lines will be discussed later). Most wounds will be conducive to elliptical closure. However, elliptical closure becomes difficult in cases where there is incomplete or nonadjacent skin laxity, when functional anatomic sites are in the way or may be disrupted by tension, or when a long linear scar puts cosmesis at risk. These complicating factors often arise when operating on the face. When a simple linear closure in the form of an elliptical excision is not appropriate due to one of these challenges, alterations to closure design are available. These include several variations on the ellipse, which allow for simple adaptations based on the site of the defect; flaps, which utilize an adjacent tissue reservoir in more complex ways; and grafts, which utilize a distant tissue reservoir. This section will explore the ellipse, elliptical variations, and some special circumstances specific to pediatrics in which the tissue reservoir is particularly limited. Flaps will be touched on briefly; further discussion of flaps and grafts are beyond the scope of this text.

10.3.2 Principles of Wound Closure Design

Cosmesis is an important part of cutaneous surgery, especially in pediatrics. Once the excision itself is complete, the central goal of wound closure design is to create a surgical scar that is as close as possible to near invisible. The three most important means of achieving an optimal scar are minimization of tension, camouflage, and prevention of postoperative complications. All three can be addressed with good closure design.

Minimizing tension will generally require sufficient undermining. This should be done carefully in any direction in which tissue needs to be freed to allow for easy closure. To undermine, blunt or sharp dissection may be used; however, blunt dissection should be used in danger zones, in particularly vascular regions, and when anatomy is not absolutely certain. Undermining is complete when forceps or skin hooks can bring the edges of the wound together with minimal force. Undermining must be done in the right tissue plane; in general, above the avascular galea on the scalp, subdermal on the face, and just above the fascia for extremities [5]. In addition to undermining, applying dermal sutures in such a way as to achieve optimal eversion also minimizes tension on the wound edges. Everted epidermal edges provide leeway for the processes of scar contraction and skin stretch. An everted wound edge will settle into a flat scar, whereas a flat noneverted wound edge will settle into a more noticeable depressed scar (details on how to create optimal eversion are discussed in Chapter 9).

When possible, wounds should be closed with regard to relaxed skin tension lines, or Langer's lines. This will help reduce tension and in some cases help to camouflage the surgical scar within skin folds. Relaxed skin tension lines are relatively constant from body to body. These lines represent natural axes of tension. If a circular wound is made along one of these axes, it will naturally be stretched into an elliptical shape in the direction of the axis. When skin has good elasticity, these can be difficult to see. While they are easy to see in older adults, they will not be readily apparent in children. In some cases, they may become detectable when the skin around the site is gently pinched in several directions; the skin should wrinkle more easily in the direction of relaxed skin tension lines. If relaxed skin tension lines are hard to determine before excision, the surgeon can first perform a circular, rather than fusiform or otherwise designed excision; after undermining, the best orientation for closure along relaxed skin tension lines will become apparent.

Understanding dog ears and dog ear management is key for the dermatologic surgeon. Tension and compression are the two major forces playing a role in wound closure. While tension occurs due to the displacement of adjacent skin into the wound (such as centrally), compression occurs at rotational points due to redundant tissue (such as at corners). A dog ear is outward and upward protrusion of tissue formed by the compressive forces of adjacent skin [6]. Dog ears only become apparent once elastic properties of the skin are exceeded [6]. Inherent skin properties as well as extent of undermining determine elasticity. Wounds under excessive tension create more prominent dog ears, due to depression of the central portion of the wound and vertical displacement of apices [6]. Wound geometry is the most important influence on dog ear formation, and the management of dog ears is at the cornerstone of wound closure design. The ideal placement of dog ears will be discussed below.

For the sake of camouflage, the surgeon should be familiar with the cosmetic subunits of the face and the concept of free margins. Cosmetic subunits are structural divisions of the face based on the way the eye breaks up and recognizes facial features. They tend to be separated by topographic boundaries, such as the melolabial fold or the nasofacial sulcus. Within each subunit, skin tends to have similar properties such as thickness, color, hair density, sebaceous gland density, and actinic damage. Optimal cosmetic outcomes can be achieved by treating cosmetic subunits as separate entities during wound closure. For example, in general, a longer scar that stays in one cosmetic subunit will be less noticeable than a shorter scar that crosses the border between two units. In addition, a separate repair may be required for each cosmetic subunit involved in a single wound to preserve facial shapes and appropriate skin characteristics. When possible, scars are most effectively hidden in topographical junctions between subunits. This is because in this area, the eye of an observer will group the surgical scar with the natural lines of the face.

In respecting anatomical boundaries on the face, the surgeon must also be aware of free margins. These are structures that are "free" from or discontinuous with the rest of the contour of the face, and can therefore be easily distorted by tension, even by that of a distant wound. They include the helices, eyelids, nasal rims, and to a lesser extent, the nasal tip and brows. Specifically, these areas need to be protected from excessive tension by designing the vector of tension for closure parallel to the free margin.

10.4 The Perfect Ellipse

The ellipse is the prototypical method for primary side-to-side closure. The fusiform shape comes from a circular or oval defect and its dog ears. Alternatively, it can be thought of as the shape needed to produce a linear closure without creating dog ears. The perfect ellipse minimizes the two main forces acting on a wound: tension, which is greatest at the central portion, i.e. the site of greatest tissue displacement, and compression, which is greatest at the apices due to rotational force and which causes the skin to buckle into a dog ear [6]. In a quantitative analysis of wound tension, it was found that closing an elliptical wound produces less tensile and compressive stress on the skin than closing a circular wound [7]. Besides the poor cosmesis associated with bunching of skin at redundant sites, removing dog ears also creates a more tension-free wound [7].

On a flat surface, the apices of a fusiform structure should be about 30° angles to prevent skin buckling. A larger angle can exceed the ability of the skin to accommodate the compressive rotational forces at the apex and adds undue tension to the central axis of wound closure. A 30° angle corresponds to a length to width ratio of between 3:1 and 4:1. It is more intuitive to think in terms of length to width ratio when designing a closure, so classical teaching advises the surgeon to design her ellipses with a 3:1 ratio and the angle will be appropriate. Quantitative analysis shows that the stresses along the edge of an elliptical wound become more uniform as the ratio of long axis to short approaches 3:1 and above, which theoretically produces a more uniform healing process [7].

On very flat surfaces, such as the back, slightly smaller ratios, such as 2.5:1 should suffice, especially given the good skin elasticity in pediatric patients. The 3:1 ratio can be diminished on concave surfaces as well, since some vertical displacement of apices of the ellipse can be tolerated in these settings. On convex surfaces, however, in order to maintain a convex contour, larger ratios will be needed, often up to 5:1. In convex areas, such as on the extremities or over the jaw or chin, the surgeon must unfortunately plan to create much longer linear scars when performing an elliptical closure. This is because a scar designed to lie flat, compounded by the effect of horizontal wound contraction, will actually appear as a depression on a convex surface, with accentuated tissue elevation at the apices. A longer length minimizes central tension and allows for smaller apical angles, which overall reduces apical vertical displacement. Interestingly, dog ears tend to resolve on their own in areas of minimal subcutaneous fat [6], so ellipses on the convex surfaces of the dorsal hand and scalp often do not need to be so long. Conversely, dog ears left on areas with significant subcutaneous fat, such as the cheek, will often require surgical revision and correction.

When excising an ellipse, the blade should be kept vertical and perpendicular to the skin surface at all times. The blade should be brought smoothly from one point to the other in one motion, ideally down to subcutaneous fat on the first pass. The point of the blade makes the initial and final contact at the apices while the sharper belly of the blade should do the majority of cutting along the arc. Traction of the surrounding area is critical to a smooth incision, either with the help of an assistant, or by "three-point traction", i.e. holding tension with one's non-dominant hand in one axis while the fifth finger of one's cutting hand pulls in the other axis. It is important that the incision is made perpendicular to the skin all the way to the tip. If the scalpel blade is tilted inward at the tips, which is a common mistake, the protruding dermis and subcutis will further lift the apices, accentuating the dog ears, and prevent precise approximation of the wound edges.

Once the ellipse is cut, the tips should be freed with the scalpel. Then, using a scalpel or tissue scissors, the lesion is transected at the base. It should be transected on a horizontal plane with care to avoid "diving" deeper. This may happen unintentionally if the surgeon is "peeling off" the ellipse, so it may be helpful to hold the excised tissue in place as this is done.

Once undermining is complete, the ellipse should be closed in two layers (suturing technique is discussed in Chapter 9). Because tension is highest in the middle of an ellipse, many choose to close in a "zipper" technique, whereby sutures are placed first in the area of lowest tension at one apex and advanced toward the other apex. This technique can only be used in ellipses with symmetric wound edges otherwise skin redundancy will be pushed to one end and require excision.

10.5 Variations on the Standard Elliptical Excision

10.5.1 Crescentic Excision

For elliptical excisions along surfaces with curvilinear relaxed skin tension lines, such as the cheek and chin, or within cosmetic subunit boundaries, such as the melolabial fold, an ellipse can be curved into a crescent shape in order to better hide the scar. In this case, apices are arranged curving slightly into each other, creating a half-moon shape. It is important to remember when closing these that one side is longer than the other. The price of varying the ellipse, so to speak, is tissue redundancy on the longer side. This tissue redundancy should be sutured out incrementally or it will bunch at one end and necessitate excision. These wounds are therefore closed with "the rule of halves", whereby each suture is placed in the center of the available wound edge. The wound is first halved, then quartered, and so on. In this way, the tissue redundancy is parsed out evenly along the entire edge and is absorbed by the elasticity of the skin.

10.5.2 M-Plasty

When a linear closure with a classic ellipse would disrupt a neighboring anatomic structure, such as the eye, or would cross into a second cosmetic subunit, the ellipse can be shortened with an M-plasty. It can also be useful to shorten an unappealingly long scar, such as on the convex surface of the cheek. When designing the ellipse, at the side to be shortened, one inverts the tip to create an "M". The central apex of the "M" should extend to about one quarter the length of the ellipse. When excising along these lines, redundant tissue is split in half and partially redistributed lateral to the main axis of the ellipse. The final scar takes the shape of a "Y" at this end instead of a simple line.

10.5.3 Lazy S Closure

For elliptical excisions on highly convex surfaces, when ellipses will have to be extended in length to maintain contour, one may use an S-plasty or Lazy S. The jaw and chin, lateral forehead, malar cheek, and extremities are sites particularly conducive to this method. Essentially, rather than extending a classic ellipse to a 5:1 length to width ratio to accommodate a highly convex surface, the length of the wound can be extended in an S-shaped fashion that keeps the distance between apices constant. This technique reorients the ends of the wound away from areas of maximal convexity and redirects horizontal wound contraction into straightening the S before producing scar depression [6]. In some cases, this shape will also allow the scar to be hidden better in curvilinear relaxed skin tension lines. It can be created similar to the crescentic ellipse (above), but in this case, one apex turns slightly out while the other turns slightly in to create a spindle shaped ellipse that will close in a gentle S-shaped scar. Another method is to create a typical ellipse that is then obliquely sutured in order to produce redundancy on opposite sides of each apex; these dog ears can then be excised to create an upturn and downturn of opposite corners and thus the desired spindle shape [6].

10.6 Partial Closures

10.6.1 Purse String Closure

Some consider the purse string closure to be a fifth major category of closure options for dermatologic surgical defects [8]. The purse string closure is used to decrease the size of a circular wound, generally to create a smaller area for secondary intention healing, but in some cases to undergo further primary repair. As discussed, wounds left to heal by secondary intention can do extremely well on the right anatomic site. In other cases, secondary intention healing may be less than ideal; in these cases as well, a purse string closure may be useful to minimize poor cosmetic outcome. After undermining minimally around a circular wound, the surgeon threads an absorbable suture in a subcuticular plane around the entire perimeter of the clean wound edge. The suture is then pulled taut and tied to its tail, causing traction evenly on all sides of the wound and shrinking the area of exposed subcutis. The redundant skin bunches evenly around the perimeter of the wound, and no dog ear needs to be taken. In larger wounds or those under high tension, two layers of subcuticular suture may be required (one in the deeper dermis or subcutis and the second in the dermis).

A slight alternative to the purse string is the cerclage. This is a similar concept, except that a non-absorbable is used in an epidermal fashion along the perimeter of the wound. The knot ultimately lies on top of the skin and is not buried like in a purse string closure. For both methods, monofilament suture, either non-absorbable or absorbable, is best, since it reduces tissue drag and allows for easier tightening. Interestingly, with either method, there is often excellent tissue movement with little to no undermining, minimizing the potential morbidity and time taken for extensive undermining [8].

After a defect is partially closed with purse string or cerclage, the remaining wound can be left to heal by secondary intention, grafted, or closed side to side. While purse string has traditionally been applied to large wounds that cannot be closed linearly, it may also be a good choice in certain small wounds, such as those on mobile areas of the body with little excess laxity. Examples of this would be the shoulder and back, where elliptical excisions often close well initially but then spread to leave thick scars [8]. Weisberg and Greenberg have described excellent cosmetic results from purse string closure with subsequent side to side closure using vertical mattress sutures; which help to place the final axis of the scar along relaxed skin tension lines even if there is not enough laxity to close the wound completely this way [8]. Deep vertical mattress sutures can also be used. The dog ears that arise on either end, due to side-to-side closure of a circular wound, tend to flatten out over time once sutures are removed [8]. In these cases, purse string with subsequent side to side closure can minimize the final length of the scar, compared with elliptical excision [8].

Some authors have described the use of purse string closure in large facial hemangiomas. This method can avoid grafts in some cases and large flaps on the face. If resection is indicated, an additional benefit of circular excision with purse string closure is that it utilizes the redundant skin inherent in a large hemangioma, thereby diminishing the size of an excisional defect [9]. The defect is tightened until there is no longer distortion of surrounding facial structures by the hemangioma [9]. At this point, the defect can be left open or closed with a small graft. The repair of large facial wounds with purse string and subsequent full-thickness skin graft has also been reported to be successful in Mohs surgery patients [10].

10.6.2 Guiding Sutures

Wounds under high tension may be left open to heal by secondary intention as discussed above. The scalp and legs are two areas where defects are often under high tension. It is better to plan for secondary intention healing than to force skin closed and risk dehiscence. "Guiding sutures" can be used to direct healing along desirable axes, such as relaxed skin tension lines. In these cases, sutures are not placed with the intent of closure but simply to shape the final wound. This is often done with strong non-absorbable sutures, such as polypropylene, which span the wound in order simply to cinch it. Polypropylene causes minimal tissue damage and reactivity and has good plasticity. Alternatively, a wound can be sutured at either end, where there is less tension, and left open in the center. Even if a surgical wound, for example an ellipse, is not closed completely, the final scar will typically take on the linear conformation of the sutured ends.

10.7 Simple Flaps

Flaps allow the surgeon to harness nearby areas of laxity in order to repair a defect. Flaps can also displace areas of redundancy created by wound closure to areas more convenient for dog ear excision. They can be used to optimize cosmesis and feasibility on more complex sites.

10.7.1 A-T Closure

An A-T flap is a simple flap that can be helpful in certain specific anatomic sites. When defects directly about a functional facial structure or cosmetic subunit boundary, such as in the preauricular area or just above the brow, this simple flap should be considered. It can be thought of as a variation on a typical ellipse. A standard dog ear is removed from one side of the wound where there is tissue available, while on the other side, the redundant skin is split in two and brought away from the wound perpendicular to the axis of the ellipse. This allows the surgeon to halt the ellipse at an anatomic border and finish it at right angles from the central axis. Redundant tissue can then be excised as dog ears at the ends of this perpendicular incision, parsed out along the incision to be absorbed by skin elasticity, or excised crescentically along this incision.

10.7.2 Other Flaps

Basic flaps can be grouped into five major categories: advancement, rotation, transposition, interpolation, and island pedicle. All involve shifting tissue into a wound in different ways. Advancement flaps, of which A-T closure above is an example, involve sliding tissue in vertically or horizontally. Rotation flaps similarly harness nearby tissue but do so in an arc, along a rotational axis. Further discussion of flaps is beyond the scope of this text.

10.8 Large Lesions

There are some instances in pediatric dermatology where large lesions require full excision. The most commonly excised large lesions are congenital melanocytic nevi; others include areas of alopecia, tattoos, or scars [5]. Excision of large congenital melanocytic lesions is controversial [1]. It has not yet been determined whether excision reduces melanoma risk, as studies are difficult due to the low prevalence of large congenital melanocytic nevi and the low incidence of melanoma [1]. Large lesions have been reported to carry a 2–2.8% risk of melanoma occurring in the early teen years on average [1]. Routine full-thickness excision is controversial due to the idea of persistent melanocytes in subcutaneous fat, fascia, and muscle as well as the small risk of melanoma arising in sites outside of the large nevus excision of large congenital nevi may not produce satisfying results for the patient and family. Whereas the vast majority of patients with small nevi and those with nevi on the head and neck reported satisfaction after excision, 14% of patients with large nevi elsewhere felt surgery worsened their appearance [1, 11]. Whether to excise large lesions should be decided on a case-by-case basis.

If excision is planned, some dermatologic surgeons feel that lesions should be excised as early as possible, as skin elasticity is greatest in infancy and declines with age [12]. Two methods for excising such large lesions, where the size of a defect will far surpass available tissue, are staged excision and tissue expansion.

10.8.1 Staged Excision

Staged excision refers to excision of a large lesion with the use of multiple more manageable smaller excisions over time, allowing the skin to stretch after each stage to accommodate the next. Staged excision allows for a shorter final scar than if excision is done in a single stage and allows for reorientation of the scar into relaxed skin tension lines [13]. Usually, serial elliptical excisions are used. All excisions, until the final excision, should ideally fall entirely within the lesion in order to preserve normal tissue [5]. This is especially important for pigmented lesions as pigment cells within a nevus can migrate across suture into nonlesional skin [14]. To ensure this and to minimize the number of necessary excisions, the final scar should be considered before planning even the first excision [5]. The surgeon may wish to close initial excisions with dermal sutures that are non-absorbable. Leaving non-absorbable dermal sutures has been shown to prevent scar stretching when left in for six months, at which point they are excised with a subsequent stage [15]. Any scar stretching of initial stages will widen the lesion and thereby compromise the efficacy of a staged excision.

One particular technique for staged excision is called the “cake flap” [16]. The lesion is first divided into four segments – like cutting a cake into four slices –along and perpendicular to either the axis of the lesion or the axis of relaxed skin tension lines [16]. Two diagonal quadrants are excised, and the remaining two quadrants are raised as flaps and advanced into the defects, resulting in a Z-shaped closure [16]. In a relatively small and round lesion, one cake flap will produce an ellipse-shaped lesion that can be excised completely by elliptical excision at the next stage without sacrificing normal tissue [16]. Furthermore, since this Z-shaped scar redistributes forces, scar stretching will be reduced [13].

Another technique to prevent waste of normal skin is called the "cogwheel pattern" [13]. A thin central ellipse is excised with hooked extensions on opposite sides. This leaves two small flaps opposite each other that again form a Z-shaped closure in the center of the lesion. Similar to the "cake flap," this will create an elliptical shaped lesion that can be excised via ellipse at the next stage without sacrifice of normal tissue in dog ears [13].

10.8.2 Tissue Expansion

If more than two or three procedures in a staged excision are anticipated, tissue expansion should be discussed and considered [5]. Tissue expansion is commonly used among plastic surgeons for excision of large congenital melanocytic lesions. An inflatable expander is placed beneath the skin and inflated over time to create a large tissue reservoir prior to excision and closure of the wound. Downsides to tissue expansion include the inconvenience of weekly injections and cosmetic unacceptability of the expander prior to excision. Some worry that activating the skin to grow via expanders may adversely affect the nevus. Kinsler and colleagues reported that full or partial excision with tissue expanders was associated with new satellite nevi; some suggest this is due to "activation" of remaining melanocytes [1, 11]. If tissue expansion is considered, referral should be made to a pediatric plastic surgeon.

10.9 Complications and Poor Outcomes

Surgical excision and repair are associated with risks. These will be discussed in detail in Chapter 14. However, particular complications and poor outcomes may result from errors in wound closure technique. Defects that are closed under excessive tension may result in wound dehiscence, skin necrosis, scar stretch, hypertrophic scarring, or atrophic scarring. The principles above, such as sufficient undermining, designing closure along relaxed skin tension lines, and managing dog ears appropriately, can help minimize wound tension. Poor wound closure design can lead to unappealing or conspicuous scars that are overly long, cross cosmetic subunits, or fall oblique to natural skin folds and relaxed skin tension lines. Ellipses that are too short can leave concave scars in areas of convexity or prominent dog ears that must be later corrected. Finally, misplaced tension vectors can disrupt anatomic free margins, such as those of the eye or lips.

10.10 Conclusion

For lesions requiring excision or excisional biopsy, there is a range of wound closure techniques available to the pediatric dermatologist to effectively manage surgical wounds of many sizes and sites.

References

1 Mann, J.A. (2014). Update on pediatric dermatologic surgery from tots to teens. *Curr. Opin. Pediatr.* 26 (4): 452–459.

2 Thomas, R.W., Perkins, J.A., Ruegemer, J.L., and Munaretto, J.A. (1999). Surgical excision of pilomatrixoma of the head and neck: a retrospective review of 26 cases. *Ear Nose Throat J.* 78 (8): 541, 4–6, 8.

3 Yencha, M.W. (2001). Head and neck pilomatricoma in the pediatric age group: a retrospective study and literature review. *Int. J. Pediatr. Otorhinolaryngol.* 57 (2): 123–128.

4 Diwan, R., Tromovitch, T.A., Glogau, R.G., and Stegman, S.J. (1989). Secondary intention healing. The primary approach for management of selected wounds. *Arch. Otolaryngol. Head Neck Surg.* 115 (10): 1248–1249.

5 Quaba, O., Shoaib, T., Durrani, A.J., and Quaba, A.A. (2008). A user's guide for serial excision. *J. Plast. Reconstr. Aesthet. Surg.* 61 (6): 712–715.

6 Weisberg, N.K., Nehal, K.S., and Zide, B.M. (2000). Dog-ears: a review. *Dermatol. Surg.* 26 (4): 363–370.

7 Chaudhry, H.R., Bukiet, B., Siegel, M. et al. (1998). Optimal patterns for suturing wounds. *J. Biomech.* 31 (7): 653–662.

8 Weisberg, N.K. and Greenbaum, S.S. (2003). Revisiting the purse-string closure: some new methods and modifications. *Dermatol. Surg.* 29 (6): 672–676.

9 Vlahovic, A., Simic, R., and Kravljanac, D. (2007). Circular excision and purse-string suture technique in the management of facial hemangiomas. *Int. J. Pediatr. Otorhinolaryngol.* 71 (8): 1311–1315.

10 Brady, J.G., Grande, D.J., and Katz, A.E. (1992). The purse-string suture in facial reconstruction. *J. Dermatol. Surg. Oncol.* 18 (9): 812–816.

11 Kinsler, V.A., Birley, J., and Atherton, D.J. (2009). Great Ormond street hospital for children registry for congenital melanocytic naevi: prospective study 1988–2007. Part 2 – evaluation of treatments. *Br. J. Dermatol.* 160 (2): 387–392.

12 Gibson, T. and Kenedi, R.M. (1967). Biomechanical properties of skin. *Surg. Clin. North Am.* 47 (2): 279–294.

13 Kang, H.G., Park, M.C., and Park, D.H. (2014). A new modality for treating congenital melanocytic nevus: "cogwheel pattern" serial excision method. *Arch. Plast. Surg.* 41 (4): 418–420.

14 Altchek, E.D. (1980). A technical consideration in the serial excision of a nevus. *Plast. Reconstr. Surg.* 66 (6): 849–850.

15 Elliot, D. and Mahaffey, P.J. (1989). The stretched scar: the benefit of prolonged dermal support. *Br. J. Plast. Surg.* 42 (1): 74–78.

16 Tang, L., MacKenzie Ross, A.D., and Nduka, C. (2011). The cake flap: a new technique for serial excision of benign cutaneous lesions. *J. Plast. Reconstr. Aesthet. Surg.* 64 (9): 1194–1196.

11

Wound Closure Material

V.M. Carlberg[1,2] and J.L. Fewkes[1,2,3]

[1] Department of Dermatology, Massachusetts General Hospital, Boston, MA, USA
[2] Harvard Medical School, Boston, MA, USA
[3] Department of Otolaryngology, Massachusetts Eye and Ear Infirmary, Boston, MA, USA

11.1 Introduction

Though historically there were few surgical options, wound closure in the new millennium may be accomplished using a variety of materials. There are now over 5000 different types including a myriad of suture materials and needles, staples, topical adhesives, tapes, and more [1]. This chapter evaluates the properties of the most commonly employed wound closure materials in pediatric dermatologic surgery.

- Sutures are the most commonly used wound closure material in dermatologic surgery.
- Each suture material has unique features (i.e. physical configuration, size, coefficient of friction) that influence suture strength, workability, and potential for complications.

Suture features are standardized by the United States Pharmacopeia (USP) and include physical configuration, tensile strength, size, plasticity, elasticity, memory, pliability, coefficient of friction, and tissue reactivity [2]. Each of these variables contributes to the knot strength, ease of handling, and potential for wound complications as outlined below.

Individual suture characteristics

Monofilament. "Mono", meaning "one" or "single", indicates a suture is composed of a single strand [1, 2]. Some advantages of this configuration include lower coefficient of friction and potentially decreased risk of infection (see below for more details). On the other hand, monofilament sutures tend to be stiffer and have decreased knot security.

Multifilament. As implied by the name, multifilament (sometimes called polyfilament) suture is composed of multiple strands that are braided, spun, or twisted [1, 2]. This configuration lends itself to increased pliability, strength, knot security, and easier handling. However, multifilament sutures also have higher capillarity, and this may increase risk for wound infection (see Capillarity below).

Tensile strength. Tensile strength is defined as the measured force (in pounds) that a suture may withstand before breaking [1]. It is calculated by dividing the weight necessary to break the suture by its cross-sectional area [3]. Sutures with larger diameters have greater tensile strength, whereas sutures with smaller diameters have lower tensile strength.

Pediatric Dermatologic Surgery, First Edition. Edited by Keyvan Nouri, Latanya Benjamin, Jasem Alshaiji, and Jan Izakovic.

Size. The size of suture is determined by the cross-sectional diameter and is designated in descending order (i.e. 1-0 is larger than 11-0) [1]. As previously mentioned, size contributes to tensile strength and is therefore relevant when considering anatomic location and the degree of tension placed on a wound. Ideally, one should select the finest gauge suture compatible with the natural strength of the tissue [1]. For example, the face and neck generally have lower tension, thus 5-0 and 6-0 sutures are typically used [3]. For wounds on the trunk and extremities, where there is more dynamic motion and increased wound tension, 3-0 and 4-0 sutures may be used. Lastly, deeper sutures bear more tension compared to their superficial counterparts, so one might use larger-gauge sutures to approximate the tissue and close dead space while selecting finer gauge sutures for epidermal closure.

Knot Strength and Security. Knot strength is defined as the force required to cause a knot to slip [1, 3]. Knot security is the quality of a suture that allows it to be tied with a minimum number of throws per knot [1, 3]. Both features depend on suture memory, coefficient of friction, and pliability (see individual definitions below). A suture with high memory (i.e. Prolene®) tends to return to its original shape, and thus resists being tied in a knot and offers low knot security. A suture with a high coefficient of friction (i.e. silk) generally has good knot security. A suture that is pliable (i.e. silk) is able to bend, thus favors the knot configuration. When working with suture with low knot security, consider placing additional knots [1].

Plasticity. The ability of suture to stretch and maintain new length is called suture plasticity [1, 3]. If a suture is too plastic, it may stretch when skin is swollen but fail to correctly appose wound edges after edema resolves [1].

Elasticity. Suture elasticity is characterized by a suture's ability to stretch and return to its original form [1, 3]. Suture with high elasticity permits tissue edema without cutting through tissue, and then maintains wound edge approximation after the edema resolves.

Memory. Memory is characterized by the tendency of suture to retain its natural configuration after removal from packaging and to remain free of other contortions [1–3]. Suture with high memory (i.e. Nylon) is good for retaining surface approximation; however, it is also more difficult to handle and has poor knot strength.

Pliability. Pliable sutures are those that are easily bent [2]. Highly pliable suture is easiest to tie in knots. Braided sutures (i.e. silk) are most pliable.

Capillarity. Suture capillarity relates to the ability of suture to absorb fluid [2]. Capillarity is significant, as bacteria and other contaminants may also be absorbed and transported through tissue via suture. Multifilament sutures (i.e. Vicryl®) have greater capillarity due to increased interstitial space [1]. Natural sutures (i.e. plain and chromic gut) also have more capillarity than synthetic sutures (i.e. Prolene), which tend to be hydrophobic [1].

Coefficient of friction. The coefficient of friction describes the ease with which suture pulls though tissue [2]. Sutures with low coefficient of friction slide easily through tissue. However, knot strength is proportional to coefficient of friction and a low coefficient of friction equates to low knot strength. For example, polypropylene (Prolene) has a low coefficient, making it an ideal choice for running subcuticular closure, yet requiring additional knots for security.

Handling characteristics. Suture handling, or workability, depends on elasticity, plasticity and memory (discussed above) [3]. For example, suture with high memory (i.e. Nylon) may be more difficult to handle and hold knots. However, the smaller the size or caliber of the suture, the easier it is to handle regardless of other characteristics. Silk has exceptional handling and is the standard with which all other material is compared [1].

Tissue reactivity. Suture material is foreign to the body, thus elicits an inflammatory response when used to close a wound. The degree of inflammation in response to suture is known as suture tissue reactivity. Highly reactive suture interferes with normal wound healing and increases risk for infection. Natural and multifilament sutures (i.e. surgical gut, silk) tend to produce robust reactions, whereas synthetic or monofilament sutures (Nylon®) are less reactive [1, 3]. Sutures with the least reactivity are nonelectrolytic, noncapillary, nonallergenic, and noncarcinogenic [1].

11.2 Suture Material

Key Points

- The biggest distinction between sutures is whether the material is absorbable or non-absorbable.
- Absorbable sutures are primarily use for buried stitches in a layered closure; though in pediatric dermatologic surgery they may offer advantages for both deep and superficial sutures.
- Non-absorbable sutures are primarily used as superficial sutures in a layered closure or for simple full-thickness repair of a smaller defect.

In addition to the suture characteristics already discussed, perhaps the clearest distinction between suture materials is whether the material is absorbable or non-absorbable. By definition, absorbable sutures are broken down via enzymatic digestion or tissue hydrolysis; thus, are most often utilized for buried deep stitches to close the wound and reduce wound tension [1, 3]. Non-absorbable sutures resist degradation, and they are used to approximate epidermal wound edges. The most commonly used absorbable sutures in dermatology include polyglactin 910 (Vicryl), polydioxanone (PDS®), poligelcaprone (Monocryl®), surgical gut, and polyclocolic acid (Dexon®) (See Table 11.1) [2, 4–6]. The most commonly used non-absorbable sutures include nylon (Ethilon®, Surgilon®), polypropylene (Prolene, Surgilene®), polyester (Ethibond®, Dacron®), polybutester (Novafil®), and silk (See Table 11.2) [2, 4–6].

11.3 Suture Selection

Key Points

- Select the smallest suture that will achieve the required strength for a given closure [2].
- Consider the location on the body (i.e. face, trunk, mucosa, hair-bearing region) and individual wound characteristics (i.e. degree of tension, risk of infection) to further guide suture selection and ensure optimal outcomes.

Surgeons must select sutures that adequately close a wound while balancing this need with their own preferences for suture workability. As mentioned, absorbable sutures are often used for buried stitches, while non-absorbable sutures are used superficially. Suture selection is further guided by the anatomic location and individual wound characteristics.

One should select the finest gauge suture that will provide sufficient strength for the wound tension [2]. Deep sutures bear the brunt of wound tension, thus, they typically are larger gauge than the sutures used for epidermal closure. Additionally, wound tension varies depending on anatomic location. For example, for facial repairs 4-0 or 5-0 absorbable sutures are used for buried stitches and 5-0 or 6-0 non-absorbable sutures are used for the surface [2]. For repairs on the trunk, 3-0 or 4-0 absorbable sutures may be used for buried stitches, while 3-0, 4-0, or 5-0 non-absorbable sutures are used superficially. Sutures with high tensile strength and slow degradation (i.e. PDS, Maxon) may be used for truncal defects requiring long-term support. Poliglecaprone 25 (Monocryl) results in less tissue reactivity, though polyglactin 910 (Vicryl) is easier to handle.

Table 11.1 Absorbable sutures used in dermatologic surgery [2, 4–6].

Suture (Trade Name)	Configuration	Tensile Strength	Absorption Complete By	Knot Security	Ease of Handling	Tissue Reactivity	Uses
Fast-absorbing gut	Monofilament	Low; 50% at 3–5 days	20–40 days (falls off by 1 week)	Poor	Fair	Low	Punch biopsy closure; surface sutures for mucosa and skin; skin graft closure
Plain surgical gut	Monofilament	Low at 1 week	60–70 days	Poor	Fair	Moderate-High	Rarely used
Chromic surgical gut	Monofilament	Low at 3 weeks	80 days	Poor	Poor	Moderate-High	Surface sutures for mucosa and skin; skin graft closure
Polyglactin 910 (Vicryl Rapide)	Polyfilament	Low; 50% at 5 days; none by 2 weeks	40 days (falls off by 1 week)	Fair	Good	Moderate	Punch biopsy closure; surface sutures for mucosa and skin
Polyglactin 910 (Vicryl, Polysorb®)	Polyfilament	High; 75% at 2 weeks; 50% at 3 weeks; 25% at 4 weeks	90 days	Fair	Good	Moderate	Subcutaneous closure; vessel ligation
Polyglycolic acid (Dexon)	Polyfilament	Moderate; 20% at 3 weeks		Good	Good	Low	Subcutaneous closure; vessel ligation
Polydiaxanone (PDS, PDO®)	Monofilament	High; 70% at 2 weeks; 50% at 4 weeks; 25% at 6 weeks	180 days	Poor	Poor	Low	Subcutaneous closure in high-tension areas
Polyglyconate (Maxon®)	Monofilament	High; 74% at 2 weeks; 60% at 4 weeks	180 days	Good	Fair	Low	Subcutaneous closure in high-tension areas
Polycaprone 25 (Monocryl)	Monofilament	Moderate-High; 50–70% at 1 week; 20–40% at 2 weeks	20–120 days	Good	Good	Low	Subcutaneous closure; vessel ligation; when low reactivity is important
Glycomer 631 (Biosyn®)	Monofilament	High; 75% at 2 weeks; 40% at 3 weeks	90–110 days	Poor	Good	Low	Subcutaneous closure in high-tension areas

Table 11.2 Non-absorbable sutures used in dermatologic surgery [2, 4–6].

Suture (Trade Name)	Configuration	Tensile Strength	Memory	Knot Security	Ease of Handling	Tissue Reactivity	Uses
Nylon (Ethilon, Dermalon, Monosof®)	Monofilament	High	High	Poor	Fair-Good	Low	Surface closure on face, trunk and extremities
Nylon (Surgilon, Nurolon)	Polyfilament	High	Moderate	Fair	Fair-Good	Low	Surface closure on face, trunk and extremities
Polypropylene (Prolene, Surgilene, Surgipro)	Monofilament	Moderate-High	High	Poor	Fair-Good	Very low	Surface closure on face, trunk, or extremities; running subcuticular sutures; when low reactivity is important
Polybutester (Novafil)	Monofilament	Very high	Low	Poor	Fair-Good	Low	Skin closure on face, trunk, or extremities; running subcuticular sutures; when edema is anticipated
Polyester (Ethibond, Dacron, Mersilene)	Polyfilament	High	Moderate	Good	Good	Moderate	Mucosal surfaces, intertriginous areas, scalp
Silk (Sofsilk®, Perma-Hand®)	Polyfilament	Low	Low	Good	Excellent	High	Mucosal surfaces

Regarding epidermal closures, nylon (Ethilon, Dermalon®, Surgilon, Nurolon®), polybutester (Novafil), and polypropylene (Prolene, Surgilene, Surgipro®) are all appropriate choices for the face, trunk, and extremities. Both silk and polyester (Ethibond, Dacron, Mersilene®) are soft, thus good choices for mucosal, intertriginous surfaces, and scalp. Due to its low coefficient of friction, polypropylene (Prolene) is an excellent choice for running subcuticular sutures. Though non-absorbable sutures are often used to close the wound superficially, absorbable sutures may be considered in children to obviate the need for suture removal. Several studies show equivalent cosmetic outcomes between wounds closed with absorbable and non-absorbable top sutures [7–12]. Some absorbable sutures, such as fast-absorbing gut and partially hydrolyzed polyglactin 910 (Vicryl Rapide®), spontaneously dissolve within 7–14 days, thus avoiding the need for suture removal all together. These fast-absorbing sutures are also good for full-thickness skin grafts. As an alternative to sutures, staples, adhesives, and tapes may be used for epidermal closure and will be reviewed later in this chapter.

11.4 Needles

Key Points

- The most commonly used needle in dermatologic surgery is a 3/8 circle with a reverse cutting edge [2].
- Smaller needles (i.e. P-3 or PS-3) are used for precision work, especially on the face, or when working in tight spaces.
- Larger needles (P-2) are best for deep wounds and areas with thick dermis, such as on the back.
- Needle drivers with smaller jaws are appropriate for finer needles and those with larger jaws are best for larger needles [2].

Surgical needles are sharp, strong, stainless steel instruments designed to carry suture material through skin [2, 3]. Needles have three distinct parts including the shank, body, and point [2, 3]. The shank connects to the suture material. The body can be circular or straight and is where the surgeon grasps the needle using the needle driver. In dermatologic surgery, the curvature of circular needle bodies may range from 1/4 of a full circle to 5/8 of a full circle; however, the 3/8 circle is most commonly used. The needle point should be sharp and with either a rounded or triangular shape.

Triangular needles are advantageous, as the sharp edges more readily pass through tissue [2, 3]. Triangular needles are thus called "cutting" needles. Depending on the orientation of the sharp edge, the needle will be conventional cutting or reverse cutting. Conventional needles have the sharp edge oriented on the inside of the needle arc. With reverse cutting needles, the sharp edge is on the outside. With the later configuration, there is less tissue trauma and the risk of cutting previously placed sutures is minimized.

The nomenclature for surgical needles is not standardized, thus each brand has their own labels. Ethicon is a prominent manufacturer and Davis and Geck is another. Ethicon produces for skin (FS), plastic skin (PS), precision point (P), and precision cosmetic (PC) needles [3]. In dermatologic surgery, the PS, P, and PC are commonly employed. The PS is a reverse cutting needle. The P is a sharper version of the PS. Finally, the PC is a conventional cutting needle which is considered superior for cosmetic work. Davis and Geck produce cutting (CE), plastic reverse (PRE), skin closure (SC), slim blade (SBE), and diamond point (DP) needles [3]. Of these, the PRE is most similar to Ethicon's PS and P needles.

Regardless of manufacturer, the needles sizes used in dermatologic surgery are uniformly two or three, with two being larger [2]. Larger needles (i.e. PS-2) are typically used to close deep wounds on the trunk – particularly the back – where the dermis is thicker and the defect is deeper. Their sturdy shape is able to make larger passes through the tissue and also avoids bending. Finer needles (i.e. P-3 or PS-3) are good for more delicate work on the face or in wounds within tight spaces, such as the ear or scalp. Needle drivers with smaller jaws should be used to grasp finer needles, while those with larger jaws are used with larger needles.

11.5 Staples

Key Points

- Staples provide the highest tensile strength of available wound closure materials.
- They are good for wounds on the scalp or areas with high tension.

Delivered via lightweight, easy-to-grip cartridges, staples may be placed quickly with diminished risk of sharps injury, making them a convenient option for some wound closures in children. Additionally, they provide excellent wound eversion and may confer lower risk of wound infection compared to sutures [1]. Furthermore, staples are available in non-absorbable or absorbable options.

Non-absorbable staples (Proximate®) are made of steel and provide high tensile strength, making them a good selection for wounds on the scalp or in other areas of high tension. In at least one study [13] comparing wounds closed with silk versus stainless steel staples, there were similar esthetic outcomes on the day of removal and at 15 and 30 days after removal. Staples were certainly faster to apply, but they were at least twice as expensive. However, when considering labor and time spent suturing, the cost differential may be negligible. Other outcomes (patient comfort, pain on removal, complications) were similar between the two groups. Steel staples also have lower tissue reactivity [1]. On the downside, non-absorbable staples must be removed using a staple extractor or hemostat, which children may not tolerate. In this setting, absorbable staples may be a better option.

Absorbable staples (Insorb®) are composed of polylactide and polyglycolid and absorb within months [1]. They are placed subcuticularly, further reducing risk for needle sticks, tissue strangulation, and track marks as may occur with conventional suturing. Though less commonly an issue for routine dermatologic surgery, absorbable staples do not interfere with magnetic resonance imaging.

11.6 Adhesives

Key Points

- Tissue adhesives form a strong polymer bond across apposed wound edges.
- Adhesives are a convenient and less traumatic alternative to sutures and staples, but should be used with caution in higher tension wounds.

Compared with sutures, staples, and tapes, tissue adhesives can be quickly applied, require minimal training on the part of the practitioner and little wound care by the patient, and result in similar cosmetic outcomes [1]. These attributes make them a convenient treatment option for children with small, superficial lacerations. They have also been marketed to replace sutures 5-0 and smaller in diameter for incisional repair [14]. Evidence for use in larger wounds is lacking, but may indicate increased risk for wound dehiscence; thus, surgeons must use this wound closure modality with caution – particularly those wounds typically closed with 3-0 or 4-0 suture [15–19].

Cyanoacrylates, the active ingredient in tissue adhesives, were originally manufactured in the late 1940s; however, original formulations resulted in undesirable tissue toxicity [14]. More recent technology has resulted in tissue adhesives (i.e. Dermabond®) with less toxicity and improved bonding strength. An additional advantage, cyanoacrylates may have antibacterial properties [20].

For use in a layered closure, the surgeon must ensure buried sutures approximate the tissue edges securely and evenly. The wound is then cleaned in preparation for the adhesive. The adhesive is packaged as a sterile single-use vial, which must be crushed and then spread over the wound via the applicator tip. Crushing is required to initiate polymerization and moisture on the skin surface acts as the final catalyst, forming a strong bond across apposed wound edges [14]. Though relatively easy to apply, the surgeon must avoid getting adhesive into the wound, as this can result in a foreign body reaction or interfere with wound healing. Maximum strength is achieved at 2.5 minutes and is retained at seven days post repair. If not applied within minutes of crushing, the adhesive will solidify within the vial. No additional dressing is required, though in children a bandage may provide a barrier against excoriation or other trauma to the area.

After closure using tissue adhesive, children may shower and pat the area dry, but should avoid baths as prolonged moisture may loosen the adhesive. Antibiotic ointments should also be avoided, as they may breakdown the polymer bonds. Adhesives are not good candidates for wounds on mucosa or in areas of high moisture content (i.e. groin or axillae) [14]. They may be used on the scalp, if the surgeon meticulously avoids spreading the sticky substance throughout the hair. They may also be used on skin overlying joints, but only if immobilized. Other contraindications may not apply to elective pediatric dermatologic surgery, but are worth noting and include: animal bites, contaminated wounds, ulcers, and puncture wounds.

11.7 Tapes

Key Points

- Tapes may be use in lieu of epidermal sutures or staples during wound closure, as an adjunct to running subcuticular sutures, or to provide longer-lasting support following suture or staple removal.
- When used as the only material to secure the epidermis in a layered closure, tape should be reserved for low-tension wounds.

Tissue tapes (Steri-Strips®) offer an atraumatic alternative to epidermal sutures and staples during layered closure in which the buried sutures achieve excellent tissue approximation [2]. Ideally, closure with tape is reserved for small linear wounds under little tension [1]. Tape may also be used in conjunction with running subcuticular suture to further reduce tension and/or assist in epidermal closure/approximation. Lastly, tape can be applied after suture or staple removal to provide continuing support without risk for track marks if sutures were left in for a longer time. These later points are important to consider in active children who may be at risk for wound dehiscence.

To correctly apply tissue tape, the surgeon first applies a liquid adhesive (Mastisol®) and then orients parallel strips of the tape perpendicular to the wound [2]. Compared to sutures and staples, tape may offer improved cosmesis at the time of closure and within the first few weeks of the procedure [21]. Thereafter, cosmetic outcomes are similar [21–23], corroborating the idea that undermining and placement of deep buried sutures are the primary determinants of final wound appearance [1].

Unfortunately, tissue tapes have several disadvantages. First, they offer less precise wound approximation and have lower tensile strength compared to sutures. Unsurprisingly, this correlates with a higher rate of dehiscence [23]; hence they are reserved for small, shallow, low-tension wounds. During application, they require the use of adhesive adjuncts, which may be irritating to the skin and are not effective in hair-dense regions. If applied to moist surfaces, sites of movement (i.e. overlying a joint), or on a wound that later becomes edematous, they may fall off [1, 23].

11.8 Complications

Key Points

- Suture related complications are generally due to improper suture placement or due to tissue reactivity.

- Staples result in fast closure, but still require removal which can be uncomfortable.
- Tissue adhesives and tapes may increase risk for wound dehiscence if buried sutures do not provide adequate strength for the degree of wound tension.

Each wound closure material has advantages and disadvantages. With regards to suture complications, suture placement is often the leading factor [2]. If the suture is too tight, the tissue will be strangulated and necrose. If the suture is too loose, the wound may dehisce. Furthermore, the inherent properties of suture can lead to tissue reactivity. This is particularly a problem if the suture is a buried and left in place to absorb. In these settings, the inflammation may result in a sterile pustule, suture abscess, granuloma, or expulsion of the suture (a.k.a. "spitting suture") via a sinus track [2]. Inflammation also predisposes to infections and less cosmetically acceptable scars. If top sutures or steel staples are removed too early, a wound may dehisce. If removed too late, they may leave track marks.

With regards to needle size, if a large needle is improperly selected to close a narrow space, this may create difficulty during wound closure. Similarly, small needles will be unable to create large passes through thick dermis. Conventional cutting needles may cause undesired tissue trauma or accidentally slice though knots that have already been placed, taking the surgeon back a step.

Tissue adhesives and tapes may also predispose to wound dehiscence if used in a high-tension wound where buried dermal sutures aren't secured in children who are very active. These closure materials are also susceptible to falling apart in the setting of prolonged moisture or topical antibiotic use. Ultimately, there are numerous ways to close a wound, but the cost of a complication does not justify the use of less expensive, lower quality, or more convenient closure materials.

11.9 Conclusion

Selection of wound closure material is dictated by patient demographics, type of procedure, anatomic location, wound surface area and depth, and preferences of the surgeon. Closing a wound in an infant or child differs from that in an adult who may have atrophic skin or co-morbidities that influence wound healing. While sutures are most commonly utilized in dermatologic surgery, pediatric patients may also have difficulty cooperating with a prolonged procedure (unless sedated), thus quicker closure techniques (i.e. tissue adhesives, staples) may be attractive options. In contrast, some of these applications (particularly tissue adhesives and tapes) may offer inferior wound closure in areas of tension. Pediatric patients may have difficulty with suture or staple removal, further influencing wound closure choice. All of these factors must be considered on an individual basis.

References

1. Hochberg, J., Meyer, K.M., and Marion, M.D. (2009). Suture choice and other methods of skin closure. *Surg. Clin. North Am.* 89 (3): 627–641.
2. Ammirati, C.T. and Goldman, G. (2012). Wound closure materials and instruments. In: *Dermatology*, 3e, vol. 2 (ed. J.L. Bolognia, J.L. Jorizzo and J.V. Schaffer), 2353–2363. Philadelphia, PA: Elsevier Saunders.
3. Bogle, M.A., Fisher, V.T., and Joseph, A.K. (2010). Instruments and materials. In: *Surgery of the Skin: Procedural Dermatology*, 2e (ed. J.K. Robinson, C.W. Hanke, D.M. Siegel, et al.), 65–72. Philadelphia, PA: Elsevier Mosby.
4. Weitzul, S. and Taylor, S. (2010). Suturing technique and other closure materials. In: *Surgery of the Skin: Procedural Dermatology*,

2e (ed. J.K. Robinson, C.W. Hanke, D.M. Siegel, et al.), 65–72. Philadelphia, PA: Elsevier Mosby.
5 Ethicon (2016) http://www.ethicon.com/healthcare-professionals/products/wound-closure (accessed 17 May 2016).
6 Medtronic (2016) http://www.medtronic.com/covidien/products/wound-closure (accessed 17 May 2016).
7 Al-Abdullah, T., Plint, A.C., and Fergusson, D. (2007). Absorbable versus nonabsorbable sutures in the management of traumatic lacerations and surgical wounds – a meta-analysis. *Pediatr. Emerg. Care* 23 (5): 339–344.
8 Fosko, S.W. and Heap, D. (1998). Surgical pearl – an economical means of skin closure with absorbable suture. *J. Am. Acad. Dermatol.* 39 (2 Pt 1): 248–250.
9 Holger, J.S., Wandersee, S.C., and Hale, D.B. (2004). Cosmetic outcomes of facial lacerations repaired with tissue-adhesive, absorbable, and nonabsorbable sutures. *Am. J. Emerg. Med.* 22 (4): 254–257.
10 Luck, R., Tredway, T., Gerard, J. et al. (2013). Comparison of cosmetic outcomes of absorbable versus nonabsorbable sutures in pediatric facial lacerations. *Pediatr. Emerg. Care* 29 (6): 691–695.
11 Tejani, C., Sivitz, A.B., Rosen, M.D. et al. (2014). A comparison of cosmetic outcomes of lacerations on the extremities and trunk using absorbable versus nonabsorbable sutures. *Acad. Emerg. Med.* 21 (6): 637–643.
12 Xu, B., Xu, B., Wang, L. et al. (2016). Absorbable versus nonabsorbable sutures for skin closure- a meta-analysis of randomized controlled trials. *Ann. Plast. Surg.* 76 (5): 598–606.
13 Batra, J., Bekal, R.K., Byadgi, S. et al. (2016). Comparison of skin Staples and standard sutures for closing incisions after head and neck cancer surgery – a double-blind, randomized and prospective study. *J. Maxillofac. Oral Surg.* 15 (2): 243–250.
14 Bruns, T.B. and Worthington, J.M. (2000). Using tissue adhesive for wound repair- a practical guide to dermabond. *Am. Fam. Physician* 61 (5): 1383–1388.
15 Bernard, L., Doye, J., Friedlander, S.F. et al. (2001). A prospective comparison of octyl cyanoacrylate tissue adhesive (Dermabond) and suture for the closure of excisional wounds in children and adolescents. *Arch. Dermatol.* 137: 1177–1180.
16 Devrukhkar, V.N., Hegde, R.J., Khare, S.S. et al. (2015). Evaluation of isoamyl 2-cyanoacrylate tissue adhesive in management of pediatric lacerations- an alternative to suturing. *Ann. Maxillofac. Surg.* 5 (1): 49–54.
17 Dumville, J.C., Coulthard, P., Worthington, H.V. et al. (2014). Tissue adhesives for closure of surgical incisions. *Cochrane Database Syst. Rev.* 28 (11): CD004287.
18 Farion, K.J., Osmond, M.H., Hartling, L. et al. (2003). Tissue adhesives for traumatic lacerations: a systematic review of randomized controlled trials. *Acad. Emerg. Med.* 10: 110–118.
19 Quinn, J., Wells, G., Sutcliffe, T. et al. (1998). Tissue adhesive versus suture wound repair at 1 year: randomized clinical trial correlating early 3 month and 1 year cosmetic outcomes. *Ann. Emerg. Med.* 32: 645–649.
20 Eiferman, R.A. and Snyder, J.W. (1983). Antibacterial effect of cyanoacrylate glue. *Arch. Ophthalmol.* 101: 958–960.
21 Yang, S. and Ozog, D. (2015). Comparison of traditional superficial cutaneous sutures versus adhesive strips in layered dermatologic closures on the Back – a prospective, randomized, Split-scar study. *Dermatol. Surg.* 41 (11): 1257–1263.
22 Custis, T., Armstrong, A.W., King, T.H. et al. (2015). Effect of adhesive strips and dermal sutures vs dermal sutures only on wound closure – a randomized clinical trial. *JAMA Dermatol.* 151 (8): 862–867.
23 Zempsky, W.T., Parrotti, D., Grem, C. et al. (2004). Randomized controlled comparison of cosmetic outcomes of simple facial lacerations closed with Steri strip skin closures or Dermabond tissue adhesive. *Pediatr. Emerg. Care* 20 (8): 519–524.

12

Dressings

Grace Sun

Dermatology Medical Group, Oxnard, CA, USA

12.1 Introduction

A dressing is any material applied to a wound to facilitate protection and healing. The most basic dressings provide a barrier to maintain a clean, moist environment while there is a myriad of specialized dressings that function in different ways to modify the healing process. Dressings have been used for centuries, with the earliest dating back to more than 4000 years ago. Maintaining a moist, slightly hypoxic environment accelerates wound healing and should be the goal of wound care. The ideal wound dressing would keep micro-organisms from entering, allow some oxygen in, allow carbon dioxide and water vapor out, and wick away excess moisture to create a warm, moist wound bed environment. In this chapter, we will review the many different types of available dressings and the appropriate situations in which to apply them.

12.2 Types

12.2.1 The Basic Wound Dressing

There are two different types of wound healing that can occur following a procedure. Healing via primary intention is for clean wounds that are sutured after an excision or biopsy. Healing via second intention is for wounds left open to slowly close by granulation and re-epithelization after a shave biopsy, small punch biopsy, curettage, cryosurgery, laser surgery or excision. After a procedure, petrolatum or paraffin wax is applied and then the dressing.

The basic wound dressing has three parts, all of which allow air to pass through. The first layer, closest to the wound, is called the "contact layer" which is typically made of a non-adherent material that is fluid-permeable, allowing exudate to pass through (e.g. Telfa®). The second layer is for absorbing exudate, such as gauze, cotton pads (e.g. Kerlix®). And the final outer most layer is to hold the first two in place such as tape, wraps or netting (e.g. Bandnet®, Surgilast®).

A standard post-surgical "pressure dressing" consists of a basic wound dressing with a thicker absorbent layer for areas that may have a bleeding diathesis like the scalp or digits. The addition of an elastic self-adhesive wrap (e.g. Coban®) provides the benefit of added compression of the "pressure dressing". Care must be taken not to fasten the dressing too tightly in which venous flow is compromised. This is particularly of importance on the digits, where it is important to keep the distal tip visible so the parent can ensure proper circulation is flowing to the digit.

Pediatric Dermatologic Surgery, First Edition. Edited by Keyvan Nouri, Latanya Benjamin, Jasem Alshaiji, and Jan Izakovic.

The basic wound dressing is also applicable to wounds that may not have resulted from a procedure. For example, children with blistering disorders such as epidermolysis bullosa and linear IgA will have acute and chronic superficial to partial-thickness ulcers that would benefit from ideal healing conditions.

12.2.2 Occlusive Dressings

There follows a review of the five types of occlusive dressings that are commercially available.

12.2.2.1 Films

Films are thin, transparent polyurethane or synthetic polymer adhesive dressings that are gas-permeable but not fluid-permeable. Films will keep bacteria and frank fluid from entering the wound site. Because water vapor easily passes through a film, sweat and small amounts of moisture do not become trapped and cause skin maceration. The transparent nature of films also allows one to visual the healing wound without having to dislodge the dressing to inspect it. Films are non-absorbent and therefore not suitable for wounds producing copious amounts of exudate. The adhesive nature is quite helpful for anchoring objects like catheters or topical anesthetic creams prior to procedures in children (Figure 12.1), but is not advised for use on the most fragile skin types.

Films are most often used to cover superficial wounds, split–thickness skin graft donor sites, skin abrasions and intravenous catheter sites.

Examples – Tegaderm® (3M) Opsite® (Smith and Nephew), Polyskin II® (Kendall), Window Transparent Film Dressing® (Kendall), MEPORE® film (Mölnlyche), REPARA® (Select Medical), Suresite® Transparent Film (Medline), Dermview II (Dermrite), McKesson Transparent Film Dressing (McKesson).

12.2.2.2 Foams

Foams are composed of a thick polyurethane absorbent layer with an overlying polymer layer that is gas-permeable but only semi-permeable for fluids. The inner foam layer absorbs exudate and the outer layer keeps the underlying wound from desiccating, prevents leakage, and keeps bacteria and contaminates outside the dressing. Most foams are non-adhesive (Figure 12.2) and need to be secured in place using another dressing. Many manufacturers are now marketing foam dressings with an adhesive border around the edge to eliminate the need for a secondary dressing. Foams are designed for wounds draining a moderate amount of fluid. If there is a dry wound bed, the foam will

Figure 12.1 An example of a film dressing used to occlude a topical anesthetic. Tegaderm (3M).

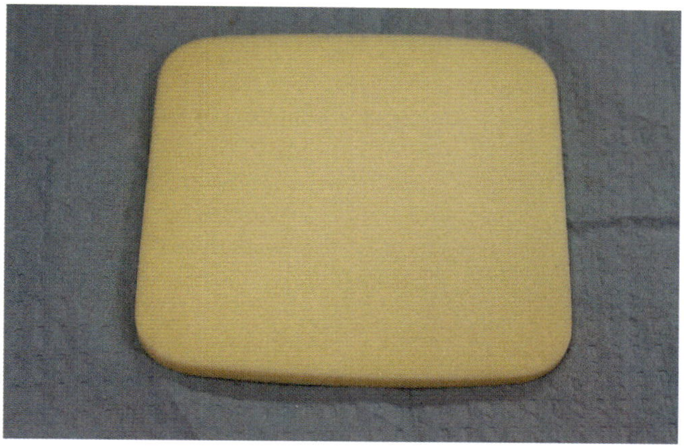

Figure 12.2 An example of a foam dressing. Hydrasorb (Dukal).

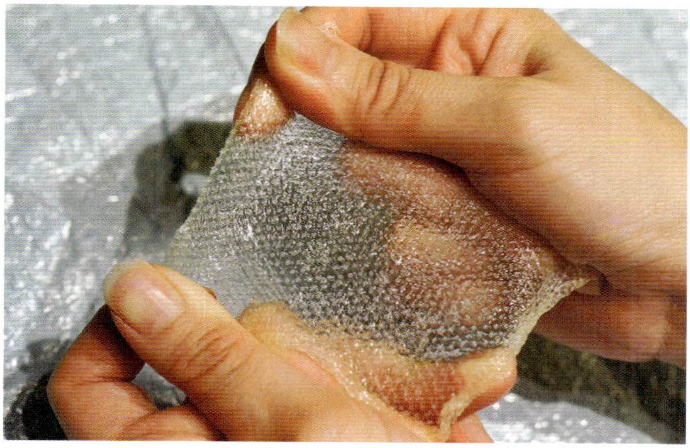

Figure 12.3 An example of a hydrogel dressing. 2nd Skin (Spenco).

overly dry the area and adhere to the wound; if the wound produces large amounts of fluid, the foam may become soaked and need to be changed frequently. There are also thinner foam dressings that are not as absorbent but serve as a gentle contact layer (Mepilex transfer®). Because foams are opaque, direct visualization of the wound is not possible with these dressings.

Foams are ideal for chronic wounds, ulcers, post-surgical/laser wounds, exudative epidermolysis bullosa erosions, and may be used to pack deep ulcers.

Examples – with adhesive – Mepilex border® (Mölnlyche), Allevyn® (Smith and Nephew), Optifoam® (Medline), Optiva® (Medline); without adhesive – McKesson Hydrocellular Foam Dressing Non-Adhesive with Film-Back® (McKesson), McKesson Hydrophilic Foam Dressing™, Non-Adhesive, Tegaderm Foam Dressing (3M), Copa® (Kendall), Biatain® (Coloplast™), Dermafoam® (Dermarite), Cutimed® (BSN Medical), Hydrasorb™ (Dukal).

12.2.2.3 Hydrogels

Hydrogels are composed of mostly fluid in a hydrophilic polymer mesh and are sold as dry or partially hydrated sheets or in a tube. Depending on the type of hydrogel, some are semi-adherent or non-adherent (Figure 12.3), can absorb a large amount of exudate and

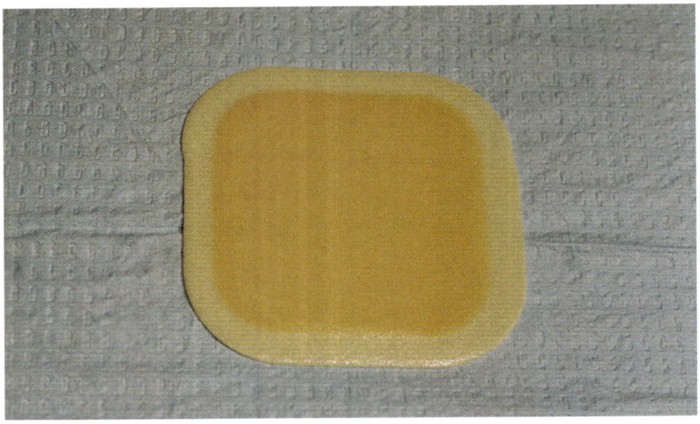

Figure 12.4 An example of a hydrocolloid dressing. Hydrocolloid dressing (McKesson).

may need an outer dressing to hold them in place. Unfortunately, hydrogels are not good antimicrobial barriers and allow gram-negative bacteria to enter the wound. To prevent infection an antibiotic ointment and an outer dressing can be used along with the hydrogel. Hydrogels maintain a moist environment and provide ideal healing conditions.

Applications include superficial erosions, pediatric burns, split–thickness skin graft donor sites, shallow ulcers, post-laser resurfacing and post-dermabrasion.

Examples – hydrogel sheets – Aquaflo® (Kendall), Allevyn Hydrogel® (Smith and Nephew), Reliamed Hydrogel sheet® (Reliamed), 2nd Skin® (Spenco); hydrogel in a tube – Coloplast 7690® (Coloplast), Carrasyn® (Carrington), Curasol® (HealthPoint), Intrasite® (Smith and Nephew); impregnated gauze – Curafil® (Kendall), Restore® (Hollister), Amerigel® (Amerigel), Hydrogel Dressing™ (McKesson).

12.2.2.4 Hydrocolloids

The term "colloid" is used to describe an insoluble particle dispersed throughout another substance. Hydrocolloid dressings are made of hydrophilic polymers and polysaccharides dispersed throughout a base composed of gelatin, pectin, and carboxymethyl cellulose. When the hydrocolloid comes in contact with an exudative wound, the exudate forms a gel with the hydrocolloid. There are often multiple layers to the hydrocolloid dressing including a waterproof layer to prevent exudate from soaking through the dressing or external water from entering. Hydrocolloids are similar to hydrogels in the sense that they are very absorbent and semi-gas permeable and promote wound healing. Additionally, hydrocolloids may act as additional protection from trauma and may be left in place up to a week at a time depending on the amount of exudate generated from the wound. Some hydrocolloids come with an adhesive border (Figure 12.4) and do not require a secondary dressing. Hydrocolloids are opaque and direct visualization of the wound bed is not possible and may also lead to a specific odor.

Hydrocolloids are useful in the pediatric population for chronic wounds, blistering disorders, surgical or traumatic wounds and burns.

Examples – Tegaderm hydrocolloid® (3M), DuoDERM® (Convatec), Restore™ (Hollister), Comfeel Plus® (Coloplast), Nu-Derm® (Johnson & Johnson), Hydrocolloid Dressing™ (McKesson), Exuderm® (Medline).

12.2.2.5 Alginates

Alginates are dressings made with a polysaccharide from different types of seaweed or algae that have a high capacity for absorption.

The alginate dressings are produced in a manner in which the sodium ions have been replaced by calcium ions. Once in contact with a wound, the calcium in the dressing is exchanged with the sodium in the exudate and blood, forming a sodium alginate gel at the point of contact. The calcium exchange is also helpful in achieving hemostasis by facilitating the clotting cascade and is sometimes used for this express reason. Alginate dressings are non-adherent and must be secured by an outer dressing. Because alginate dressings have a large capacity for absorption, dressing changes can be deferred for several days at a time. Alginates have a specific odor and a yellow-brown color. If an alginate has dried in a wound bed, normal saline should be applied first to assist with dressing changes.

Alginates are helpful in exudative chronic wounds, deep burn wounds, and surgical wounds requiring hemostasis.

Examples – Curasorb Calcium Alginate® (Kendall), Restore Calcium Alginate™ (Hollister), High-integrity Alginate Dressing™ (3M), Medihoney Calcium Alginate™ (Derma Sciences), Coloplast Biatain Alginate Dressing and Coloplast Seasorb® (Coloplast), Silvercel® (Systagenix).

12.2.2.6 Silver-Impregnated Dressings

Of the above-mentioned types of dressings, many brands have added silver as an antimicrobial agent. With the basic standard dressing, the application of silver sulfadiazine rather than petrolatum would be an option. There have been a few small studies in the burn literature that tout similar outcomes comparing petrolatum and silver sulfadiazine [1]. Films, hydrogels [2], hydrocolloids, foams, alginates likewise have similar silver – impregnated products.

12.2.3 Wound Classifications Based on Depth

Superficial: These wounds only involve damage to the epidermis and are called erosions. These heal easily with keratinocyte migration from the wound edges.

Partial-thickness: These wounds involve damage to the epidermis and part of the dermis and are called ulcers. These heal with keratinocyte migration from the wound edges and adnexal structures.

Full-thickness: These wounds involve damage to the epidermis, dermis and adnexa down to the fat and deeper. These wounds heal more slowly as keratinocytes can only migrate from the wound edges as the adnexal structures in the wound are damaged as well. Wound contraction with scar formation often occurs.

12.2.4 Wound Classifications (Based on the American College of Surgeons and Center of Disease Control)

Clean: Operative wounds that do not involve the respiratory, gastrointestinal, urinary, genital tract with no signs of local inflammation.

Clean-contaminated: Operative wounds that enter the respiratory, gastrointestinal, urinary, and genital tract in a controlled manner with no overt signs of local inflammation.

Contaminated: Open, fresh, wounds from trauma or operative wounds with a breach in sterile technique or signs of local inflammation.

Dirty: Chronic traumatic wounds with dead tissue and clear signs of infection.

Superficial wounds heal well with basic wound care and a simple dressing with a commercially available self-adhesive bandage and an ointment. Wound dressings including films, hydrogels, hydrocolloids, foams and alginates are all suitable for partial-thickness wounds. However, depending on the degree of exudate of the wound some are more preferable. For full-thickness wounds, foams and alginates may be utilized.

12.3 Conclusion

Most surgical wounds from pediatric office procedures would be considered clean wounds and depending on the procedure performed range from superficial to full-thickness as mentioned above. Ulcers can vary from superficial to partial thickness based on the type of skin disorder (such as in epidermolysis bullosa) or pressure ulcer. Given the diverse range of available wound dressings, one can successfully tailor it to the type of wound being treated and the ability to firmly secure it on, oftentimes young, mobile pediatric patients.

References

1 Genuino, G.A., Baluyut-Angeles, K.V., Espiritu, A.P. et al. (2014). Topical petrolatum gel alone versus topical silver sulfadiazine with standard gauze dressings for the treatment of superficial partial thickness burns in adults: a randomized controlled trial. *Burns* 40 (7): 1267–1273.

2 Boonkaew, B., Barber, P.M., Rengpipat, S. et al. (2014). Development and characterization of a novel, antimicrobial, sterile hydrogel dressing for burn wounds: single-step production with gamma irradiation creates silver nanoparticles and radical polymerization. *J. Pharm. Sci.* 103 (10): 3244–3253.

13

Nail Surgery

Jane Sanders Bellet

Duke University School of Medicine, Durham, NC, USA

13.1 Introduction

Nail surgery is required in a number of situations: in order to make a diagnosis via biopsy; to definitively remove a lesion; or to relieve pain such as in ingrown toenail surgery; removal of a foreign body or evacuation of a hematoma. Nail surgery in children and adolescents requires a number of special considerations, both in pathologic diagnoses as well as in the performance of the procedure itself.

13.2 Nail Anatomy

Understanding nail anatomy is crucial for success in performing nail procedures. Equally critical is understanding the disease pathology being biopsied or excised, as that informs exactly where in the nail unit a procedure should be done.

The nail unit includes the nail matrix, nail bed, proximal nail fold, and the hyponychium, in addition to the nail plate [1]. The proximal nail fold and lateral nail folds form the borders around the nail plate. The cuticle runs along this border, and covers the nail plate just as it emanates from the proximal nail fold. This is an adherent barrier to moisture and infectious agents. The nail matrix is present underneath the proximal nail fold and includes the white half-moon lunula. The matrical horns extend laterally and proximally from the proximal nail fold. These are important to note, especially when causing permanent ablation of a nail – the horns must be ablated in addition to the central matrix, otherwise spicules will develop with regrowth of the lateral nail plate. The nail bed is the pink portion visible through the nail plate. Under the nail bed, no subcutaneous tissue is present, therefore bone is directly beneath and many procedures do extend to the periosteum. The free edge of the nail plate is not attached to the nail bed and the onychodermal band marks this transition.

The digits are vascularized by the proper digital arteries, which run along each digit laterally on both sides, which in turn supply the nail unit. Veins follow the arterial supply except that collecting veins are in the lateral nail folds and also run through the proximal nail fold. Innervation is supplied by a branch of the dorsal digital nerve which runs across the DIP to the proximal nail fold, in addition to the palmar digital nerve which trifurcates distal to the DIP and supplies the nail unit, tip and pulp of the distal digit. Extensor tendons run across the DIP and attach proximal to the matrix. Lateral flexor tendons connect the base of the distal phalanx to the ungual spines [2].

Pediatric Dermatologic Surgery, First Edition. Edited by Keyvan Nouri, Latanya Benjamin, Jasem Alshaiji, and Jan Izakovic.

13.3 History and Pre-Operative Evaluation

When evaluating a patient for possible nail surgery, there are a number of considerations. Examination of all 20 nails is critical as this may aid in diagnosis even without a biopsy. If the condition affects more than one nail, then a toenail would be chosen over a fingernail and one of the smaller nails (4th or 5th) versus the larger nails (1st, 2nd and 3rd) as this will be less of a functional problem post-operatively as well as having diminished appearance concerns once healed. Inquiring as to past medical history and whether other family members have the same nail condition is useful in forming a diagnostic differential.

As with any pre-operative patient, inquiring as to: past surgeries performed on the nails; past procedures requiring general or local anesthesia; allergies; medications (including prescription, over-the-counter and herbals); past medical history of coagulation disorders such as von Willebrand factor deficiency; and whether a pacemaker or defibrillator is in place all must be ascertained.

Photographs prior to the procedure to document the lesion as well as the appearance of the entire nail unit are useful.

13.4 Preparation Prior to Nail Surgery

Once it has been determined that a nail procedure needs to be done, the decision as to whether it should be performed in the office under local anesthesia or will require general anesthesia needs to be made. For many children, the experience of a digital block can be quite scary and painful and they will require general anesthesia in order to perform the procedure in a safe manner [3]. As a general rule, children under age 12 will require general anesthesia and in certain circumstances, even older adolescents may also require general anesthesia. All patients have local anesthetic injected, even those patients under general anesthesia, so that when they awaken they are not in immediate pain. Informed consent should be obtained prior to any nail procedure and should include the possibility of permanent nail dystrophy, in addition to the standard surgical risks of bleeding, pain, scarring, infection and potential need for additional procedures.

Often, both a digital and wing block are placed, although for some procedures a wing block is sufficient. These blocks are placed using a local anesthetic. Some providers prefer plain 1% lidocaine; some prefer 1% lidocaine with epinephrine [4]. Still others prefer a mixture of short- and long-acting local anesthetics such as 0.5% lidocaine and 0.25% bupivacaine, which provides for further anesthesia after the procedure. The actual volume of local anesthetic injected must be monitored carefully, as there is a risk of ischemia due to pressure of the volume, especially if the anesthetic is inadvertently infiltrated as a total ring block [5]. The smallest volume possible should be used. Most digital and wing blocks are fully functional with only 1 ml or less of local anesthetic. If more anesthesia is needed, very careful attention should be paid to the total volume.

For awake patients, the injections of a digital and wing block are much better tolerated with the use of ethyl chloride spray prior to each injection [4, 5], as well as the use of a vibrating massager, which uses the gate theory in reducing pain perception [6].

There are multiple techniques for digital blocks. One of the simplest and safest is to use a 30-gauge needle on a 3 cc syringe, with the first injection of the digital block placed in the interdigital web space into the subcutaneous fat in the middle of the proximal phalanx [5]. This then is repeated on the other side of the digit. Then a wing block is placed, with the first injection 2–3 mm proximal to the lateral proximal nail fold; this is then repeated on the opposite side. Then, a point 1–2 mm proximal to the center of the proximal nail fold is infiltrated. Each side of the lateral nail fold more distally is injected and then finally the eponychium in three separate sites. At this point, the functionality of the blocks should be checked in an awake patient.

Once the digit is fully anesthetized, the entire hand or foot is cleansed with surgical scrub. This can be done using a chlorhexidine scrub brush. The hand or foot is then draped sterilely. In an older child or adolescent, a sterile glove can be pulled over their entire hand [7]; however, this technique does not work well in smaller patients, nor very well for toenails. A fenestrated drape is often useful, in order to isolate the single digit on which the procedure will be done.

Marking the nail lesion (dystrophy, onychoschizia, melanonychia, etc.) with a marking pen on the proximal and distal cutaneous skin is often useful as sometimes no lesion, pigment or other identifying features can be seen once the nail plate has been removed.

Nail surgery must be performed in a bloodless field; therefore a tourniquet is quite useful. There are a number of different ways in which to apply a tourniquet. One way is to snip the tip of the sterile glove that is already in place on the patient's hand and roll back the finger of the glove to the base of the digit [7]. The residual material of the glove finger can then be clamped with a hemostat [8]. Alternatively, the flat side of a small Penrose drain can be wrapped from the most distal aspect of the digit to the base of the digit and then clamped using a mosquito or Halsted hemostat. The more distal portion is then unwrapped, effectively exsanguinating the digit. Even more effective is the proprietary "T ring" tourniquet (Figure 13.1) (Precision Medical Devices, LLC, Thousand Oaks, California), which provides equal pressure circumferentially, as well as a more predictably bloodless field [9].

The biggest risk with the use of a tourniquet is ischemia due to lack of oxygen delivery, leading to acidosis. The shorter the amount of time a tourniquet is in place, the better. Monitoring the exact amount of time a tourniquet is in place is very important; therefore an assistant should mark the starting and ending time. In general, 20 minutes should be sufficient for most nail procedures and clinically important ischemia is unlikely at times less than this, as long as a small volume of local anesthetic was used. Procedure times longer than 30 minutes often require release of the tourniquet and then reapplication, often at 20 minutes [10].

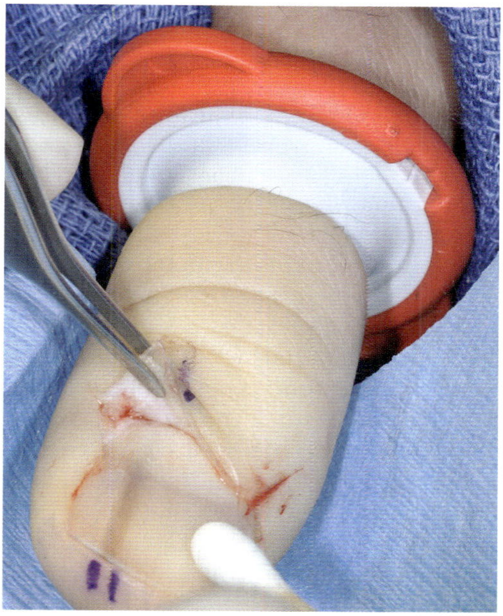

Figure 13.1 T ring tourniquet (Precision Medical Devices, LLC, Thousand Oaks, California).

13.5 Nail Procedures

13.5.1 Nail Avulsion

Nail avulsion is performed for two reasons: visualization of a biopsy or excision site or for therapeutic reasons (pachyonychia congenita, severe onychomycosis, ingrown toenail). Either full or partial nail avulsion techniques can be employed.

13.5.1.1 Chemical Nail Avulsion

For full nail avulsions, chemical avulsion can be performed with application of 40–50% urea cream or gel under full occlusion (Tegaderm [3M, St. Paul Minnesota] or secured plastic wrap) for one to two weeks [11]. Care must be taken to protect the surrounding skin, as urea can also cause desquamation of the skin. The nail is then very soft and easily removed. For some children and adolescents, this technique can be preferable to surgical avulsion.

13.5.1.2 Full Nail Avulsion, Distal Approach

A Freer septum elevator is introduced under the free edge of the nail plate and gently, but firmly pushed proximally along the nail bed. The same technique is performed along the entire free edge of the nail plate and then under the proximal nail fold, taking care not to push with too much force as the underlying soft tissue and nail bed more proximally can be disrupted. Then, the initial action is repeated at the free edge of the nail plate until a "give", that is usually felt, occurs. Next, a straight Halsted or mosquito hemostat is securely attached to the free edge of the nail. The handle of the hemostat is gently twisted side to side until the nail becomes loose. There are some attachments at the proximal and lateral nail folds that sometimes require cutting with iris scissors or a 15 blade scalpel.

13.5.1.3 Partial Avulsion

The advantage of a partial avulsion is that at least part of the nail is left in anatomic position, so that there is less trauma to the soft tissue. Additionally, the presence of the nail plate aids in the healing process as a natural "bandage" lying over a wound [12].

There are multiple partial avulsion techniques and the one chosen depends on the location of the nail unit requiring visualization, see Figure 13.2 [13].

13.5.1.4 Trapdoor Avulsion

For visualization of the entire nail bed, as well as the distal matrix and hyponychium, the trapdoor avulsion is optimal. Just as in a full nail avulsion, a Freer septum elevator is introduced under the free edge of the nail plate and gently, but firmly, pushed proximally along the nail bed. The same technique is performed along the entire free edge of the nail plate, but *not* under the proximal nail fold. Then the initial action is repeated at the free edge of the nail plate. A "give" will occur that is usually felt and then a straight Halsted or mosquito hemostat is securely attached to the free edge of the nail, see Figure 13.3 [12]. The hemostat can be held by an assistant to hold the nail plate up and away from the bed, while the biopsy or excision is performed.

13.5.1.5 Window Nail Plate Avulsion

For foreign body removal, evacuating a subungual hematoma, or excision of a well-delineated tumor, a window nail plate avulsion is useful. Two methods can be used: Method 1. A square or rectangle is scored using either an 11 or 15 blade, then the small piece of plate is pried off the bed. Method 2. A 5 or 6 mm punch trephine is used to score the plate. An 11 blade is used to lift the circular piece of plate off the bed. In both of these methods, the bed can then be biopsied using either a small punch trephine or a Teflon-coated 15 blade scalpel. The "window" of nail plate can either be sent for histopathology if needed, or replaced and secured using either a Steri-Strip (3M, St. Paul Minnesota) or suture [12].

13.5.1.6 Partial Distal Plate Avulsion

An English anvil-action nail splitter is placed into the lateral sulcus and used to cut transversely across the nail plate. A Freer septum nail elevator can then be used under the free edge of the nail plate to release the nail bed connections. This technique can be used to remove the entire distal nail plate, or alternatively only a quadrant, which is useful for tumor visualization or removal of dermatophytoma [12].

13.5.1.7 Lateral Nail Plate Avulsion

The lateral plate is cut using an English anvil-action nail splitter. A Freer septum elevator is then used under the free edge of the nail plate and along the lateral nail fold, as well as under the proximal nail fold just in alignment with the piece of nail plate desired to be removed. A Halsted hemostat can then be attached to the piece of nail plate distally and gently rocked from side to side. The piece is then removed. This technique is useful for treatment of ingrown, as well as pincer nails [12].

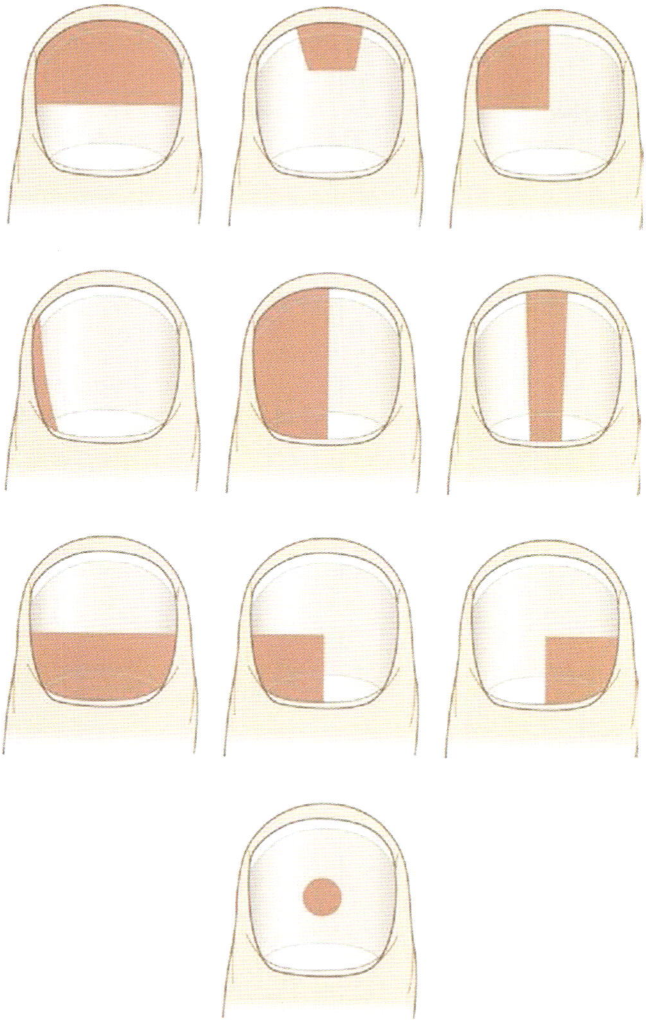

Figure 13.2 Location of partial nail avulsions [13].

13.5.1.8 Lateral Nail Plate Curl Avulsion

The lateral nail plate curl is an alternative to a full nail avulsion. It provides exposure of a portion of the nail bed, the distal and proximal matrix, as well as lateral structures. The proximal nail fold is reflected back, by making a diagonal incision with a 15 blade scalpel at the junction of the lateral and proximal nail fold and then cutting parallel to the nail plate. The plate is then released using a Freer septum elevator, by inserting first under the free edge of the nail plate which is then gently pushed. The elevator is then used along the lateral nail fold. A Halsted or mosquito hemostat is then attached to the distal-lateral plate and "curled" toward the center of the nail [12].

13.5.1.9 Partial Proximal Nail Plate Avulsion

To visualize the entire matrix without full nail avulsion, this technique is ideal. The proximal nail fold is reflected as described

(a)

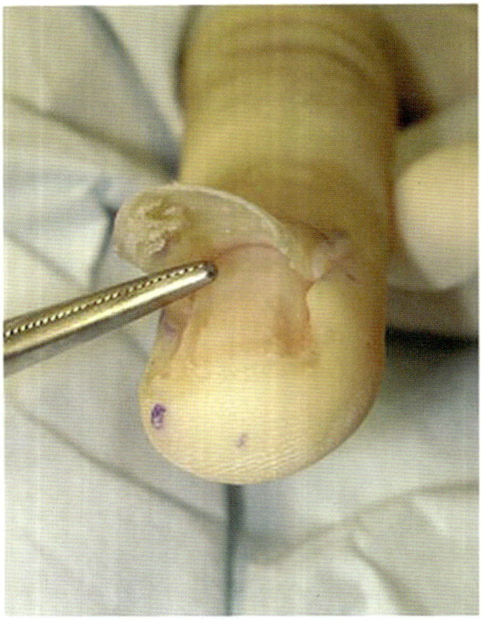

(b)

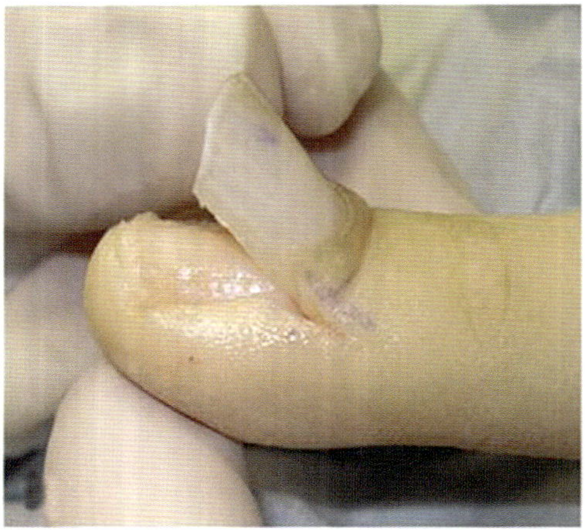

Figure 13.3 (a) End on view of trap door partial nail avulsion. (b) Lateral view of trap door partial nail avulsion [12].

above. An English anvil-action nail splitter is then placed in the lateral sulcus underneath the nail plate. A horizontal cut is then made. This can go across one quadrant, or the entire width of the nail. A hemostat is then attached laterally and then "rolled" over the bed, allowing excellent visualization of the matrix as well as the proximal nail bed. If needed for histopathological evaluation, this piece of plate can be removed completely [12].

13.5.1.10 Replacement of Nail After Avulsion

Unless there is concern for infection, malignancy, or the nail is dystrophic, replacement of the nail plate after avulsion is preferable. The plate can be secured using either 5-0 polypropylene or 5-0 fast-absorbing 910 polyglactin suture, taking care to suture the skin side first and then through the nail plate to avoid the possibility of a foreign body reaction secondary to nail plate being embedded in the skin. Alternatively, Steri-Strips and Mastisol (Ferndale Laboratories Inc., Ferndale, Michigan) can be used to secure the plate. The patient/parent should be advised that this nail will eventually be shed. Replacement of the nail allows for greater comfort, protects the underlying tissue, and leads to more rapid healing [12].

13.5.2 Punch Biopsy

A punch biopsy of the nail matrix or bed can be done to obtain tissue for histopathologic evaluation of melanonychia striata, for example, in the pediatric population. This can be done with or without nail avulsion. Sometimes it is preferable to submit the nail plate for histopathologic evaluation, in which case a punch biopsy directly through nail plate to matrix or bed is performed. Otherwise, once a full or partial nail avulsion is done, adequate visualization of the area in question must be ascertained. In order to visualize the matrix, reflecting incisions at the junction of the proximal and lateral nail folds are often required bilaterally. These incisions run from the lateral proximal nail fold more proximolaterally on a diagonal. The proximal nail fold is then gently loosened with a 15 blade scalpel or iris scissors and then a skin hook can be used to reflect the proximal nail fold and visualize the matrix. A 3 mm punch trephine is recommended to be used for a punch biopsy of the matrix or bed, see Figure 13.4 [5]. Closure

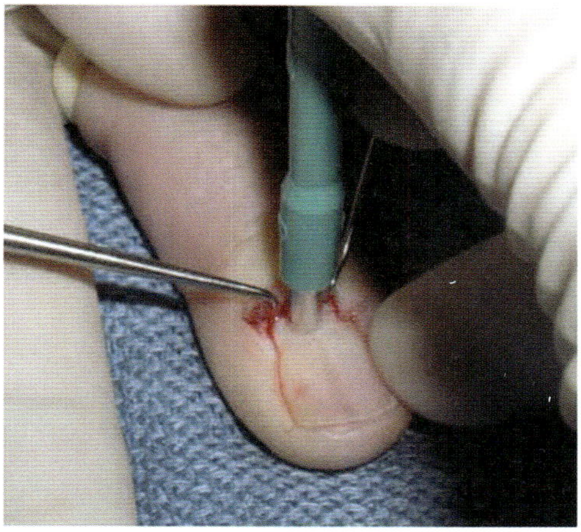

Figure 13.4 Punch biopsy of the distal matrix [5].

of this small defect is usually not required, especially when the site is more distal. If reflecting incisions were placed, then the skin flaps should be returned to anatomic position and each side sutured using either 5-0 polypropylene or 5-0 fast absorbing 910 polyglactin suture. Absorbable suture is usually preferable as the patient does not need to return for suture removal. A larger size of trephine runs the risk of causing permanent dystrophy, especially if taken from the proximal matrix without careful approximation of the edges. If the lesion is larger than 3 mm, a different biopsy technique should be used [14].

13.5.3 Matrix Shave

For lesions larger than 3 mm, the matrix shave is often a good option, as the nail matrix can be very superficially excised using the nail matrix shave technique as described by Haneke [15]. The matrix is scored using a Teflon-coated 15 blade scalpel and then the specimen is cut at the base using the scalpel in a parallel fashion to the specimen, while gentle pressure is applied with a cotton-tipped applicator. The specimen is then oriented either directly on a nail diagram and/or inked and placed in a pathology cassette so that the orientation is preserved, see Figure 13.5. A matrix shave does not require suture placement. The specimen

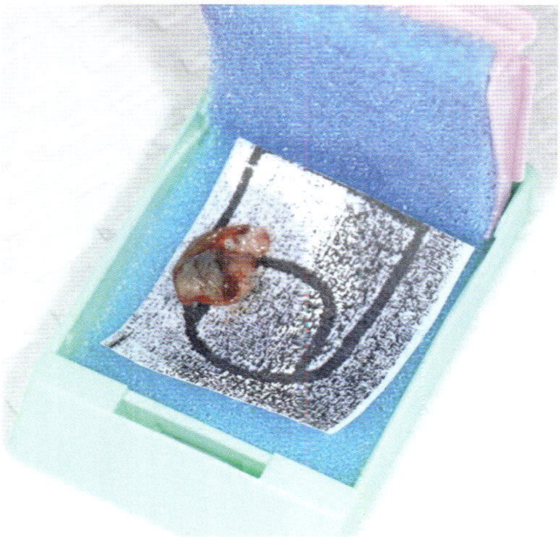

Figure 13.5 Placement of specimen in pathology cassette.

is so superficial that there is not usually resultant dystrophy, particularly if the location is in the distal matrix [16].

13.5.4 Nail Excisions

It is often preferable to perform the definitive procedure during the first nail procedure, if possible. For some longitudinal melanonychias, erythronychias or nail bed tumors that are centrally located in the nail unit, this can be accomplished via elliptical excision, with subsequent repair of the matrix and second intention healing of the bed or raising of flaps laterally.

13.5.4.1 Lateral Longitudinal Excision

For lateral melanonychia, erythronychia, or a laterally based tumor, a lateral longitudinal excision may be performed. The planned excision should be marked using a surgical marking pen, taking care to extend the excision proximally and laterally so that all components of the nail unit including the matrical horns, are included in the excision. A Teflon-coated 15 blade scalpel is then used to score along the marked lines, including directly through the nail plate. Care should be taken not to inadvertently cut through the digit and injure the surgeon. Soaking the digit prior to

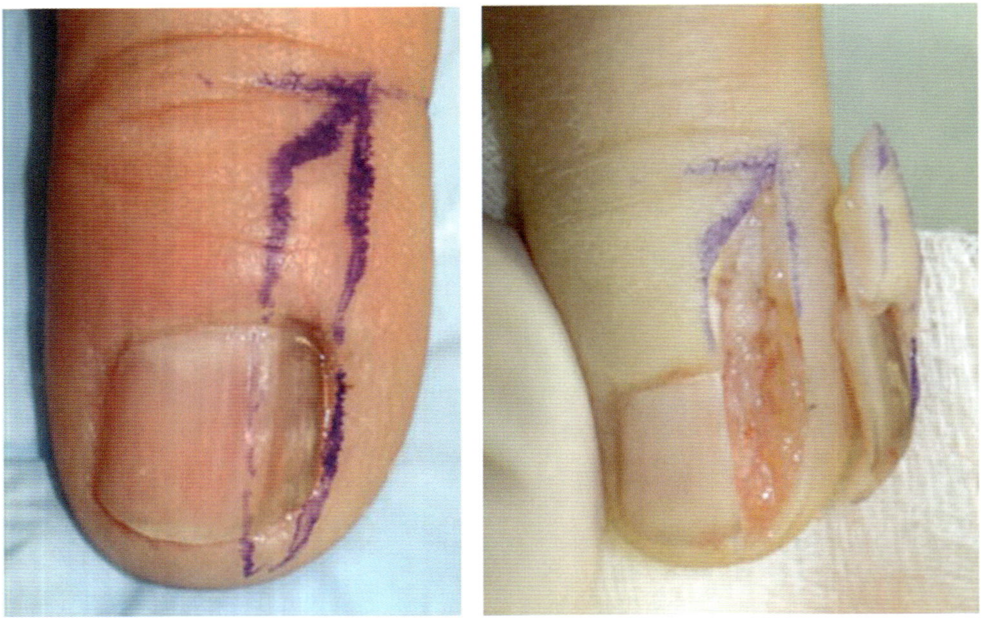

Figure 13.6 (a) Surgical marking for the planned lateral longitudinal excision. (b) Completed lateral longitudinal excision [17].

surgery in either warm water or a chlorhexidine soak often aids in the cutting of the plate. Alternatively an English anvil-action nail splitter can be used to cut the nail longitudinally without avulsing it from the bed. A 15 blade scalpel can then be used to complete the excision, see Figure 13.6 [17]. The entire specimen is then cut using scissors in the deep plane at the periosteum. The defect is repaired by first suturing the hyponychium and proximal nail fold. Undermining may be required laterally, especially in large thumbnail or great toenail excisions. The lateral nail fold is then sutured skin to nail. Rapidly absorbing polyglactin 910 suture can be used. Sometimes too much tension is present and the lateral portion is allowed to heal by second intention [17].

13.6 Post-Operative Management

Once the nail procedure is complete, the tourniquet is released and the time noted for "tourniquet time". Blood flow should be immediate. Depending on the extent of the procedure, and whether or not epinephrine was used, this may be a significant amount or not. Electrocautery is to be avoided if possible, as destruction of the nail matrix can cause nail dystrophy [18]. Even with active bleeding, the digit can usually be bandaged. This is in contrast to cutaneous excisional surgery. If the bleeding seems excessive, pressure can be held for 10 minutes before bandaging and then a piece of Gelfoam (Pharmacia and Upjohn Company, Kalamazoo, Michigan) can be placed over the site and then bandaging can proceed. Pressure should be held by compressing the DIP joint laterally on both sides, so that the digital arteries are occluded.

For procedures of the nail unit, many different bandaging methods exist. One method includes application of a small piece of petrolatum gauze or bismuth tribromophenate-impregnated gauze (Xeroform, Covidien LP, Mansfield, Massachusetts), followed by regular gauze, and then tape. Another technique includes application of plain petrolatum then a non-stick pad such as Telfa (Covidien LP, Mansfield, Massachusetts), then regular gauze, and then tape. Tape application often requires an adhesive such as Mastisol and should only be done in a longitudinal fashion to prevent post-operative ischemia of the digit [4, 5]. Since the patient is either under general anesthesia or cannot sense how much pressure is being applied due to a digital block, circumferential bandaging is not advisable. Tubular gauze or stockinette can provide a snug cohesive final layer, see Figure 13.7. The patient is then monitored for approximately 15–20 minutes to ensure there is no bleeding through the bandage. For general anesthesia patients, they are rechecked in recovery prior to discharge. If there is excessive bleeding through the bandage at this point, a new bandage should be reapplied. If there is just a small area of bleeding, that part of the bandage can be reinforced with further gauze. Finger or toe splints can also be used and in certain situations are more useful a few days after the procedure to help protect the digit from unintended trauma. An orthopedic shoe can be used if needed for toenail procedures.

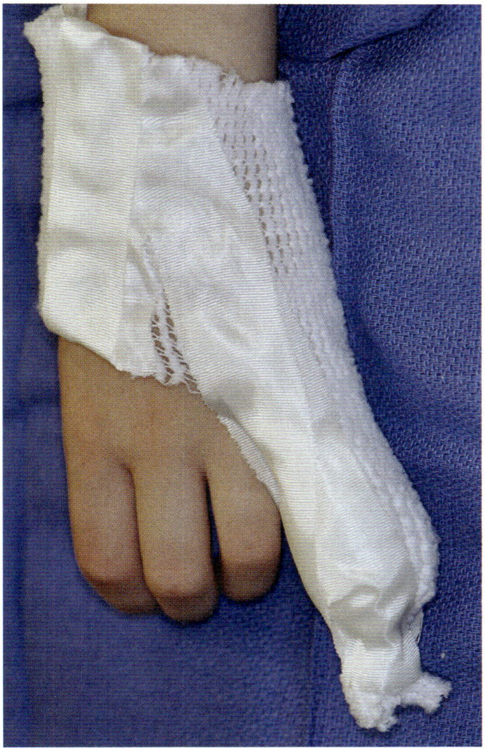

Figure 13.7 Bandaging after nail procedure, 5th fingernail.

13.7 Home Care

Patients should keep their hand or foot elevated on the way home. For those older adolescents who may be able to drive, it is important that someone else drive them home. Sometimes there is already bleeding through the bandage on the day of the procedure, in which case the patient should either reinforce that portion of the bandage if possible or reapply the entire bandage.

Post-operative pain management is very important. Nail procedures can be very painful post-operatively as the blocks wear off. Acetaminophen should be given on arrival at home. Narcotic pain medications such as acetaminophen with codeine may be required for one to three days, as there can be significant throbbing for the first 36 hours post-operatively. Alternating these two agents often works well. For one to three weeks post-operatively there can be dull pain at the surgical site.

Daily wound care is required, usually starting 48 hours after the nail procedure. Soaking the bandage off in a bath or bowl of warm water facilitates the process. Epsom salts or regular table salt can be added to the water if desired. The finger or toe should be gently dried and Vaseline applied to the nail unit. The entire nail unit should then be bandaged. At this point, the patient can bandage circumferentially as they have full sensation and can tell if the bandage is too tight and potentially causing ischemia. Bandaging daily is done for a number of reasons: to prevent infection; collect drainage; and to provide protection from inadvertent trauma and subsequent pain. More padding will be required the first week as there usually is more drainage, which diminishes with time. Often, bandaging is necessary for three to four weeks, due to drainage, especially of the great toe. A splint or orthopedic shoe for toenail procedures can be used.

13.8 Potential Complications

Despite the surgeon's planning and meticulous attention to detail, complications can still occur in nail surgery.

Bleeding is to be expected after the tourniquet is released and is unlikely to be excessive, except in the case of a patient on multiple anticoagulants or an underlying coagulation defect. In those instances, having a frank discussion with the patient and/or parent prior to the procedure regarding expectations and measures that will be taken is necessary. Usually all anticoagulants are continued as they are important for the patient's underlying condition (mechanical valve, etc.) and therefore health. For von Willebrand's disease, desmopressin (DDAVP) can be given intranasally 60 minutes prior to surgery.

Ischemia of the distal digit is a very serious complication that at its most severe leads to gangrene and possible amputation, and more commonly can cause digital parasthesias [19]. Meticulous attention to the volume of anesthetic used (as outlined above), as well as using the absolute minimum of tourniquet time, in addition to bandaging in a longitudinal fashion, will all reduce the risk to as low as possible. Removal of the tourniquet only by the operating surgeon will help to avoid inadvertently leaving it in place, which can lead to infarction [20].

Pain should not be present during the procedure if an adequate digital and wing block was placed. If an awake patient is still feeling pain, then the procedure must cease until adequate analgesia is obtained. Post-operatively, pain should be managed as outlined above. If pain is not under good control and continues to be significant, the patient should be re-evaluated to assess for causes of pain, including a subungual hematoma that is under increased pressure.

Infection can usually be avoided with careful attention to anti-sepsis. The hand or foot can be soaked in chlorhexidine wash for 10 minutes prior to the procedure [21]. As outlined above, the entire hand or foot is scrubbed and draped prior to the procedure and all procedures are done under sterile conditions. The importance of keeping the digit bandaged after the procedure while the nail unit heals cannot be over-emphasized. Despite this, some patients will develop a soft tissue infection requiring oral antibiotics. Erythema signifying inflammation should not be confused with an infection, as inflammation is very common after nail surgery and is treated with cold soaks and topical steroids. Additionally, drainage from the wound is very common after nail surgery and is often sero-sanguinous for the first few days and then becomes clear or yellow serous drainage. Purulent drainage always signifies infection and should be treated with oral antibiotics. Septic arthritis or osteomyelitis can develop if the joint space is violated, as frequently the periosteum is reached during nail bed procedures [2].

Either the flexor or extensor tendons can be injured if the procedure extends beyond the nail unit. The only case in which tendon injury is unavoidable is in the case of a malignant tumor. If extensive involvement of a tumor is known prior to surgery and possible injury to the tendon is expected, this should be discussed with the patient and/or parent and coordinated with an orthopedic surgeon as needed.

After a nail procedure, the nail may regrow with dystrophy. This is usually predictable, as injury to the proximal matrix is most likely to lead to permanent nail dystrophy. In the worst case scenario, when the matrix was fully ablated, a full split nail will occur. Sometimes this is unavoidable. Superficial and distal matrix procedures usually heal quite well with minimal dystrophy. Nail bed procedures often heal well, with non-adherence to the nail plate being one possible result if a very large area of nail bed was removed. Spicules can form if the lateral matrical horns were not adequately ablated or removed during surgery.

13.9 Conclusion

Nail procedures are frequently required to diagnose and treat nail disorders. These surgeries are successful as long as careful preparation, execution and subsequent post-operative care are employed.

References

1 Baran, R. and Dawber, R.P.R. (2012). *Baran & Dawber's Diseases of the Nails and their Management*, 4e. Chichester: Wiley.
2 Fleckman, P. and Allan, C. (2001). Surgical anatomy of the nail unit. *Dermatol. Surg.* 27 (3): 257–260.
3 Haneke, E. and Baran, R. (1992). Nail surgery. *Clin. Dermatol.* 10 (3): 327–333.
4 MacFarlane, D.F. and Scher, R.K. (2007). The nail. In: *Roenigk's Dermatologic Surgery: Current Techniques in Procedural Dermatology*, 3e (ed. R.K. Roenigk and H.H. Roenigk). New York: Informa Healthcare.
5 Jellinek, N.J. (2007). Nail surgery: practical tips and treatment options. *Dermatol. Ther.* 20 (1): 68–74.
6 Saijo, M., Ito, E., Ichinohe, T., and Kaneko, Y. (2005). Lack of pain reduction by a vibrating local anesthetic attachment: a pilot study. *Anesth. Prog.* 52 (2): 62–64.
7 McGinness, J.L. and Parlette, H.L. 3rd. (2005). Versatile sterile field for nail surgery using a sterile glove. *Dermatol. Online J.* 11 (3): 10.
8 Harrington, A.C., Cheyney, J.M., Kinsley-Scott, T. et al. (2004). A novel digital tourniquet using a sterile glove and hemostat. *Dermatol. Surg.* 30 (7): 1065–1067.
9 Lahham, S., Tu, K., Ni, M. et al. (2011). Comparison of pressures applied by digital tourniquets in the emergency department. *West J Emerg Med* 12 (2): 242–249.
10 Becerro de Bengoa Vallejo, R., Losa Iglesias, M.E., Lopez, D.L. et al. (2013). Effects of digital tourniquet ischemia: a single center study. *Dermatol. Surg.* 39 (4): 584–592.
11 South, D.A. and Farber, E.M. (1980). Urea ointment in the nonsurgical avulsion of nail dystrophies – a reappraisal. *Cutis* 25 (6): 609–612.
12 Collins, S.C., Cordova, K., and Jellinek, N.J. (2008). Alternatives to complete nail plate avulsion. *J. Am. Acad. Dermatol.* 59 (4): 619–626.
13 Abimelec, P. (2009). Tips and tricks in nail surgery. *Semin. Cutan. Med. Surg.* 28 (1): 55–60.
14 Jellinek, N. (2007). Nail matrix biopsy of longitudinal melanonychia: diagnostic algorithm including the matrix shave biopsy. *J. Am. Acad. Dermatol.* 56 (5): 803–810.
15 Haneke, E. and Baran, R. (2001). Longitudinal melanonychia. *Dermatol. Surg.* 27 (6): 580–584.
16 Richert, B., Theunis, A., Norrenberg, S. et al. (2013). Tangential excision of pigmented nail matrix lesions responsible for longitudinal melanonychia: evaluation of the technique on a series of 30 patients. *J. Am. Acad. Dermatol.* 69 (1): 96–104.
17 Jellinek, N.J. and Rubin, A.I. (2011). Lateral longitudinal excision of the nail unit. *Dermatol. Surg.* 37 (12): 1781–1785.
18 Haricharan, R.N., Masquijo, J., and Bettolli, M. (2013). Nail-fold excision for the treatment of ingrown toenail in children. *J. Pediatr.* 162 (2): 398–402.
19 Pedowitz, R.A. (1991). Tourniquet-induced neuromuscular injury. A recent review of rabbit and clinical experiments. *Acta Orthop. Scand. Suppl.* 245: 1–33.
20 Jellinek, N.J. (2013). Commentary: how much is too much? Tourniquets and digital ischemia. *Dermatol. Surg.* 39 (4): 593–595.
21 Bibbo, C., Patel, D.V. Gehrmann, R.M. et al. (2005). Chlorhexidine provides superior skin decontamination in foot and ankle surgery: a prospective randomized study. *Clin. Orthop. Relat. Res.* 438: 204–208.

14

Complications of Surgery and Invasive Procedures

Yoon Cohen[1] and Harper N. Price[2,3]

[1] Alta Dermatology, Phoenix, AZ, USA
[2] Phoenix Children's Hospital, Phoenix, AZ, USA
[3] Department of Child Health, University of Arizona College of Medicine, Phoenix, AZ, USA

14.1 Postoperative Pain

Postoperative pain assessment and management in children are a vital component of postoperative care. A key to managing postoperative pain is anticipation. The approach to postoperative pain varies according to the anticipated intensity and duration of expected pain, the context and meaning as seen by the child and family, the coping style and temperament of the child, the type of procedure, the child's history of pain, and the family support system [1]. Inadequate pain control has significant negative implications for children, including long-term consequences regarding their reactions to later painful events and acceptance of subsequent health care interventions [2]. Therefore, an approach to children that makes them as comfortable as possible and minimizes pain is crucial [2].

Pain assessment in children can be extremely challenging. Pain is a subjective experience. An accurate pain assessment is the most important and critical component of pain management. Currently, the gold standard of pain assessment is the child's self-report with aid of parent's own assessment of their child's discomfort. Cognitive and emotional developments, together with psychological defense mechanisms are important variables to be considered with pediatric pain [3]. Unfortunately, the self-report method cannot be utilized with infants and young children, as they have not yet developed sufficient cognitive and communicative abilities. In children with cognitive or physical impairments, self-report is not always an option either. Therefore, observational assessment in the form of behavioral or biological methods can be as equally important as the self-report pain evaluation. A widely adopted assessment of pain is the "Q.U.E.ST." assessment that can be easily learned and applied in a clinic setting by physicians and their support staff [4]. Q.U.E.S.T. for pain assessment consists of the following components:

Q: Question the child
U: Use pain rating scales
E: Evaluate child's behavior
S: Secure parent's involvement
T: Take action

The child's response to either the faces pain scale or numeric pain rating scale is commonly used in practice. Children ages three to seven years can use standardized visual (pictorial) scales. The Wong-Baker-FACES® has been endorsed and widely utilized by

Pediatric Dermatologic Surgery, First Edition. Edited by Keyvan Nouri, Latanya Benjamin, Jasem Alshaiji, and Jan Izakovic.

accreditation organizations and large health care institutions [4, 5]. Children eight years and older can use a 0–10 numeric scale [6]. It is important to explain to the child and the parents the detailed aspects of the scales before using them. Children do not always understand the words "pain" or "discomfort". Thus in appropriate cases it is more effective to use a variety of words such as "owie", "ouchy", "boo-boo" or "hurt" when a child may not understand the concept of pain [3]. There are also a variety of pain scales that are designed for assessment of a combination of physiological and behavioral changes in infants. A few examples include CRIES (crying; change in transcutaneous oxygen saturation, heart rate, blood pressure, facial expression and alteration in sleep pattern); Pain Assessment Tool (PAT); Premature Infant Pain Profile (PIPP); Scale for Use in Newborns (SUN) [7]. CRIES is one of most commonly used as a neonatal PAT [8]. It is a 10-point scale similar to the APGAR score (Appearance, Pulse, Grimace, Activity, Respiration) that can be easily adopted.

The involvement of parents should be encouraged to achieve an accurate pain assessment, as parents are most familiar with their child's behavior. Once the pain is assessed, the earliest action to relieve the pain should be followed as soon as possible to prevent prolonged suffering from pain and to avoid long-term consequences of reactions to later painful events. Likewise, the management of pain should be addressed immediately once postoperative pain is identified. There are many different modalities to treat pediatric pain, however, it is crucial to evaluate the relative risks and benefits of various treatments.

14.1.1 Non-Pharmacologic Pain Management

Nonpharmacologic approaches for the treatment of pain in children include psychological strategies, education, and parental support [9]. Simple distraction techniques that divert attention away from painful stimuli, praising the child no matter how poorly the procedure went, or positive incentive techniques that provide a small reward (e.g. stickers or gifts) for attempts at mastery of their responses, can be effective for children undergoing occasional procedures. For children undergoing repeated painful procedures, cognitive-behavioral therapy can decrease anxiety and distress. These techniques are designed to decrease anxiety, but are not adequate as the sole means of pain relief for most painful procedures [9].

14.1.2 Pharmacologic Pain Management, Non-opioid Analgesics

Most dermatologic procedures in pediatric patients usually do not require opioid analgesics because of their relatively less invasive nature. Therefore, non-opioid analgesics such as acetaminophen and non-steroidal anti-inflammatory drugs (NSAIDs) have become popular choices and many times first line for treating postoperative pain in children. NSAIDs inhibit cyclooxygenase (COX) enzymes and reduce inflammation in the peripheral tissues, while the mechanism for acetaminophen is less well understood but likely involves multiple pain pathways [10]. Appropriate *weight-based dosing* for pain medications should be provided to caretakers to avoid under-treatment of pain or potential overdose (Table 14.1). Non-opioid analgesics are effective, with few side effects, and produce an opioid-sparing action through decreasing the inflammatory mediators generated at the site of tissue injury. NSAIDs may cause gastrointestinal upset, and uncommonly gastrointestinal bleeding, renal dysfunction, and hypersensitivity reactions. Administration with food and avoidance in patients with dehydration and history of hypersensitivity reactions should be emphasized. NSAIDs should be used with caution in patients with liver dysfunction, renal dysfunction, coagulopathies, thrombocytopenia and active bleeding [12]. Excessive doses of acetaminophen may cause hepatic failure that can be fatal. Children with the

Table 14.1 Commonly used non-opioid analgesics and their dosages [11]. Further dose adjustments must be made for patients with renal and hepatic impairment.

Drug	Age	Dosing	Frequency	Max Daily Dose
Acetaminophen	Term neonate <10 days	10–15 mg/kg/dose	Every 6 hours	60 mg/kg/day
Acetaminophen	Term neonate >10 days	10–15 mg/kg/dose	Every 4–6 hours	≤75 mg/kg/day; do not exceed 5 doses in 24 hours
Acetaminophen	Infants, children & adolescence	10–15 mg/kg/dose	Every 4–6 hours	≤75 mg/kg/day; do not exceed 5 doses in 24 hours; do not exceed 4000 mg/day
Ibuprofen	Infants and children 6 months to 12 years[a]	4–10 mg/kg/dose	Every 6–8 hours	40 mg/kg/day Max single dose: 400 mg
	Children and adolescence ≥12 years	200 mg/dose, may increase to 400 mg/dose if no response	Every 4–6 hours	1200 mg/day
Naproxen	Children >2 years	5–7 mg/kg/dose	Every 12 hours	
	Children >12 years	200 mg/dose	Every 8–12 hours	600 mg/day

[a] Limited data available in infants <6 months.

following conditions may be more at risk for developing acetaminophen toxicity: diabetes, concomitant viral infections, family history of hepatotoxic reactions, obesity, and chronic malnourishment [13].

Non-opioid analgesics are suitable for treatment of mild to moderate pain or as adjuncts to opioid analgesics. Scheduled administration of non-opioid analgesics in the post-operative period may help to further limit the need for narcotic usage [14]. Combined use of acetaminophen and NSAIDs has shown benefits (lower pain scores, fewer side-effects, and improved patient satisfaction) in the treatment of post-operative surgical pain in adults and children post-tonsillectomy [15, 16]. The authors commonly recommend combination therapy with both acetaminophen and ibuprofen in the post-operative period and send instructions on administration and dosing home with the patient.

Acetaminophen is one of the most commonly used non-opioid analgesics in the pediatric patient. It is available over the counter as an oral suspension and chewable tablets for children who cannot swallow tablets or capsules (Table 14.2). The oral formulation is manufactured as a 160 mg/5 ml suspension, and chewable tablets are supplied as 80 mg/tablet and 160 mg/tablet. Maximum daily dose varies based on age and weight, and due to the narrow therapeutic index of acetaminophen, overdose can easily occur which can lead to acute liver failure or even death. Dosage should be based on ideal body weight in obese and overweight children (Table 14.1). Ibuprofen is a commonly used over-the-counter NSAID and comes in concentrated drops, chewable tablets, oral suspension, tablets and caplets (Table 14.2). *For both acetaminophen and NSAIDs, weight-based dosing is always preferred.* Providing caretakers with the appropriate dose as well as frequency, duration of therapy, and specific strength and formulation of over-the-counter non-opioid analgesics for their child during the post-operative period is essential.

Table 14.2 Common formulations of acetaminophen and NSAIDs available over the counter [11].

Drug	Formulation	Concentration
Acetaminophen	Liquid	160 mg/5 ml 500 mg/5 ml 500 mg/15 ml 80/0.8 ml (drops)
	Chewable tablet ODT	80 mg 80 mg, 160 mg
	Caplet/tablet/capsule	325 mg, 500 mg
Ibuprofen	Concentrated oral drops for infants and children	50 mg/1.25 ml
	Liquid	100 mg/5 ml 40 mg/ml 50 mg/1.25 ml
	Chewable tablets	50 mg, 100 mg
	(Junior strength) Caplet and tablet	100 mg
	Capsule/Tablet	200 mg
Naproxen	Liquid	125 mg/5 ml
	Capsule Tablet	220 mg 220 mg, 250 mg, 375 mg, 500 mg, 550 mg

14.1.3 Pharmacologic Pain Management, Opioid Analgesics

Pediatric patients seldom need opioid analgesics for post-operative pain following dermatologic surgery. Patients undergoing nail procedures or excisions requiring extensive undermining or tissue rearrangement may require short-term usage of opioid analgesics in combination with non-opioid analgesics or as needed for breakthrough pain. However, when opioid medications are used for pain relief, their efficacy, safety, side effects, cost and the course of recovery should be thoroughly assessed before administering [3]. The World Health Organization (WHO) recommends opioid medications in combination with non-opioid analgesics for treatment of moderate to severe pain in the post-surgical period [17, 18]. Opioid pain medications used in the post-operative period in the pediatric population can be found in Table 14.3, but prescribers should be aware of important drug–drug interactions and differences in metabolism of these drugs in this population and counsel patients and families appropriately when prescribed.

There are several factors to consider when prescribing an opioid analgesic for pain relief in the pediatric population, especially in young children. Common opioid medication options available include codeine, hydrocodone and oxycodone. The Food and Drug Administration (FDA) black box warning for codeine use following outpatient tonsillectomy and adenoidectomy was issued in May 2013 following several deaths in this population [19]. Variability in rates of metabolism of codeine may result in little to no analgesic effect or the risk of severe respiratory depression. For non-metabolizers, no analgesic effect will occur, but with ultra-rapid metabolizers, codeine is rapidly converted to morphine, leading to high drug levels that could ultimately result in respiratory depression and death. Thus the use of codeine and hydrocodone (also a prodrug that uses CYP2D6 enzyme to produce its active form) should be done with extreme caution. Because of the black box warning, many

Table 14.3 Oral dosing of opioid analgesics in infants ≥6 months, children and adolescents [11]. All dosing should be titrated to lowest possible dose to provide appropriate analgesic effects. Dosing should be adjusted for patients with hepatic and renal impairment.

Drug	Dose	Frequency
Codeine[a,b]	0.5–1.0 mg/kg/dose	Every 4–6 hours
Hydrocodone[c]	<50 kg: 0.1–0.2 mg/kg/dose ≥50 kg: 5–10 mg/dose	Every 4–6 hours
Hydromorphone[b] (Immediate release)	Infants >10 kg (> 6 months of age): 0.03 mg/kg/dose, range 0.03–0.06 mg/kg/dose	Every 3–4 hours
	Children and adolescents <50 kg: 0.03–0.08 mg/kg/dose	Every 3–4 hours
	Children and adolescents ≥50 kg: 1–2 mg/dose	Every 3–4 hours
Oxycodone[a] (Immediate release)	Infants >6 months, children and adolescents <50 kg: 0.1–0.2 mg/kg/dose	Every 4–6 hours
	Children and adolescents ≥50 kg: 5–10 mg/dose	Every 4–6 hours

[a] Available as individual drugs and in combination with acetaminophen. When combined with acetaminophen, refer to Table 14.2 for maximum daily dosing of acetaminophen.
[b] Limited data available in children.
[c] Limited data available in infants and children <2 years.

children's hospitals have removed codeine from their formulary. Oxycodone is an active drug and does not require biotransformation to produce an effect, but slow metabolizers may experience increased side effects. The use of oxycodone and certain other drugs, specifically macrolide antibiotics, antifungal agents, and antiviral agents, has also caused the FDA to issue a black box warning due to risk of enhanced opioid side effects when co-administered [10]. Also, codeine and oxycodone are available in combination with acetaminophen and caution should be taken to limit risk of potential acetaminophen overdose as a side effect of therapeutic opioid dosing.

Addressing the side effects of opioid use, such as nausea, vomiting, constipation, sedation, respiratory depression, urinary retention and pruritus, is important to minimize distress and unwanted or dangerous complications [1]. Opioid analgesics should be used as needed for breakthrough for moderate to severe pain and given on an as-needed basis along with regularly schedule non-opioid analgesics when indicated.

14.1.4 Other Techniques for Pain and Anxiety Relief

There are a variety of techniques that can improve postoperative pain. Preoperatively, it is important to make sure that the child is in a comfortable position with parental presence nearby when procedures are done with local anesthesia. Topical anesthetics can be applied pre-procedure such as EMLA® cream (AstraZeneca, London, United Kingdom) and LMX® (Ferndale Laboratories, Ferndale, Michigan) to limit pain from injection of local anesthetics or prior to other less invasive procedures. Physical tapping or vibration analgesia as well as teachable breathing techniques can be helpful to distract the patient from the injection or painful stimuli [20]. Oral sucrose solution (Sweet-Ease®, Philips, Amsterdam, Netherlands) has traditionally been used for reducing pain in neonates. When procedures are done in an operating room setting with general anesthesia, the presence of a parent during the induction process can also be helpful and reassuring to the child when possible. Preoperative administration of oral midazolam can be useful for pre-operative anxiety and may be needed for repetitive procedures such as laser treatment of port-wine stains as the child ages. Post-operative pain prevention techniques include icing, strict limitations on activity, and elevation of the affected site, appropriate wound dressing and regularly scheduled analgesics.

14.2 Postoperative Bleeding and Hematoma

Postoperative bleeding and hematoma are early postoperative complications that occur uncommonly in pediatric dermatologic surgery. Any history of significant bleeding during low-risk surgical procedures should be elicited and noted during the preoperative evaluation. Previous history of excessive or prolonged bleeding during or after surgery can indicate congenital coagulopathies including von Willebrand disease and hemophilia in pediatric patients. Although anticoagulant use is a common cause of postoperative bleeding in adults, this group of medications is not commonly administered in children and it is thus rarely a cause of postoperative bleeding and hematoma in children. It is still advisable to review dietary supplements in the form of herbal medicines, vitamins, and non-prescription medications as they can interfere with coagulation. Although aspirin can increase the risk of postoperative bleeding, there appears to be no significant increased risk of bleeding with NSAIDs [21]. Therefore, obtaining a thorough preoperative history of the child for bleeding risk is an important first step.

During the surgical procedure, careful control of bleeding is crucial to minimizing bleeding complications postoperatively. In children, the most common location of the postoperative bleeding and hematoma is the scalp [22]; therefore, ensuring adequate hemostasis before completing wound closure is imperative. Acute bleeding may also occur with post-operative trauma or with rebound vasodilatation after the effect of epinephrine dissipates in the perioperative period [23]. The risk of postoperative bleeding is greatest within the first 48 hours following the procedure, and especially in the first several hours. Mild drainage from a wound can be normal; however, if the wound dressing is soaked with blood, it requires immediate attention.

Timely management must follow once postoperative bleeding is properly identified. Direct pressure, cold packs, elevation, and rest are an important first step. Cold packs are useful to stimulate vasoconstriction and reduce edema, and elevation and rest will reduce dependent blood flow and risk of further bleeding [23]. For active bleeding, parents should be advised to apply direct and firm pressure for 15–20 minutes over the dressing and then re-evaluate. It is important not to constantly lift up the dressing while applying the pressure during this time. If the patient's wound dressing appears saturated with blood, it should be removed and a clean dressing applied, followed by another 15 minutes of compression. This will allow for better absorption and compression of the tissues. If the bleeding continues despite these measures, the patient should be referred for urgent evaluation in the office or urgent care/emergency room setting. The actively bleeding area may need exploration of the wound, to achieve hemostasis with suture ligation or electrocoagulation.

Postoperative hematoma in pediatric patients is not common, but when it occurs it is often caused by trauma from vigorous physical activity or insufficient closure of dead space. Hematomas are most likely to occur within the first 24–72 hours postoperatively and can present with an increased pressure sensation, throbbing pain, ecchymosis, and fluctuation of the tissues [24, 25]. Hematomas can be easily evaluated and diagnosed clinically as an expansible fluctuant mass under a recent surgical site. They become increasingly gelatinous and firm over time, with the formation of clots. Hematomas evolve through four stages [23]. In the first stage (early development, within hours) the wound appears swollen and warm due to active hemorrhage and blood accumulation. During the second stage (gelatinous phase), the wound becomes more fluctuant and develops a purplish hue. Subsequently, the third stage involves organization into a firm rubbery mass within several days. During the final and fourth stage (liquefaction), the organized hematoma begins to liquefy (after 7–10 days).

Management of hematomas depends on the size, stage, associated symptoms and risk to surrounding tissues [23]. If a hematoma is noted early in the development stage, intervention is recommended, which usually consists of partial or complete suture removal to identify areas of bleeding and achieve hemostasis. Re-suturing may be done in non-contaminated wounds after irrigation and re-examination for bleeding. Hematomas in the gelatinous stage that are smaller than a ping-pong ball should be left to reabsorb if viable tissues are not at risk [22]. In the case of larger size, symptoms, or injury to viable tissues at this stage, it is important to evacuate the hematoma with replacement of a pressure dressing to prevent reformation. During the organization stage of a hematoma, deferring intervention until the fourth stage is often best. Once a hematoma starts to liquefy, total resorption can take weeks to months. Often evacuation may be done via needle aspiration at this stage [26].

Bleeding and hematoma formation in the postoperative period resulting from trauma at the site, due to the tendency of children to attempt to resume their normal activity immediately after surgery. Postoperative methods to minimize the risk of bleeding and hematoma should include giving the caregiver and patient (when applicable) both written and verbal postoperative wound care instructions at the end of the procedure. A pressure dressing should be applied and left in place for a minimum of 48 hours, especially for wounds on the scalp and extremities where physical activity and trauma are more likely. An adequate compressive dressing should immobilize the wound, prevent trauma and provide additional hemostasis. Bulky and exaggerated wound dressings also serve as a reminder to both the patient and the parent that the child had a recent procedure and needs to limit physical activities [27] (Figure 14.1). Strict limitations on physical activity should be discussed and written down for patients and their families. It is advisable to avoid any excessive physical activities (such as gym class, recess, recreational swimming and contact sports) for at least the first two to three weeks of the post-operative period.

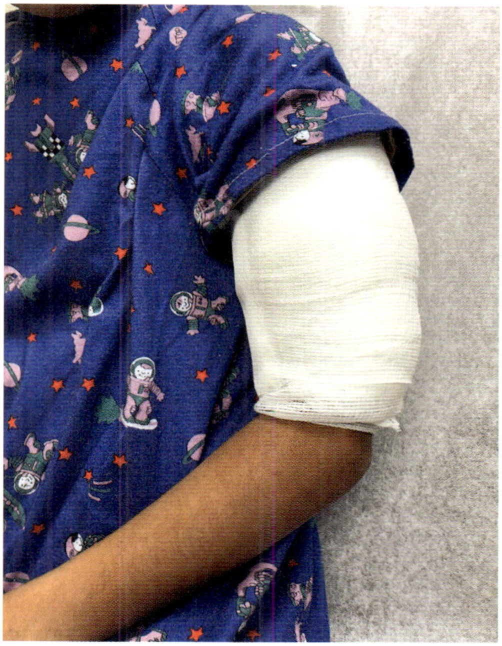

Figure 14.1 Large and bulky dressings are useful as a reminder of the recent surgery, to limit activity and serve as padding for potential future trauma.

14.3 Postoperative Seroma

An accumulation of serous fluid can occur after surgery due to excessive leakage from blood vessels and lymphatics into large spaces generated during surgery due to extensive dissection. The incidence of seroma in pediatric dermatologic surgery is not known but is likely quite uncommon. Seromas have been described as a surgical complication after excision of lymphatic malformations, neck surgery and lymph node biopsies and dissections. In a series of 193 pediatric surgery patients with lymphangiomas, the incidence of seromas was 3.5% of all resections [28].

Clinical evaluation of the post-operative wound may reveal swelling, redness and warmth at the surgical site, leakage of clear fluid from the incision, and tenderness. Small seromas will often self-resolve and some may calcify if left untreated. Larger seromas may require drainage via needle aspiration. Infection of a seroma can occur and may require antibiotic therapy. Post-operative immobilization, adequate compression dressings, and drain placement may help prevent the development of a seroma in those higher risk procedures.

14.4 Postoperative Infections

Postoperative wound infection is a relatively uncommon complication of cutaneous surgery that usually presents between postoperative days four and 10. The Center for Disease Control (CDC) defines a surgical wound infection as the development within 30 days of a surgical procedure of any one or more of the following: purulent drainage; isolation of organisms obtained aseptically from fluid or tissue near the surgical site; development of signs or symptoms (pain or tenderness, heat, localized redness, swelling) of infection unless the site is culture-negative; superficial incision deliberately opened by surgeon, unless culture is negative; diagnosis of superficial incisional skin or soft tissue infection by surgeon or attending physician [29]. Most bacterial infections are thought to result from the presence of bacteria on the patient's skin or mucosa [30]. Infection may also occur in the post-operative period due to improper wound care. Improper hygiene and soiled and bloodied dressings can serve as a source of bacterial contamination of the healing wound. A classification system of surgical wounds based on the associated risk of infection is well accepted and utilized in the literature (Table 14.4). Most cutaneous surgical procedures result in class I and II wounds which have a low risk of developing infection [31].

Overall, dermatologic surgery in the adult population (including Mohs micrographic surgery) is known to have a low postoperative infection rate, ranging from less than 1% up to 2.29% of cases [33–37]. No significant data exists on infection rates in pediatric dermatologic surgery, but the incidence is thought to be similar to that published in the adult literature [38]. Wound infection rates in pediatric general surgery involving procedures requiring skin incision (e.g. herniorrhaphy, central venous access, gastric tube placement) have ranged from 2.5 to 5.43% but these studies include hospitalized patients, critically ill patients, higher frequencies of contaminated and clean-contaminated wounds and more complicated/emergent procedures [39–42]. In pediatric surgery cases involving skin incisions, some factors found to be significantly associated with a postoperative wound infection were the amount of contamination at operation and the duration of the operation [41].

Known risk factors for postoperative wound infection in the adult population undergoing dermatologic surgery include contaminated and dirty-infected wounds or sites, remote site infections, cigarette smoking, advanced age, poor nutritional status, certain body locations (e.g. the ear, groin, below the knee, acral surfaces) and inadequate aseptic and surgical technique [31]. Risk factors for surgical site infections in the pediatric population are not well defined.

Table 14.4 CDC surgical wound classification system, modified [29, 31, 32].

Classification	Description	Example	Infection risk
Class I – Clean	Operative wound without inflammation or violation of respiratory, alimentary, genital, or urinary tract	Wound created on normal (clean, intact) skin using clean or sterile technique	Very low
Class II – Clean-contaminated	Operative wound with controlled violation of the respiratory, alimentary, genital, or urinary tract without unusual contamination	Wound created on contaminated skin or any mucosal or moist intertriginous region	Low
Class III –Contaminated	Fresh traumatic wounds or operative wounds with either break in sterile technique or gross spillage from alimentary tract	Wound created on visibly inflamed skin with or without purulence	Moderate
Class IV – Dirty-infected	Old traumatic wounds with devitalized tissue or operative wounds involving existing clinical infections	Wound created on dirty and/or infected skin with presence of purulence	High

Care should be taken to review the patient's medical history for conditions that may put the patient at higher risk for overall infection (e.g. immunosuppression, immunodeficiency). Performing a procedure in the groin area when a child is still in diapers puts the patient at great risk of postoperative wound infection [22, 43]. The feet are also a region with a higher risk of wound infection in pediatric patients [22]. Avoidance of preoperative hair removal via shaving is recommended as the resultant small abrasions can compromise skin integrity and allow bacterial growth, increasing the risk of infection.

Common organisms isolated in surgical site infections include gram-positive organisms – *Staphylococcus aureus*, coagulase-negative staphylococci, *Enterococcus* spp. – and gram-negative organisms – *Escherichia coli*, and *Pseudomonas aeruginosa*, *Enterobacter* spp., *Proteus mirabilis* and *Klebsiella pneumonia* [44]. The most common causative organism for superficial skin infections is *S. aureus*. The prevalence of methicillin-resistant *S. aureus* (MRSA) as a source of post-operative wound infections in dermatologic surgery is unknown, but knowledge of local resistance patterns can be helpful. Gram-positive organisms are responsible for most surgical site infections in class I (clean) wounds, except in the groin, where gram-negative organisms predominate [32]. In class II–III wounds gram-positive organisms predominate but gram-negative organisms have an increasing contribution [32].

Recognizing the early symptoms and signs of surgical site infection is important to achieve a good outcome. Postoperative infection usually does not become evident until four to eight days after the procedure. It is imperative to differentiate between a normal healing wound and an actual skin infection as mild redness, wound-site edema, mild tenderness, and serosanguinous discharge can be seen in the first few days of a normal healing wound [31]. In contrast, in an infection, increasing redness and warmth at the surgical site will be seen. The wound site often becomes more painful or tender, and localized swelling, redness or heat can be more obvious as the wound-site infection progresses (Figure 14.2). Spreading redness may

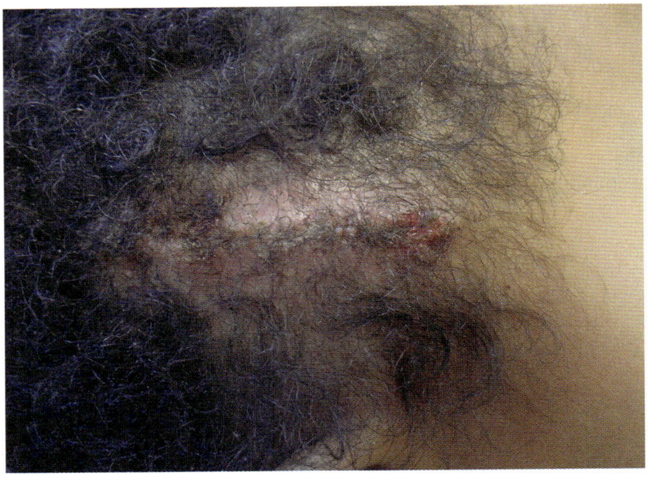

Figure 14.2 *Staphylococcus aureus* infection of a surgical wound on the scalp noted at post-operative day six. Patient presented with mild tenderness, purulent drainage, erythema, edema and crust along the suture line.

represent lymphangitis. Drainage of malodorous and purulent material may occur as well as formation of pustules. Development of fever and chills are uncommon but may represent a sign of spreading infection.

When wound infection is suspected, it is important to obtain a wound culture from the exudate or affected tissues at the wound site to identify the causative organism(s). If the infection appears more severe (fluctuance, ischemia or necrosis, or signs of dehiscence) consider partial suture removal to allow drainage or complete suture removal and leaving the wound site open to drain and heal by secondary intention. Initiating treatment of suspected wound infection with empiric antibiotics is usually recommended until culture and sensitivities are resulted [22, 45]. Worsening signs and symptoms of infection despite empiric antibiotics may indicate MRSA, highlighting the need for culture and sensitivities to guide treatment choice.

Antibiotics used in the pediatric population for wound infections and dosing regimens can be found in Table 14.5. A 7- to 10-day course of antibiotics is often all that is needed for simple skin infections. The most likely causative organism should drive appropriate antibiotic choice (Table 14.6). Empiric treatment with drugs that cover gram-positive organisms, mainly *Staphylococcus aureus*, will often be effective for most surgical site infections. Cephalosporins such as cephalexin are the most commonly used class of antibiotics currently used to treat skin infections, particularly because of their broad-spectrum activity and safety profile, as well as due to the increasing resistance among strains of group A streptococci and *S. aureus* to macrolides like erythromycin. The third-generation agent cefdinir also has good coverage against a broad range of likely pathogens, including staphylococci. It is administered twice daily and offers a favorable efficacy and tolerability profile in pediatric patients with an oral suspension [46]. MRSA infection is often treated with trimethoprim-sulfamethoxazole, clindamycin, or doxycycline (when age-appropriate). When a MRSA abscess is present surgical drainage should also occur. Suspected or proven gram-negative organisms, which may be present in the groin, perineum, lower legs, moist intertriginous areas and ear, are treated with some third- or fourth-generation cephalosporins, expanded spectrum penicillins, quinolones or aminoglycosides [31]. If systemic symptoms are present, admission to the hospital for intravenous antibiotics is often indicated.

Although overall infection rate in pediatric dermatologic surgery is likely low, prevention of infection is key and should

Table 14.5 Oral dosing for commonly used antibiotics for mild to moderate pediatric skin infections [11]. Drug choice should be based on culture and sensitivity whenever possible. Dosing adjustments may be needed in patients with hepatic and renal impairment.

Drug	Dosing	Frequency	Max dose
Cephalexin	25–50 mg/kg/day	Divided every 6–8 hours	4 g/day
Cefdinir	Infants >6 months and children: 14 mg/kg/day	Divided twice daily for 10 days	600 mg/day
	Adolescents: 300 mg/dose	Every 12 hours for 10 days	
Clindamycin[a]	Infants, children and adolescents: 10–25 mg/kg/day	Divided every 8 hours	1800 mg/day
Trimethoprim-sulfamethoxazole	Infants >2 months, children and adolescents: 8–12 mg TMP/kg/day	Divided every 12 hours	Max single dose: 160 mg TMP
Doxycycline	Children ≥8 years: 2–4 mg/kg/day	Divided every 12–24 hours	200 mg/day
Dicloxacillin[b]	Children <40 kg: 25–50 mg/kg/day	Divided every 6 hours	2 g/day
	Children >40 kg: 125–500 mg	Every 6 hours	2 g/day
Azithromycin	5–12 mg/kg/dose (typical dose 10–12 mg/kg/dose on day 1 followed by 5 to 6 mg/kg once daily for remainder)	Daily	Total course 1500 to 2000 mg

[a] Clindamycin therapy has been associated with severe colitis.
[b] Only available in oral capsules.

Table 14.6 Common agents used for skin infections and targeted organisms.

Antimicrobial agent	Targeted organism
Cephalexin Cefdinir Dicloxacillin	First-line agents for *Staphylococcus aureus*
Azithromycin	Alternate for *S. aureus* coverage in penicillin allergic patients
Trimethoprim-sulfamethoxazole	MRSA[a] and genitourinary organisms
Clindamycin	MRSA[a] and oral surgery

[a] Treatment of MRSA should be based on sensitivity results whenever possible.

include perioperative counseling to restrict excessive activities during the post-operative period to prevent trauma (subsequent hematoma or dehiscence), with the use of a bulky pressure dressing and explicit wound care instructions to adequately keep the surgical site clean, with the mention of the signs and symptoms of infection. Caretakers should be instructed to wash hands before and after dressing changes. Wound dressings should be kept dry and intact for the first 48 hours after surgery. Office contact information for any after-hours concerns should be provided to families. Generally, prophylactic antibiotics are not recommended unless there is evidence of infection (class IV wound) or the surgical site is considered contaminated (class III). The need for prophylactic antibiotics in pediatric patients with high-risk cardiac conditions or orthopedic prostheses should be discussed with the patient's subspecialist prior to the surgical procedure.

14.5 Suture Reactions and Granulomas

All suture materials will exhibit some type of inflammatory response in the skin; however, the degree of this response is variable based on suture properties. When the inflammatory response to suture materials is excessive, the likelihood of dehiscence, infection and delay in healing is increased [47]. Suture complications include inflammatory reactions to suture, pustules or suture abscesses, granulomatous foreign body reaction, suture extrusion, and rarely true allergy to suture material (Figure 14.3). Incidence of suture reactions in pediatric dermatologic surgery is currently unknown, but they seem to occur more in the childhood and early adolescence years.

When choosing appropriate suture materials, understanding of the caliber of the suture and its configuration (monofilament or multifilament) are important to limit reactivity [48]. Larger-caliber (diameter) and multifilament sutures have a greater chance of tissue reactivity; likewise, natural materials such as surgical gut and silk will induce more tissue reactivity as compared to synthetic (such as nylon, polypropylene) suture [49]. Absorbable sutures of any type will induce an immune response, necessary for dissolution, while non-absorbable sutures cause less of a host response [48]. True suture allergy is rare, but is often to surgical gut suture and may be attributed to their foreign collagen or chromic salts [50]. Bovine collagen that may be found in surgical gut suture could also cause an immediate hypersensitivity reaction, and this may be confirmed via skin-prick testing [51]. Silk suture has been described to cause a suppurative and granulomatous response [52].

Knowledge of clinical appearance of suture reactions is helpful to identify when they occur. Placement of highly reactive epidermal sutures such as silk or surgical gut may cause inflammation consisting of erythema and edema along the length of the suture line or around each epidermal suture. As digestion

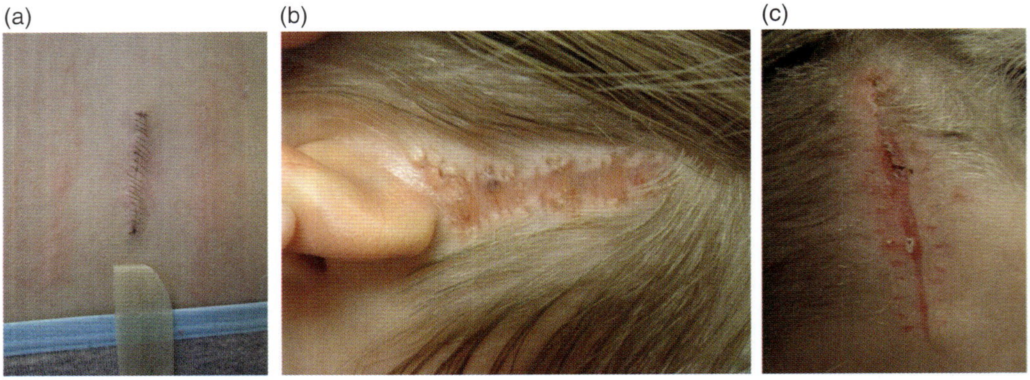

Figure 14.3 Suture reactions. Erythema surrounding chromic gut sutures at post-operative day 10 (a). Widened surgical incisions with small sinus tracts extruding suture material, small pustules and crusted pink papules (b,c).

of sutures takes place, pustules or deeper red papules with superimposed pustules may be seen. Visualization of an extruding suture with surrounding erythema or purulence, or formation of a sinus tract along the suture tract represents a "spitting" or extruding suture. This is often noticed approximately one to four months after surgery, with an average of six weeks postoperative at time of onset [53]. A tender indurated red papule or nodule may represent a granulomatous foreign body reaction to buried suture. Suture reactions may cause mild–moderate tenderness at the site when palpated.

Reassurance can be given to patients and caregivers when suture reactions occur as oftentimes healing and scar formation is not impeded. Definitive removal of the offending suture will alleviate the inflammatory response. Remove visualized suture with sterile forceps. A sterile needle to open pustules or red papules and inspection and gentle pressure will often facilitate removal of deeper sutures. Mechanical massage at home can be used for firm, deeper papules. A punch biopsy can also be used to remove a deeper and/or larger papule or nodule that may represent a granulomatous reaction to a buried suture.

Suture selection is important to prevent unwanted suture reactions. Less reactive suture materials should be chosen whenever possible. Often times, polyglactin 910 (Vicryl®) or poliglecaprone (Monocryl®) are chosen for buried sutures due to their ease of use in the tissue, tensile strength and low reactivity. Buried running subcuticular sutures or simple interrupted sutures using polypropylene (Prolene®) will be non-reactive and can be removed post-operatively quite easily. When an absorbable suture is needed for epidermal closure for situations where suture removal may be difficult or not feasible, more rapidly dissolving absorbable sutures such as polyglactin 910 (Vicryl Rapid®) or chromic gut may be the least reactive choices. Also, the smallest-caliber suture with adequate strength to adequately close the excision, based on location, skin thickness and wound tension, should be chosen. Avoidance of placing buried sutures too close to the surface of the wound may help prevent "spitting" sutures, although this is somewhat controversial as deeper placed buried sutures can certainly extrude post-operatively. Lastly, smaller size suture can be used at the end of the excision where tension is less, and fewer throws can be used when knotting suture to keep knot size as small as possible at the apices of the excision.

14.6 Wound Dehiscence

The separation of a previously apposed wound edges, or dehiscence, most often occurs due to a surgical wound infection; other causes of dehiscence include improper wound apposition, tissue necrosis, premature suture removal and excessive tension on wound edges. It is commonplace to close wounds under tension in cutaneous surgery. Thus, proper suture choice, placement of secure buried sutures, sufficient undermining, wound edge approximation, the use of special suture techniques, and strict limitations on post-operative activity may all help limit the risk of wound dehiscence. Dehiscence most often occurs at the time of suture removal but can occur both prior and after this time.

Evaluation of an abnormal appearing wound should include assessing for signs of infection such as erythema, edema, purulent drainage and pain. In the absence of infection, wound dehiscence in small areas of the suture line or complete wound dehiscence may be seen. Areas of tissue necrosis or hematoma may also be seen in the setting of dehiscence.

In an otherwise clean wound, if dehiscence occurs within the first 24 hours, the wound may be re-sutured, especially if deep sutures are intact and the wound is under minimal to no tension in a clean location [54]. Otherwise, in clean dehisced wounds, healing by secondary intention may be best, especially if the wound is under high tension or necrosis has occurred. Necrotic wounds should be left alone, avoiding significant debridement and allowing the formation of eschar and healing underneath. If hematoma formation has caused dehiscence or tissue necrosis, evacuation and irrigation of the wound bed is recommended (see section of postoperative bleeding and hematoma).

Ideal timing of suture removal should be followed, and if a surgeon is unsure of potential wound dehiscence, sutures may be removed in a gradual and temporal manner. Often times, removing every other suture may be first attempted and subsequent close monitoring for further dehiscence. For small areas of dehiscence on clean wounds, especially after suture removal, the placement of skin closure tapes with tactifiers, such as tincture of benzoin (Mastisol® Ferndale laboratories, Ferndale, Michigan) for further wound support can be placed and should last one to two weeks. Discussion regarding reinforcement of activity limitations with the patient and caregiver is essential.

When a wound infection is diagnosed, cultures and appropriate antibiotic therapy should be initiated (see section on postoperative infection). Many infected wounds that result in dehiscence will heal in via granulation and still end up with a cosmetically suitable scar. The use of dressings on dehisced wounds that will heal by secondary intention will help prevent further infection and allow the proper environment to facilitate wound healing. Depending on the location of the wound and wound bed characteristics such as moisture level and presence or absence of infection, an ideal dressing should be chosen (refer to chapter 12 on dressings). Clear and repetitive instructions should be given to the patient (when age-appropriate) and caregiver regarding wound care including cleansing of the wound and dressing placement when healing by secondary intention. Frequent office visits are also helpful to assure at-home instructions are being followed and that adequate healing has occurred.

14.6.1 Pre-Operative Considerations to Prevent Dehiscence

The timing of elective excisional surgery is pediatric patients should be taken into account when attempting to minimize wound dehiscence. Scalp skin of a neonate or infant is especially flexible and mobile as compared to the scalp skin in a teenager, which tends to have significantly less stretch. Thus removal of a large nevus sebaceous of the scalp is preferred earlier in life and could result in a smaller scar than waiting until the patient is a teen. Once a child begins to ambulate, frequent falls and trauma are much more likely. In active children and teenagers, the need for strict limitations on activities (such as gym class, sports, and recess) in the post-operative period should be discussed and emphasized.

14.6.2 Intraoperative Techniques to Decrease Risk of Dehiscence

When surgical procedures occur in the operating theater, modifications can be done to minimize the risk of wound dehiscence, one of the most effective method being "over sewing" [27]. Lesesky et al. recommend doubling the number of deep dermal sutures when excisions are performed over or near a joint or in areas of high tension or frequent movement [27]. Few permanent (non-dissolvable) deep sutures may also be used for some of the deep dermal sutures in areas of high movement or tension such as the knee [27]. Additional techniques include choosing a larger suture size for buried sutures, using a buried pulley stitch for closures under high tension, and utilizing a running subcuticular suture which can be left in place longer during wound healing than simple interrupted sutures [27].

Undermining 2–3 cm from the wound edges will typically relieve wounds under high tension. To prevent tissue necrosis, avoid the over-tightening of epidermal sutures and crush injury of wound edges with forceps, and ensure adequate blood flow to flap tips and wound edges. In particular for scalp excisions, ensure that adequate hemostasis has been achieved before closing the wound to prevent hematoma formation.

14.6.3 Post-Operative Techniques to Minimize Wound Dehiscence

After surgery has been completed, there are several techniques that may decrease the risk of wound dehiscence in the postoperative period. The placement of large bulky dressings can impair attempts by children to resume normal activity soon after surgery or removal of the dressing. Bulky dressings also serve as a reminder to the child and caretaker to restrict movement and add additional padding to protect against trauma. They may also restrict movements themselves. Some authors also recommend the use of crutches and removable splints when surgery occurs at or near a joint to further restrict motion and over-activity [27]. The use of skin tape and adhesive perpendicular to the wound edges may help alleviate wound tension if additional support is needed. Strict adherence to physical activity limitations should be emphasized in the post-operative instructions.

14.7 Postoperative Scar Formation

Many myths surround the idea of scarring in children. Many parents assume that minimal to no scarring in children is possible, whether from a biopsy procedure in clinic or an excision performed in the operating room. For many dermatologists comfortable with surgical procedures on the adult and elderly population, performing surgical procedures in the pediatric population can be more frustrating and disappointing, as scars tend to widen over time. Additionally, children may tend to be more reactive to suture material, and tend to extrude sutures and form suture granulomas, especially in those patients of mid-childhood and prepubertal ages. Older children and teens are also prone to developing hypertrophic scars and keloids. Chapter 15 will address both non-invasive and invasive techniques to improve scars in pediatric patients.

Acknowledgements

Many thanks to Dr Raj Singhal and Mark Popenhagen for their review and input in the post-operative pain section as well as to Kathy Zeblisky for her help with the literature search and reference materials.

References

1 American Academy of Pediatrics. Committee on psychosocial aspects of child and family health; Task force on pain in infants, children, and adolescents (2001). The assessment and management of acute pain in infants, children, and adolescents. *Pediatrics* 108 (3): 793–797.

2 Metz, B.J. (2013). Procedural pediatric dermatology. *Dermatol. Clin.* 31: 337–346.

3 Gehdoor, R.P. (2004). Post operative pain management in pediatric patients. *Indian J. Anaesth.* 48: 406–414.

4 Baker, C.M. and Wong, D.L. (1987). Q.U.E.S.T.: a process of pain assessment in children. *Orthop. Nurs.* 6: 11–21.

5 Wong-Baker FACES Foundation Resources: Qualities of the Wong-Baker FACES® Pain Rating Scale www.wongbakerfaces.org (accessed 5 January 2015).

6 Kraemer, F.W. and Rose, J.B. (2009). Pharmacologic management of acute pediatric pain. *Anesthesiol. Clin.* 27 (2): 241–268.

7 Mathew, P.J. and Mathew, J.L. (2003). Assessment and management of pain in infants. *Postgrad. Med. J.* 79: 438–443.

8 Krechel, S.W. and Bildner, J. (1995). CRIES: a new neonatal postoperative pain measurement score. Initial testing of validity and reliability. *Paediatr. Anaesth.* 5 (1): 53–61.

9 American Medical Association. Module 6 Pain Management: Pediatric Pain Management: AMA. http://ama-cmeonline.com (accessed 24 December 2014).
10 O'Donnell, F.T. and Rosen, K.R. (2014). Pediatric pain management: a review. *Mo. Med.* 111 (3): 231–237.
11 Lexicomp Online®, UpToDate® (2015) Safety review update of codeine use in children; new boxed warning and contraindication on use after tonsillectomy and/or adenoidectomy. http://www.fda.gov (accessed 24 May 2015).
12 Kokki, H. (2003). Nonsteroidal anti-inflammatory drugs for postoperative pain: a focus on children. *Paediatr. Drugs* 5 (2): 103–123.
13 Dlugosz, C.K., Chater, R.W., and Engle, J.P. (2006). Appropriate use of nonprescription analgesics in pediatric patients. *J. Pediatr. Health Care* 20 (5): 316–325.
14 Wong, T., Stang, A.S., Ganshorn, H. et al. (2013). Combined and alternating paracetamol and ibuprofen therapy for febrile children. *Cochrane Database Syst. Rev.* 10: CD009572. https://doi.org/10.1002/14651858.CD009572.pub2.
15 Merry, A.F., Edwards, K.E., Ahmad, Z. et al. (2013). Randomized comparison between the combination of acetaminophen and ibuprofen and each constituent alone for analgesia following tonsillectomy in children. *Can. J. Anaesth.* 60 (12): 1180–1189.
16 Ong, C.K., Seymour, R.A., Lirk, P. et al. (2010). Combining paracetamol (acetaminophen) with nonsteroidal antiinflammatory drugs: a qualitative systematic review of analgesic efficacy for acute postoperative pain. *Anesth. Analg.* 110 (4): 1170–1179.
17 Vargas-Schaffer, G. (2010). Is the WHO analgesic ladder still valid? Twenty-four years of experience. *Can. Fam. Physician* 56 (6): 514–517, e202–5.
18 Pergolizzi, J.V. (2011). Quantifying the impact of drug-drug interactions associated with opioids. *Am. J. Manag. Care* 17 (Suppl 11): S288–S292.
19 Safety review update of codeine use in children; new boxed warning and contraindication on use after tonsillectomy and/or adenoidectomy. www.fda.gov (accessed 24 May 2015).
20 Jacobs, A., Price, H.N., and Popenhagen, M.P. (2014). Blowing away the pain: a technique for pediatric pain management. *Pediatr. Dermatol.* 31 (6): 757–758.
21 Krishna, S., Hughes, L.F., and Lin, S.Y. (2003). Postoperative hemorrhage with nonsteroidal anti-inflammatory drug use after tonsillectomy. *Arch. Otolaryngol. Head Neck Surg.* 129: 1086–1089.
22 Cunningham, B. and Wagner, A.M. (2011). Surgical techniques. In: *Pediatric Dermatology*, 4e (ed. L.A. Schachner and R.C. Hansen), 211–298. Philadelphia, PA: Mosby Elsevier Ltd.
23 Robinson, J.K., Hanke, C.W., Siegel, D.M. et al. (2010). Hemostasis: postoperative care. In: *Surgery of the Skin: Procedural Dermatology*, 2e (ed. T.H. Nguyen and Q.L. Erickson), 235–237. London: Mosby.
24 Roenigk, R.K., Ratz, J.L., and Roenigk, H.H. (2007). *Roenigk's Dermatologic Surgery: Current Techniques in Procedural Dermatology*. New York: Informa Healthcare.
25 Delaney, A., Diamantis, S., and Marks, V.J. (2011). Complication of tissue ischemia and in dermatologic surgery. *Dermatol. Ther.* 24: 551–557.
26 Salasche, S.J. (1986). Acute surgical complications: cause, prevention, and treatment. *J. Am. Acad. Dermatol.* 15 (6): 1163–1185.
27 Lesesky, E.B., Cunningham, B.B., and Makkar, H.S. (2007). Pediatric surgical pearls: minimizing complications. *Semin Cutan Med Surg* 26: 54–64.
28 Hancock, B.J., St-Vil, D., Luks, F.I. et al. (1992). Complications of lymphangiomas in children. *J. Pediatr. Surg.* 27 (2): 220–224.
29 Mangram, A.J., Horan, T.C., Pearson, M.L. et al. (1999). Guideline for prevention of

surgical site infection. 1999. Centers for Disease Control and Prevention (CDC) hospital infection control practices advisory committee. *Am. J. Infect. Control* 27 (2): 97–132.

30 Altemeier, W.A., Culbertson, W.R., and Hummel, R.P. (1968). Surgical considerations of endogenous infections – source, types, and methods of control. *Surg. Clin. North Am.* 48: 227–240.

31 Wood, L.D., Warner, N.M., and Billingsley, E.M. (2011). Infectious complications of dermatologic procedures. *Dermatol. Ther.* 24 (6): 558–570.

32 Bucher, B.T., Warner, B.W., and Dillon, P.A. (2011). Antibiotic prophylaxis and the prevention of surgical site infection. *Curr. Opin. Pediatr.* 23 (3): 334–338.

33 Futoryan, T. and Grande, D. (1995). Postoperative wound infection rates in dermatologic surgery. *Dermatol. Surg.* 21 (6): 509–514.

34 Dixon, A.J., Dixon, M.P., Askew, D.A. et al. (2006). Prospective study of wound infections in dermatologic surgery in the absence of prophylactic antibiotics. *Dermatol. Surg.* 32: 819–827.

35 Maragh, S.L. and Brown, M.D. (2008). Prospective evaluation of surgical site infection rate among patients with Mohs micrographic surgery without the use of prophylactic antibiotics. *J. Am. Acad. Dermatol.* 59 (2): 275–278.

36 Cook, J.L. and Perone, J.B. (2003). A prospective evaluation of the incidence of complications associated with Mohs micrographic surgery. *Arch. Dermtol.* 139 (2): 143–152.

37 Kulichová, D., Geimer, T., Mühlstädt, M. et al. (2013). Surgical site infections in skin surgery: a single center experience. *J. Dermatol.* 40 (10): 779–785.

38 Alfageme Roldan, F., Ciudad Blanco, C., Campos Dominguez, M. et al. (2009). Risk factors in pediatric dermatologic surgery. *Dermatol. Online J.* 15 (9): 2.

39 Bhattacharyya, N. and Kosloske, A.M. (1990). Postoperative wound infection in pediatric surgical patients: a study of 676 infants and children. *J. Pediatr. Surg.* 25 (1): 125–129.

40 Davis, S.D., Sobocinski, K., Hoffmann, R.G. et al. (1984). Postoperative wound infections in a children's hospital. *Pediatr. Infect. Dis.* 3 (2): 114–116.

41 Horwitz, J.R., Chwals, W.J., Doski, J.J. et al. (1998). Pediatric wound infections: a prospective multicenter study. *Ann. Surg.* 227: 553–558.

42 Sharma, L.K. and Sharma, P.K. (1986). Postoperative wound infection in a pediatric surgical service. *J. Pediatr. Surg.* 21 (10): 889–891.

43 Hurst, E.A., Grekin, R.C., Yu, S.S. et al. (2007). Infectious complications and antibiotic use in dermatologic surgery. *Semin. Cutan. Med. Surg.* 26: 47–53.

44 (1996). National Nosocomial Infections Surveillance (NNIS) report, data summary from October 1986–April 1996, issued May 1996. A report from the National Nosocomial Infections Surveillance (NNIS) system. *Am. J. Infect. Control* 24 (5): 380–388.

45 Bucko, A.D., Hunt, B.J., Kidd, S.L. et al. (2002). Randomized, double-blind, multicenter comparison of oral cefditoren 200 or 400 mg BID with either cefuroxime 250 mg BID or cefadroxil 500 mg BID for the treatment of uncomplicated skin and skin structure infections. *Clin. Ther.* 24: 1134–1147.

46 Hedrick, J. (2003). Acute bacterial skin infections in pediatric medicine: current issues in presentation and treatment. *Paediatr Drugs* 5: 35–46.

47 Brunius, U. and Zederfeldt, B. (1970). Suture materials in general surgery. A comment. *Prog. Surg.* 8: 38–44.

48 Bennett, R. (1988). Materials for wound closure. In: *Fundamentals of Cutaneous Surgery* (ed. R.G. Bennet), 274–309. St. Louis, MO: Mosby.

49 Hurty, C.A., Brazik, D.C., Law, J.M. et al. (2002). Evaluation of the tissue reactions in the skin and body wall of koi (Cyprinus

carpio) to five suture materials. *Vet. Rec.* 151 (11): 324–328.

50 Engler, R.J., Weber, C.B., and Turnicky, R. (1986). Hypersensitivity to chromated catgut sutures: a case report and review of the literature. *Ann. Allergy* 56 (4): 317–320.

51 Mullins, R.J., Richards, C., and Walker, T. (1996). Allergic reactions to oral, surgical and topical bovine collagen. Anaphylactic risk for surgeons. *Aust. N. Z. J. Ophthalmol.* 24 (3): 257–260.

52 Hocwald, E., Sichel, J.Y., Dano, I. et al. (2003). Adverse reaction to surgical sutures in thyroid surgery. *Head Neck* 25 (1): 77–81.

53 Ammirati, C.T. and Goldman, G. (2012). Wound closure materials and instruments. In: *Dermatology*, 3e (ed. J.L. Bolognia, J.L. Jorizzo and J.V. Schaffer), 2353–2364. Philadelphia, PA: Elsevier.

54 Man, J. and Goldberg, D. (2011). Medical legal complications of cutaneous surgery. *Dermatol. Ther.* 24 (6): 515–523.

15

Improving Scars

Harper N. Price[1,2] and Maria Princesa P. Curtis[1]

[1] Phoenix Children's Hospital, Phoenix, AZ, USA
[2] Department of Child Health, University of Arizona College of Medicine, Phoenix, AZ, USA

15.1 Introduction

Surgical and laser procedures, deep tissue injuries and trauma, and burns may cause the development of scars in pediatric patients that are symptomatic, and restrictive and/or unsightly, especially if the scarring is excessive (Figure 15.1). Hypertrophic scars and keloids represent abnormal responses to wound healing. Each has its own clinical characteristics, natural history and associations (Table 15.1). The mechanism of abnormal scar formation is complex and involves a cascade of inflammatory reactions that are not completely understood to date.

Despite knowledge of risk factors, it is still difficult to predict whether a newly created scar will develop into an abnormal scar. Techniques to potentially minimize risk include avoiding closing wounds under high tension and close follow-up in the post-operative period for those scars in high-risk sites (earlobes, mandibular angle, upper back and chest, shoulders, posterior neck and upper arms) [3]. Diligent post-operative follow-up is essential in the pediatric population as patients often experience little post-operative pain and will resume normal activity quickly if allowed. It is believed that increased activity level in the acute post-operative period in children contributes greatly to complications and abnormal scar formation [2].

Excessive scarring affects a patient's quality of life. Both the caregivers and the pediatric patient may find a scar cosmetically and socially displeasing. Scars may cause pain, pruritus, and cutaneous dysesthesias, and in severe cases, contractures and functional impairment. The development and treatment of keloid and hypertrophic scars is often frustrating for both the patient/caregiver and the physician. A variety of invasive and noninvasive treatments have been evaluated to prevent or minimize scars and associated symptoms. Due to the lack of strong evidence behind most of these treatments, no single modality is defined as the gold standard. Treatment options for abnormal scarring are discussed in this chapter (Table 15.2). The use of multiple concurrent scar treatment modalities is common and often necessary to see more rapid improvement and acceptable results.

Prior to pursuing scar treatment, it is important to address the primary goals of therapy and set realistic expectations based on the treatment modalities available and age of the patient. When assessing abnormal scars, the color, texture and any functional limitations and symptoms should be noted. The easiest of the nonsurgical treatment options that can be done

Pediatric Dermatologic Surgery, First Edition. Edited by Keyvan Nouri, Latanya Benjamin, Jasem Alshaiji, and Jan Izakovic.

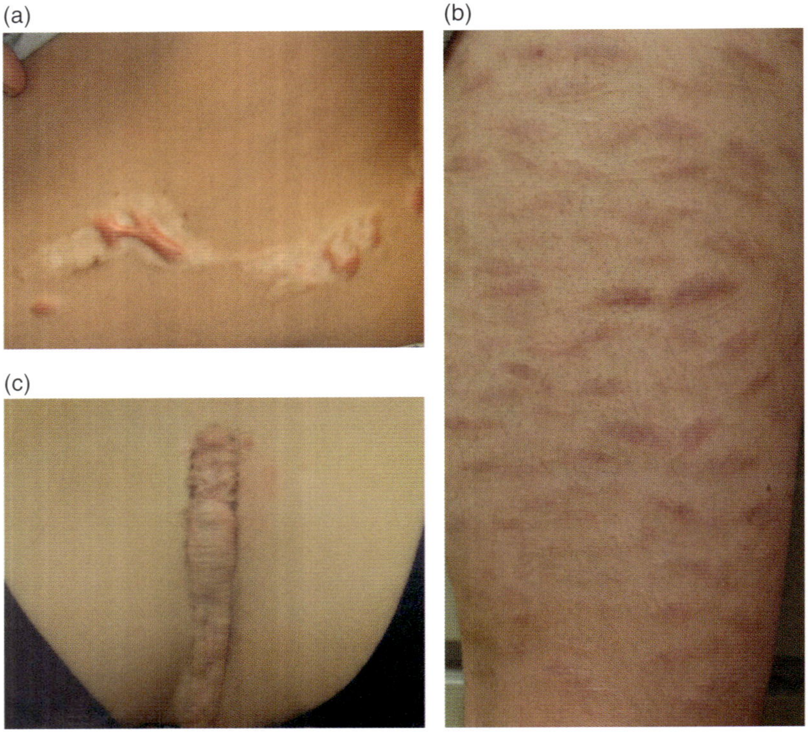

Figure 15.1 Examples of abnormal scarring in pediatric patients. (a) Development of keloids status-post carbon dioxide laser ablation of an epidermal nevus on the trunk. (b) Hypertrophic scars on the legs as a result of repetitive self-trauma. (c) Large chest keloid that developed several months after open-heart surgery.

Table 15.1 Characteristics of hypertrophic and keloid scars [1–8].

	Hypertrophic scars	Keloid scars
Timing	• Develop within 3 months of injury • Often regress over time without treatment	• Develop up to 1–3 years after injury • No spontaneous regression • Recur following therapy
Clinical features	• Contained within borders of injury • Raised, linear, firm	• Extend beyond borders of injury • Raised, hard, bosselated tumors
Associations	• Post-burn, post-excision, trauma • Pediatric age	• Any dermal injury • Darker skin types (Fitzpatrick IV, V, VI) • Hispanic, Asian, African descent • Age < 30 years • Pregnant women • Pubertal age • History of cutaneous inflammatory disorder or infection • Family history (autosomal dominant)

Table 15.2 Therapies for pediatric keloid and hypertrophic scars based on ease of use, evidence and invasiveness.

1st line: non-invasive options
• Photoprotection
• Scar massage
• Silicone sheeting/gels
2nd line:[a] may be used in conjunction with 1st line therapies
• Intralesional triamcinolone injections
• Cryotherapy and intralesional triamcinolone injections
• Pulsed-dye laser (585-nm and 595-nm)
• Pulsed-dye laser and intralesional triamcinolone injections
3rd line:[a] may be used in conjunction with 1st line therapies
• Excision of scar with post-operative triamcinolone injections
Topical therapies such as imiquimod 5% cream, 5-fluorouracil cream, vitamin E, topical retinoid creams and onion extract have little evidence to support their use in children and/or side effects are limiting in the pediatric population.

[a] The pain of these procedures in the office limits their use in children over age eight years.

at almost any age are daily photo protection and scar massage. Compliance with both home therapies and timely in-office treatments is key.

15.2 Massage

Burn centers and surgeons commonly use massage, often as an adjunctive scar therapy modality, although there is little scientific evidence to support its use. Massage is routinely used for the treatment of hypertrophic scars following burn injury. It also appears to have good efficacy when used on postsurgical scars [9, 10].

15.2.1 Appropriate Usage

There is no consensus regarding the timing of initiation, technique, frequency, and length of treatment for scar massage. For post-surgical scars, massage is generally initiated after suture removal and complete closure of the wound, and done for several minutes a day as tolerated. A bland ointment or cream, free of potential sensitizers, could be used as a lubricant. In general, clean hands should be used to apply pressure to the scar enough to cause blanching without pain or skin irritation. In the author's experience (HP), once to twice daily massage for 10 minutes with petrolatum jelly while doing another activity such as watching television or reading is an acceptable and low-cost treatment plan for most pediatric patients and their families.

15.2.2 Mechanism of Action

Although the mechanism of action of massage in scar therapy is not known, one hypothesis is that massage therapy is thought to increase the pliability of scars by mechanically disrupting fibrotic tissue [10].

15.2.3 Efficacy and Benefits

A few limited studies in children and adults with post-burn scars reported that patients had decreased pain, itching, and anxiety, and an increase in mood with massage [11–15]. Likewise, in a limited number of adults and children with post-surgical scars utilizing massage, the majority had improvement in appearance or on POSAS scar assessment scale [16, 17]. Other positive aspects of scar massage include the low-cost, direct involvement of the patient and family in their care, hastening absorption of buried dissolvable suture material, and improvement in edema and induration of the scar [10].

15.2.4 Side Effects and Contraindications

Risks of scar massage include the development of irritant or allergic contact dermatitis to the lubricant used and possible worsening of the scar due to irritation or injury. Scar massage is contraindicated in the presence of a break in the epidermis, infection, bleeding, significant pain, wound dehiscence, or graft failure [10].

15.3 Silicone Scar Products

First reported in the early 1980s for usage in burn scars, silicone-based products are now recommended as a first-line noninvasive method for both the prevention and treatment of hypertrophic and keloid scars [18]. They make an attractive option for use in children because they are painless, easy to use, and have a low risk of adverse effects. Very few studies evaluate the use of silicone products on pediatric scars but this modality has been become the mainstay of treatment in this population [2].

15.3.1 Formulations and Usage

Silicone products are manufactured in the form of sheets and gels. Sheets are soft and occlusive and contain the inert polymer polydimethylsiloxane. To provide extra durability and flexibility, some sheets contain a polytetrafluoroethylene membrane. Some silicone sheets are self-adhesive while others require taping to affix onto the skin. To be effective, they require contact with the scar for at least 12 hours per day for two to three months [19, 20]. Use for at least six months' duration should be advocated for utmost improvement. Silicone gel sheets are not suitable for use over large areas or joints where they do not conform. Patient compliance also often becomes an issue when scars are located in visible areas such as the face [19, 21]. Recently, silicone gel formulations were developed to overcome these problems. Self-drying silicone gel is applied as a thin layer on the skin where it forms a transparent, gas-permeable, and waterproof sheet [22]. It can be applied over the face, irregular skin surfaces, joints and flexures, and over any size of scar [23].

15.3.2 Mechanisms of Action

The mechanism of action of silicone on scars has not been determined, but many hypotheses have been proposed. Potential mechanisms reported include temperature alteration, hydration and occlusion, polarization of scar tissue, modulation of expression of growth factors and down-regulation of fibroblasts [20, 24–28].

15.3.3 Efficacy and Benefits

Despite their frequent use in practice, studies on the use of silicone products to prevent and/or treat hypertrophic scars and keloids are limited in quality, design and other factors and thus only limited conclusions can be drawn [19]. Perkins and colleagues first described the successful use of silicone gel sheets to treat children with scars resulting from burn injuries [18]. There is some weak evidence to support the claim that the use of silicone gel products on incisions may decrease the likelihood of development of abnormal scars in high-risk individuals [pooled studies 29–31]. In studies comparing silicone gel sheeting to a control, improvement in scar thickness favoring silicone products was found [32, 33]. Significant improvement in scar elasticity in those treated with silicone sheeting has also been reported [31, 32, 34, 35].

15.3.4 Side Effects and Contraindications

Silicone scar patches/gel are generally well tolerated. Reported adverse effects include rash, contact dermatitis, pruritus, maceration, odor, and infection. These reactions can be prevented by gradually increasing time of application, instituting good hygiene by washing the scar and gel sheet more frequently with soap and water, and avoiding hot, humid environments [20, 24, 36]. Avoid use on open wounds. To limit cost of product, individual patches can be cleansed on a daily basis and can be utilized for up to a few weeks; also, sheeting may be cut to size or in half for smaller scars.

15.4 Intralesional Corticosteroid Therapy

Intralesional corticosteroid injections have been widely used for the treatment of scars for over 50 years despite the limited number of prospective randomized studies to support their use [37]. Several corticosteroid preparations have been used for injection of hypertrophic and keloid scars, including dexamethasone, hydrocortisone acetate, methylprednisolone, and most commonly triamcinolone acetonide [38].

15.4.1 Formulations and Usage

There is no standardized protocol for treatment with intralesional corticosteroids and thus, concentration, frequency and technique vary widely. Triamcinolone acetonide suspension, the most commonly used corticosteroid, is injected into the mid-dermis and results in blanching that should not extend beyond the treatment area. Depending on the amount of scar formation, area of the body involved, and individual patient, a concentration of 10–40 mg/ml is typically used. As the scar softens and flattens, the concentration of corticosteroid can be reduced. As a general guideline, approximately 0.1 ml is injected into every linear centimeter of the keloid, with resultant blanching of the overlying skin [39]. In areas more prone to atrophy (such as facial locations) and for thin hypertrophic scars, lower doses should be used initially. Injections are usually repeated every four to six weeks until clinical improvement or development of adverse effects [38]. Injections can be used as monotherapy or in combination with silicone patches or other modalities such as cryotherapy and laser. Due to the high recurrence rate of keloids after excision, intralesional corticosteroids are commonly used intra- or post-operatively to prevent regrowth [39].

15.4.2 Mechanism of Action

Corticosteroids inhibit inflammation and mitosis while increasing vasoconstriction in scar tissue [40]. Triamcinolone prevents proliferation of normal and keloid fibroblasts, inhibits collagen synthesis, increases collagenase production in scars and down regulates collagen gene expression [41–44].

15.4.3 Efficacy and Benefits

This sole modality has a variable response rate of 50–100%, with a broad recurrence rate of up to 50% [37, 45–47]. Steroid injections can be quite effective in completely flattening early hypertrophic scars. When used on older scars and keloids, corticosteroids may only soften and flatten scars to some extent but can provide symptomatic relief [48]. Excellent efficacy (82–93% response rate) can be seen when intra-op steroid injections are used in combination with excisional surgery as well as significant improvement in symptoms such as pruritus [49, 50]. Cryotherapy has also been utilized *prior* to injection with up to an 84% success rate [45]. These two modalities are thought to have a synergistic effect as increased tissue edema during the thaw process of cryotherapy increases the overall volume of the lesion that may allow for better corticosteroid penetration into the scar tissue [51, 52].

15.4.4 Side Effects and Contraindication

Injections with corticosteroids are painful and may not be tolerated by younger children. Topical anesthetic creams used prior to the procedure can alleviate some discomfort in older children (age eight years or older). Many techniques to help minimize pain can also be utilized to make the procedure more tolerable (for example, vibratory analgesia, distraction, and ice packs). Local side effects of intralesional corticosteroids include cutaneous atrophy, capillary dilatation, telangiectasias, hypopigmentation, depigmentation, and rarely necrosis and ulceration. Many local side effects experienced will improve over time and will not require treatment. Care should be taken to avoid injecting the corticosteroid into the subcutis or surrounding unaffected dermis. Systemic effects of intralesional corticosteroids are not common, but rare cases of Cushing's syndrome have been reported. Children seem to be most at risk for Cushing's syndrome and monthly total dosage should not exceed more than 30 mg of triamcinolone [53].

15.5 Laser Therapy

Various lasers were introduced for the treatment of keloids in the mid-1980s, but the most encouraging results to date have been obtained with the 585-nm and 595-nm flash-pumped pulsed-dye laser (PDL) [4, 54]. PDL is currently considered the laser of choice and is considered to be an excellent first-line option for hypertrophic scars and keloids [55, 56].

15.5.1 Formulations and Usage

PDL therapy is best utilized in lighter-skin types and higher energy densities are not necessarily correlated with therapeutic effect [57]. Adjacent, non-overlapping pulses at energy densities ranging from 6.0 to 7.5 J/cm^2 (7 mm spot) or 4.5–5.5 J/cm^2 (10 mm spot) are recommended for hypertrophic scars and keloids [58]. Treatment should be initiated with the most effective and lowest energy density and increased only if the response is suboptimal. For the 595-nm PDL, a pulse duration of 0.45 ms was more effective in decreasing scar size and pliability than a 40 ms pulse width, whereas comparison of 0.45 and 1.5 ms pulse duration with the 585-nm PDL found no difference in outcomes between the two pulse durations [59, 60]. Significant improvement is generally noted after two to three treatments but larger and thicker scars may require additional treatments. In general, treatment intervals of six to eight weeks are recommended. Older patients may tolerate PDL treatments with a topical anesthetic cream applied prior to treatment whereas younger patients may require general anesthesia for management of larger scars. All persons must don eyewear appropriate for the wavelength of the laser device to avoid ocular damage. A small test spot or patch can be done initially if potential concerns regarding the patient's response to laser therapy exist. PDL may be used alone or in combination with other scar treatments. Intralesional corticosteroids are more easily delivered immediately *after* PDL irradiation due to the resultant edema, making the scar softer and facilitating penetration of the needle [61].

15.5.2 Mechanism of Action

The PDL works by selective photothermolysis of oxyhemoglobin molecules, resulting in microvascular damage, coagulative necrosis, and tissue hypoxia. It is possible that absorption by oxyhemoglobin in scar tissue and subsequent heating leads to thermal injury in the scar microvasculature, resulting in ischemia and reduced collagen [55]. Kuo et al. reported PDL induction of keloid regression through reduced transforming growth factor beta expression, decreased fibroblast proliferation, increased collagen III deposition and increased matrix metaloproteinase-13 activity [62, 63].

15.5.3 Efficacy and Benefits

When used for hypertrophic and keloid scars, PDL therapy will improve erythema, reduce scar volume, improve scar surface texture, and symptoms of pain and pruritus [64, 65]. In a meta-analysis on laser therapy for excessive scars by Jin et al., the majority of included studies involved the 585/595-PDL and these laser systems proved to be the most effective in improving hypertrophic scars and keloids. Reduction of scar height and improvement in erythema were significant secondary outcomes [57]. There is additional benefit provided in terms of improvement of scar height, erythema, and pain/itching when PDL is combined with intralesional corticosteroid injection for significantly proliferative scars [61].

15.5.4 Side Effects and Contraindications

Common side effects of PDL treatment include pain, post-treatment purpura (may persist up to 7–10 days) and edema. Less common and more severe side effects that may result from PDL treatment are crust formation, blistering, hyperpigmentation and hypopigmentation and superficial burn. To prevent pigmentary changes, strict sun avoidance and appropriate photoprotection should be advocated. Laser should be used with strong caution in darker skin types due to risk of competing chromophore of melanin.

15.6 Other Topical Therapies

Topical therapies such as vitamin E and onion extract (Mederma™, Merz Pharmaceuticals, Frankfurt, Germany) available over the counter are often used by patients due to previous familiarity or usage with these products. In clinical trials, these modalities have not shown any medical benefit except perhaps in combination with massage or other modalities [9]. The use of prescription topical therapies such as imiquimod 5% cream, 5-flourouracil cream and topical retinoids for abnormal scars has been studied with mixed outcomes and due to high frequency of local side-effects, these treatments are generally not recommended for use in the pediatric population [9, 66].

References

1 Lawrence, J.W., Mason, S.T., Schomer, K. et al. (2012). Epidemiology and impact of scarring after burn injury: a systematic review of the literature. *J. Burn Care Res.* 33 (1): 136–146.

2 Cunningham, B. and Wagner, A.M. (2011). Surgical techniques. In: *Pediatric Dermatology*, 4e (ed. L.A. Schachner and R.C. Hansen), 211–298. China: Elsevier Ltd.

3 Hom, D.B. (2001). Treating the elusive keloid. *Arch. Otolaryngol. Head Neck Surg.* 127 (9): 1140–1143.

4 Gauglitz, G.G., Korting, H.C., Pavicic, T. et al. (2011). Hypertrophic scarring and keloids: pathomechanisms and current and emerging treatment strategies. *Mol. Med.* 17: 113–125.

5 Lane, J.E., Waller, J.L., and Davis, L.S. (2005). Relationship between age of ear piercing and keloid formation. *Pediatrics* 115: 1312–1314.

6 Moustafa, M.F., Abdel-Fattah, M.A., and Abdel-Fattah, D.C. (1975). Presumptive evidence of the effect of pregnancy estrogens on keloid growth. Case report. *Plast. Reconstr. Surg.* 56: 450–453.

7 Marneros, A.G., Norris, J.E., Watanabe, S. et al. (2004). Genome scans provide evidence for keloid susceptibility loci on chromosomes 2q23 and 7p11. *J. Invest. Dermatol.* 122: 1126–1132.

8 Brown, J.J., Ollier, W.E., Thomson, W. et al. (2008). Positive association of HLA-DRB1*15 with keloid disease in Caucasians. *Int. J. Immunogenet.* 35: 303–307.

9 Foo, C.W. and Tristani-Firouzi, P. (2011). Topical modalities for treatment and prevention of postsurgical hypertrophic scars. *Facial Plast. Surg. Clin. North Am.* 19: 551–557.

10 Shin, T.M. and Bordeaux, J.S. (2012). The role of massage in scar management: a literature review. *Dermatol. Surg.* 38: 414–423.

11 Field, T., Peck, M., Hernandez-Reif, M. et al. (2000). Postburn itching, pain, and

psychological symptoms are reduced with massage therapy. *J. Burn Care Rehabil.* 21: 189–193.

12 Patiño, O., Novick, C., Merlo, A. et al. (1999). Massage in hypertrophic scars. *J. Burn Care Rehabil.* 20: 268–271.

13 Morien, A., Garrison, D., and Smith, N.K. (2008). Range of motion improves after massage in children with burns: a pilot study. *J. Bodyw. Mov. Ther.* 12 (1): 67–71.

14 Roh, Y.S., Cho, H., Oh, J.O. et al. (2007). Effects of skin rehabilitation massage therapy on pruritus, skin status, and depression in burn survivors. *Taehan Kanho Hakhoe Chi* 37 (2): 221–226.

15 Cho, Y.S., Jeon, J.H., Hong, A. et al. (2014). The effect of burn rehabilitation massage therapy on hypertrophic scar after burn: a randomized controlled trial. *Burns* 40 (8): 1513–1520.

16 Bianchi, F.A., Roccia, F., Fiorini, P. et al. (2010). Use of patient and observer scar assessment scale for evaluation of facial scars treated with self-drying silicone gel. *J. Craniofac. Surg.* 21 (3): 719–723.

17 Bodian, M. (1969). Use of massage following lid surgery. *Eye Ear Nose Throat Mon.* 48 (9): 542–547.

18 Perkins, K., Davey, R.B., and Wallis, K.A. (1983). Silicone gel: a new treatment for burn scars and contractures. *Burns Incl. Therm. Inj.* 9 (3): 201–204.

19 O'Brien, L. and Jones, D.J. (2013). Silicone gel sheeting for preventing and treating hypertrophic and keloid scars. *Cochrane Database Syst. Rev.* 9: CD003826.

20 Berman, B., Perez, O.A., Konda, S. et al. (2007). A review of the biologic effects, clinical efficacy, and safety of silicone elastomer sheeting for hypertrophic and keloid scar treatment and management. *Dermatol. Surg.* 33: 1291–1303.

21 Meaume, S., Le Pillouer-Prost, A., Richert, B. et al. (2014). Management of scars: updated practical guidelines and use of silicones. *Eur. J. Dermatol.* 24: 435–443.

22 Monstrey, S., Middelkoop, E., Vranckx, J.J. et al. (2014). Updated scar management practical guidelines: non-invasive and invasive measures. *J. Plast. Reconstr. Aesthet. Surg.* 67: 1017–1025.

23 Puri, N. and Talwar, A. (2009). The efficacy of silicone gel for the treatment of hypertrophic scars and keloids. *J Cutan Aesthet Surg* 2: 104–106.

24 Lyle, W.G. (2001). Plastic Surgery Educational Foundation DATA Committee. Silicone gel sheeting. *Plast. Reconstr. Surg.* 107: 272–275.

25 Musgrave, M.A., Umraw, N., Fish, J.S. et al. (2002). The effect of silicone gel sheets on perfusion of hypertrophic burn scars. *J. Burn Care Rehabil.* 23: 208–214.

26 Tandara, A.A. and Mustoe, T.A. (2008). The role of the epidermis in the control of scarring: evidence for mechanism of action for silicone gel. *J. Plast. Reconstr. Aesthet. Surg.* 61: 1219–1225.

27 Kuhn, M.A., Moffit, M.R., Smith, P.D. et al. (2001). Silicone sheeting decreases fibroblast activity and downregulates TGFbeta2 in hypertrophic scar model. *Int. J. Surg. Investig.* 2: 467–474.

28 Hanasono, M.M., Lum, J., Carroll, L.A. et al. (2004). The effect of silicone gel on basic fibroblast growth factor levels in fibroblast cell culture. *Arch. Facial Plast. Surg.* 6: 88–93.

29 Gold, M.H. (1994). A controlled clinical trial of topical silicone gel sheeting in the treatment of hypertrophic scars and keloids. *J. Am. Acad. Dermatol.* 30: 506–507.

30 Gold, M.H., Foster, T.D., Adair, M.A. et al. (2001). Prevention of hypertrophic scars and keloids by the prophylactic use of topical silicone gel sheets following a surgical procedure in an office setting. *Dermatol. Surg.* 27: 641–644.

31 Ahn, S.T., Monafo, W.W., and Mustoe, T.A. (1991). Topical silicone gel for the prevention and treatment of hypertrophic scar. *Arch. Surg.* 126: 499–504.

32 Li-Tsang, C.W., Lau, J.C., Choi, J. et al. (2006). A prospective randomized clinical trial to investigate the effect of silicone gel sheeting (Cica-Care) on post-traumatic hypertrophic scar among the Chinese population. *Burns* 32 (6): 678–683.

33 Li-Tsang, C.W., Zheng, Y.P., and Lau, J.C. (2010). A randomized clinical trial to study the effect of silicone gel dressing and pressure therapy on posttraumatic hypertrophic scars. *J. Burn Care Res.* 31 (3): 448–457.

34 Ahn, S.T., Monafo, W.W., and Mustoe, T.A. (1989). Topical silicone gel: a new treatment for hypertrophic scars. *Surgery* 106 (4): 781–786.

35 Carney, S.A., Cason, C.G., Gowar, J.P. et al. (1994). Cica-Care gel sheeting in the management of hypertrophic scarring. *Burns* 20 (2): 163–167.

36 Medhi, B., Sewal, R.K., Kaman, L. et al. (2013). Efficacy and safety of an advanced formula silicone gel for prevention of post-operative scars. *Dermatol. Ther. (Heidelb)* 3: 157–167.

37 Ketchum, L.D., Smith, J., Robinson, D.W. et al. (1966). The treatment of hypertrophic scar, keloid and scar contracture by triamcinolone acetonide. *Plast. Reconstr. Surg.* 38 (3): 209–218.

38 Jalali, M. and Bayat, A. (2007). Current use of steroids in management of abnormal raised skin scars. *Surgeon* 5 (3): 175–180.

39 Al-Attar, A., Mess, S., Thomassen, J.M. et al. (2006). Keloid pathogenesis and treatment. *Plast. Reconstr. Surg.* 117: 286–300.

40 Juckett, G. and Hartman-Adams, H. (2009). Management of keloids and hypertrophic scars. *Am. Fam. Physician* 80 (3): 253–260.

41 McCoy, B.J., Diegelmann, R.F., and Cohen, I.K. (1980). In vitro inhibition of cell growth, collagen synthesis, and prolyl hydroxylase activity by triamcinolone acetonide. *Proc. Soc. Exp. Biol. Med.* 163: 216–222.

42 Cruz, N.I. and Korchin, L. (1994). Inhibition of human keloid fibroblast growth by isotretinoin and triamcinolone acetonide in vitro. *Ann. Plast. Surg.* 33 (4): 401–405.

43 Boyadjiev, C., Popchristova, E., and Mazgalova, J. (1995). Histomorphologic changes in keloids treated with Kenacort. *J. Trauma* 38 (2): 299–302.

44 Kauh, Y.C., Rouda, S., Mondragon, G. et al. (1997). Major suppression of pro-alpha1(I) type I collagen gene expression in the dermis after keloid excision and immediate intrawound injection of triamcinolone acetonide. *J. Am. Acad. Dermatol.* 37 (4): 586–589.

45 Berman, B. and Bieley, H.C. (1995). Keloids. *J. Am. Acad. Dermatol.* 33 (1): 117–123.

46 Darzi, M.A., Chowdri, N.A., Kaul, S.K. et al. (1992). Evaluation of various methods of treating keloids and hypertrophic scars: a 10-year follow-up study. *Br. J. Plast. Surg.* 45 (5): 374–379.

47 Perdanasari, T.A., Lazzeri, D., Su, W. et al. (2014). Recent developments in the use of intralesional injections keloid treatment. *Arch. Plast. Surg.* 41 (6): 620–629.

48 Nemeth, A.J. (1993). Keloids and hypertrophic scars. *J. Dermatol. Surg. Oncol.* 19: 738–746.

49 Chowdri, N.A., Masarat, M., Mattoo, A. et al. (1999). Keloids and hypertrophic scars: results with intraoperative and serial postoperative corticosteroid injection therapy. *Aust. N. Z. J. Surg.* 69: 655–659.

50 Tang, Y.W. (1992). Intra- and postoperative steroid injections for keloids and hypertrophic scars. *Br. J. Plast. Surg.* 45 (5): 371–373.

51 Lahiri, A., Tsiliboti, D., and Gaze, N.R. (2001). Experience with difficult keloids. *Br. J. Plast. Surg.* 54: 633–635.

52 Ceilley, R.I. and Babin, R.W. (1979). The combined use of cryosurgery and intralesional injections of suspensions of fluorinated adrenocorticosteroids for reducing keloids and hypertrophic scars. *J. Dermatol. Surg. Oncol.* 5 (1): 54–56.

53 Fredman, R. and Tenenhaus, M. (2013). Cushing's syndrome after intralesional triamcinolone acetonide: a systematic review of the literature and multinational survey. *Burns* 39: 549–557.

54 Apfelberg, D.B., Maser, M.R., Lash, H. et al. (1984). Preliminary results of argon and carbon dioxide laser treatment of keloid scars. *Lasers Surg. Med.* 4 (3): 283–290.

55 Elsaie, M.L. and Choudhary, S. (2010). Lasers for scars: a review and evidence-based appraisal. *J. Drugs Dermatol.* 9: 1355–1362.

56 Alster, T.S. and Handrick, C. (2000). Laser treatment of hypertrophic scars, keloids, and striae. *Semin. Cutan. Med. Surg.* 19 (4): 287–292.

57 Jin, R., Huang, X., Li, H. et al. (2013). Laser therapy for prevention and treatment of pathologic excessive scars. *Plast. Reconstr. Surg.* 132 (6): 1747–1758.

58 Tanzi, E.L. and Alster, T.S. (2004). Laser treatment of scars. *Skin Therapy Lett.* 9: 4–7.

59 Manuskiatti, W., Wanitphakdeedecha, R., and Fitzpatrick, R.E. (2007). Effect of pulse width of a 595-nm flashlamp-pumped pulsed dye laser on the treatment response of keloidal and hypertrophic sternotomy scars. *Dermatol. Surg.* 33 (2): 152–161.

60 Nouri, K., Elsaie, M.L., Vejjabhinanta, V. et al. (2010). Comparison of the effects of short- and long-pulse durations when using a 585-nm pulsed dye laser in the treatment of new surgical scars. *Lasers Med. Sci.* 25 (1): 121–126.

61 Sobanko, J.F. and Alster, T.S. (2011). Laser treatment for improvement and minimization of facial scars. *Facial Plast. Surg. Clin. North Am.* 19: 527–542.

62 Kuo, Y.R., Wu, W.S., Jeng, S.F. et al. (2005). Suppressed TGF-beta1 expression is correlated with up-regulation of matrix metalloproteinase-13 in keloid regression after flashlamp pulsed-dye laser treatment. *Lasers Surg. Med.* 36 (1): 38–42.

63 Kuo, Y.R., Jeng, S.F., Wang, F.S. et al. (2004). Flashlamp pulsed dye laser (PDL) suppression of keloid proliferation through down-regulation of TGF-beta1 expression and extracellular matrix expression. *Lasers Surg. Med.* 34 (2): 104–108.

64 Alster, T.S. (1994). Improvement of erythematous and hypertrophic scars by the 585-nm flashlamp-pumped pulsed dye laser. *Ann. Plast. Surg.* 32: 186–190.

65 Alster, T.S. and Nanni, C.A. (1998). Pulsed dye laser treatment of hypertrophic burn scars. *Plast. Reconstr. Surg.* 102 (6): 2190–2195.

66 Gold, M.H., Berman, B., Clementoni, M.T. et al. (2014). Updated international clinical recommendations on scar management: part 1--evaluating the evidence. *Dermatol. Surg.* 40 (8): 817–824.

16

Special Dermatologic Surgery

Ramin Fathi[1], James William Behan[2], and Meena Julapalli[3]

[1]Department of Dermatology, University of Texas Southwestern Medical Center, Dallas, TX, USA
[2]Department of Dermatology, Kaiser Permanente, Pleasanton, CA, USA
[3]Department of Dermatology, Children's Hospital Colorado, University of Colorado School of Medicine, Aurora, CO, USA

16.1 Nevus Sebaceus of Jadassohn

Nevus sebaceus (NS) is a hamartoma with epithelial and nonepithelial origins that presents at birth. NS grows proportionally with the patient. Most commonly it presents as a round, oval, or linear smooth, yellowish-orange papule or plaque on the head, neck and scalp leading to alopecia [1]. While a trichoblastoma is considered to be the most common neoplasm to arise from a NS [2], malignant transformation, most commonly to a basal cell carcinoma, is a concern [3]. As a result, prophylactic excision of a NS has undergone considerable debate. The two main reasons to excise NS include concern about malignancy and undesirable cosmesis. Once a malignant lesion arises within NS, it is generally agreed that the tumor and the entire nevus should be removed. However, a review of previous literature published shows significant disagreement about prophylactic removal for malignancy [1]. In studies from the 1960–1980s, the reported incidence of BCC arising in NS ranged from 6 to 22%, but recent studies report incidence as low as 0.8% [4]. Verrucous changes are the most common reason patients and their families opt for surgical removal.

Depending on the location of the NS (i.e. in non-danger zone locations) a full-thickness excision through the subcutaneous fat with 2–3-mm margins is recommended. Technique of excision and closure depends on the location of the NS. The temporal scalp, anterior hairline, and forehead are cosmetically sensitive landmarks that can be manipulated surgically for an excellent cosmetic result [1]. Davison et al. reports the use of a rotation flap based on the superficial temporal artery as a method of reconstruction for NS located on the temporal scalp [5]. Additionally, to minimize the risk of alopecia, staples tend to be less inflammatory than absorbable sutures and are the source of closure material for some surgeons [5].

For large defects, tissue expansion may be a great option with the caveat that this requires time and multiple steps. One report discusses the use of tissue expansion with purse string closure after excision of an 11 × 13 cm NS. Initially, the authors placed an 1100 cc, 18 cm base diameter round tissue expander through an access incision in the middle of the NS between the galea and peri-cranium. After 11 weeks of expansion, the entire nevus was excised and closed with a purse string suture technique. After scar excision using another round of tissue expansion, the authors

Pediatric Dermatologic Surgery, First Edition. Edited by Keyvan Nouri, Latanya Benjamin, Jasem Alshaiji, and Jan Izakovic.

reported no evidence of alopecia with no recurrence of the tumor [6].

Some surgeons believe that the risk of malignant transformation is minimal to none and that treatment should be done only for cosmetic reasons. CO_2 laser and photodynamic therapy (PDT) have been used as a method of improving the cosmetic appearance [7–9]. These methods, however, do not remove the entire lesion, but only the part in the epidermis and papillary dermis [7].

16.2 Congenital Nevus

Congenital melanocytic nevi (CMN) appear at birth or within the first week of life and are thought to occur in 0.5–31.7% of infants [10]. They are most commonly on the trunk and extremities [11]. CMN may develop associated nonmelanocytic tumors including rhabdomyosarcoma, liposarcoma, and melanocytic tumors such as proliferative nodules and malignant melanoma. Malignant transformation, specifically melanoma risk, is stratified with CMN size placing less than 1% risk for small and medium CMNs. There is a wide range of risk for large CMNs due to heterogeneity and rarity, but it is likely less than 5% [11]. To date there is no consensus on optimal management. Most pediatric dermatologists recommend clinical monitoring of CMN and satellite nevi (including serial photography and dermoscopy), with excisional biopsy as needed for new concerning papules or nodules that appear within the nevus. Patients with large CMN should be followed for signs or symptoms suggestive of central nervous system involvement [12]. Treatment of CMN is typically undertaken for two reasons: (i) to reduce the risk of cutaneous malignant degeneration, which is controversial and unproven [13], and (ii) for cosmetic reasons [14]. Approaches can be grouped into partial or full-thickness procedures. Consideration of patient age, CMN size, location, and especially projected adult size (PAS) should help direct the choice of intervention. PAS is determined by multiplying the observed size by a factor of 2 on the head and neck and a factor of 3 on other regions [15]. Grading is typically divided into small <1.5 cm, intermediate 1.5–20 cm, large 20–40 cm, and giant CMN (GCMN) >40 cm [16]. Tromberg et al. found a significant proportion of parents felt excision worsened the appearance of the child's CMN when the PAS >20 cm; however, almost 95% of parents felt surgery was beneficial when the PAS was less than 20 cm. The same group found a 28% incidence of repigmentation at the treated wound edges [17].

When addressing both goals of reduction in malignancy risk, or more appropriately concerning phenotypic features and cosmesis, excision is considered first line [13, 14]. Timing of surgery has not been demonstrated to impact clinical or esthetic outcomes in most cases [18]. CMN <5 cm can typically be removed in one excision, whereas larger growths will require multistep procedures requiring the use of tissue expanders or serial excisions. Serial excisions for large CMN are most common on the extremities (50% of repairs) while expanded flaps are utilized more often on the head and neck (49% of repairs) [19]. Cost analysis has found equivalence between single-step excision and lifelong follow-up at four-year intervals and multistep procedures having a similar cost to a two-year interval [20]. Some recommend excisions down to fascia given sparse and controversial reports that large CMN develop melanoma at deeper levels. When approaching CMN <3 cm on the face, consideration for a multidirectional vector excision may limit the number of cosmetic units involved by reducing final scar length from a 3.00 to 4.50 ratio with traditional elliptical excision to 1.10–1.15 [21]. Key recommendations from Arad et al. include: delay of scalp excision until after the age of two to avoid undue pressure on the developing skull and possible partial involution of the CMN; the considerable risk tissue expansion on the forehead poses to developing frontal branch nerve palsy, instead using serial excision and grafts; and the importance of leaving eyebrow CMN as the removal results in substantial deformity [13].

Partial-thickness procedures include: dermatome shaving, curettage, dermabrasion, chemical peels, electrosurgery, hydrosurgery, ablative and pigment-specific lasers. These methods may reduce some of the malignant potential by removing some or most of the CMN, but the present literature does not support such claims. In fact all current reports are comparative, correlation, and case-controlled studies including expert opinion [14]. Curettage is a preferred choice among surgeons given to lower rates of bleeding and postoperative pain, but should be performed within the first eight weeks of life [12]. Similar benefits and requirements are also found with dermabrasion and hydrosurgery [12, 14, 22]. Lasers have demonstrated very good cosmesis in many situations; however, there is no consensus yet whether ablative or a combination of pigment-specific and ablative is superior [23–27]. It is important to note that there are still strong opinions regarding the danger of using lasers for CMN given the debated malignant potential, as they may make surveillance of future degeneration more difficult [25]. Use of ablative lasers as monotherapy, CO_2 and erbium-doped yttrium aluminum garnet (Er:YAG) lasers can be ideal for cosmetically sensitive and critical areas [24, 27]. Groups have also demonstrated similar success with CO_2 followed by either quality-switched (QS) ruby laser (RL), QS alexandrite laser (AL), frequency-doubled QS neodium-doped yttrium aluminum garnet laser (Nd:YAG), and pulse dye laser (PDL) followed by QSRL [23, 24, 26].

16.3 Acquired Nevi

Common acquired nevi appear after birth and increase in number over the first two decades of life [28] with an association of nevus count with phototype, sun exposure, and sun protection behavior [29]. A nevus with unusual clinical features should be considered for biopsy, which may reveal features of a dysplastic nevus [30]. The presence of dysplastic nevi confers a slightly increased overall risk for melanoma [31]. However, the risk of any individual nevus turning into a melanoma is quite small: for a dysplastic nevus the lifetime transformation risk is approximately 1 in 10 000 (varying with grade of atypia) [32]. An important theory to consider when clinically assessing dysplastic-appearing nevi is that many patients have a predominant phenotype regarded as signature nevi. Selecting nevi with atypia deviating from the signature nevi, the "ugly duckling", is a well-accepted approach [33].

Aside from excision, nevi that are cosmetically concerning have been successfully treated with lasers. However, this practice is not reported in the United States. A group from Amsterdam achieved complete clearance with adverse effects of hypopigmentation using a QSRL followed by normal mode (NM) RL [34], while a Turkish group reported short pulse Er:YAG improved cosmesis in 96% of patients with hyperpigmentation as an adverse effect [35].

16.4 Spitz Nevus

Prior to the seminal article by Sophie Spitz [36], these lesions were referred to as juvenile melanomas [37]. Spitz nevus is an uncommon, benign melanocytic neoplasm that shares many clinical and histological features with melanoma [38]. Initially described as pink [36], these lesions can range from brown to black and form a spectrum of distinct entities encompassing Spitz nevi, atypical Spitz nevi and spitzoid melanoma, which range from benign to malignant [39]. This presents clinical ambiguity that makes the diagnosis and management of the patient difficult. There is a wide variance of management depending on patient age, nevus size and whether dermatologists or general and plastic surgeons are making recommendations based on surveys [40, 41].

Most pediatric dermatologists recommend excisional biopsy for suspected Spitz nevi in post-pubertal patients and in a child of any age with atypical features (size larger than

1 cm, rapid evolution, asymmetry, pain, or ulceration) [12], whereas general and plastic surgeons recommend wide local excision with 5 mm margins as a minimum management, allowing for exceptions in cosmetically sensitive areas [39]. While some advocate for dermoscopy to aid in management [42], one study found a 13.3% incidence of melanoma in the excision of symmetric spitzoid tumors assessed with dermoscopy, with a probability that increases to 50% in patients greater than 50 years of age [43]. The role of sentinel lymph node biopsy (SLNB) is very controversial, with no defined routine benefit [44].

16.5 Hemangiomas

Infantile hemangiomas (IH) are the most common tumor of infancy, affecting 4–10% of full-term infants in the United States [45]. IH uniquely co-expresses glucose transporter protein 1 (GLUT-1) and other markers with placenta [46]. The only vascular anomaly that expresses GLUT-1 is IH, making this an important marker to histologically confirm a diagnosis of IH. The natural history of IH consists of a period of rapid postnatal proliferation followed by a phase of involution. In addition to the phase of its natural history and anatomic site, IHs are described by the degree of cutaneous involvement. Superficial IHs are limited to the superficial dermis and can be thick. Deep IHs involve the deep dermis and subcutaneous layers and without overlying skin involvement. Compound or mixed IHs involve both the superficial and deep layers. Congenital hemangiomas (CH) are grouped into rapidly involuting (RICH) and non-involuting (NICH). They are present at birth and will be covered briefly.

Management for IH can be divided into observation, medical therapy (which is outside the scope of this section), lasers, and surgery. Universal application of the "leave it alone, it will go away" approach is no longer accepted [47]. The management goal for IH is to achieve a functionally and esthetically acceptable final result with the least amount of morbidity and lowest likelihood of complications. Ideally intervention is pursued before a child's development of self-image, which begins at age 2.5–3 years, or before the social pressures of school at 5–6 years, to minimize the psychological effects of these lesions [48]. There is approximately a 16% rate of ulceration which can be lowered in some cases if kept hydrated with petrolatum [49].

The most commonly used laser is PDL, with the greatest effect on the superficial components of the tumor, with decreasing efficacy in tumors greater than 3 mm [50] and no effect in deep lesions without a superficial component [47]. There are ranges of regimens that involve serial treatments every two to six weeks, beginning during the proliferation phase, with each session proceeding until the development of purpura. There is some data that suggests the final outcome of PDL treatment is not significantly different then observation, however, there is agreement that the time course is hastened [25, 51, 52] and early initiation is reported to increase the rate of ulceration [53]. However, PDL also has a definitive role in treating ulcerated IHs and residual telangiectasias after involution [54]. An example setup used by Brauer et al. involves local anesthesia, 9.0–10.5 J/cm^2, 0.45 ms pulse, 7 mm spot size with a two-week interval for 2–12 sessions with a maximum improvement of 90% [55]. However, initiation settings with lower fluence spaced four weeks apart are more typically deployed. Nd:YAG has also gained popularity, especially during the involution phase. Care should be taken if applied during the proliferation phase, as ulceration is a common adverse event [25]. Burns et al. recommend general anesthesia in an operating room with initial settings at 80 J/cm^2, 50 ms pulse, at a frequency of 1 Hz, 6 mm spot size [25]. Contour irregularities can be further treated effectively with Fraxel [56, 57]. CHs often require no treatment but the involuted stage can be managed in a similar fashion to IH [57].

Surgical treatment and timeline is controversial [56] but is more commonly applied to the involuting rather than proliferating lesion. The use of tissue expanders or free tissue transfers is rarely needed as serial excisions spaced three to four months apart is more common place, with an average of three excisions [47]. Alternatively, circular excision on the face followed by purse string closure yields acceptable resolution, and greater than 50% of parents never elect to re-excise for a linear scar [58]. Cosmetically sensitive areas that provide additional challenge include the lip and nasal tip. When the vermilion is not crossed additional surgical principles include: (i) maintaining central fullness, utilizing a bi-lobed wedge resection rather than a lenticular wedge resection; (ii) placement of the scar in the mucosa, directing any correction or standing cone deformity toward the mucosa instead of the vermilion border to maintain contour. Hemangiomas that cross the vermillio-cutaneous (VC) junction should be staged to first re-align the VC junction, and then excise the standing cones, camouflaging the cutaneous scar in the VC junction [59].

16.6 Pyogenic Granulomas

Pyogenic Granuloma (PG) is also referred to as lobular capillary hemangioma [60]. PG is a solitary red papule that grows rapidly, forming a stalk. It initially resembles telangiectasias with a very small, flat central erythematous macule that develops into a thin papule. While PG can occur at any time in life, there is a bimodal distribution in childhood that peaks at 1 year of age and again between 11 and 12 years of age, with the great majority of the tumors developing on the head and neck and upper extremities [61].

There are numerous treatment modalities published with varying rates of recurrence and cosmesis. While excision can provide up to a 0% recurrence in some studies [62, 63], overall recurrence was noted at 3.6% [61]. PG is known to be highly recurrent with rates as high as 43.5% [62]. This is due in part to a common involvement of the reticular dermis, making excision the definitive treatment [49, 62, 64]. When first apparent, PG is amenable to the PDL (585-nmwavelength) as a very effective tool to eliminate the lesion [64]. However, many groups recommend the histopathologic diagnosis to rule out malignancies like amelonotic melanoma [61]. As PG continues to grow it is usually complicated by ulceration and bleeding; it also causes a visible deformity because it is commonly located on the face [49]. Other therapeutic approaches like shave excision followed by photocoagulation has a reported 5% recurrence rate and still maintains the ability to confirm the diagnosis [65]. Combined continuous-wave/pulsed CO_2 laser in 98 patients, had no recurrence, ~10% rate of slight textural change in skin and 100% patient satisfaction with settings starting in continuous mode at 15 W, then pulse mode: pulse length 0.6–0.9 ms, energy fluence 500 mJ/pulse [66]. Other methods of intervention include topical agents, sclerotherapy, Nd:YAG, and cryotherapy, but are reported as small case series [67].

16.7 Vascular Malformations

Unlike a vascular tumor, vascular malformations (VM) arise via dysmorphogenesis, while exhibiting normal endothelial turnover [68]. VMs have a tendency to grow with the child and after the individual has attained full growth, the VMs remain stable throughout life. Unlike hemangiomas, they do not regress, but some enlargement may occur in response to trauma or hormonal disturbances during puberty or pregnancy [69].

For venous malformations, sclerotherapy is the mainstay of treatment, including detergents sclerosants, ethanol and bleomycin. Absolute alcohol and sodium tetradecyl sulfate (STS) are most commonly used as the sclerosing agent, with success rates of 30–95% [70] in an average of two to four sessions [71]. STS agent is preferred by many due to its less toxic profile, with lower reported rates of skin necrosis, neurological complications, and systemic complications [72]; however, there are reports of anaphylaxis [73]. For treating more of the superficial component, lasers are becoming more common. Nd:YAG penetrating up to 10 mm results in deep vessel coagulation in vessels up to 3 mm, underlying prudent use since dermal damage is a risk [25]. Care should also be taken to avoid overcooling the treatment area as this might inadvertently protect the target vessel. Burns et al. recommends 10–12 °C [25].

For capillary malformations, the most common being the port-wine stain (PWS), PDL with epidermal cooling is the mainstay of treatment [25]. Most patients require multiple treatments (typically at least four to six) at four- to eight-week intervals, with each treatment bringing about interval lightening of the birthmark [12] up to an average of 40–55% reduction in color difference from unaffected skin [74]. Although PDL is effective, most PWS gradually redarken after laser treatments are discontinued, necessitating additional treatments in adolescence or adulthood [75].

16.8 Epidermal Nevus

An epidermal nevus (EN) is a developmental hamartoma that is relatively common. They present early in life with a predilection for the neck, trunk, and extremities. They may present as one to many small warty brown or pale papules or plaques, either isolated or in a pattern (e.g. linear, zosteriform, blashkoid). Typically, treatments used include topical agents such as retinoic acid or 5-fluorouracil, but small lesions can be removed by surgical excision [76]. Surgical excision was reported in a child with systematized EN with a partial-thickness skin excision. While the areas treated remained disease-free on long-term follow-up, they did heal with hypertrophic scars and keloids [77].

A study of 43 patients reported efficacy with argon-laser coagulation and carbon dioxide laser vaporization for EN. The argon laser was more effective for "soft" lesions on palpation whereas the carbon dioxide laser was more effective for "hard" lesions. The carbon dioxide laser has an increased risk of hypertrophic scarring [78, 79]. The pulsed RL has also been reported as effective in treating five patients with EN. One patient, who had dark pigmentation, experienced depigmentation as a side effect [80]. Er:YAG laser treatment has also been used with some success. In one study, after a single laser treatment, successful elimination of verrucous EN was observed in 15/20 patients, with a post-operative healing time of 7–10 days. Adverse effects included postinflammatory hyperpigmentation and hypopigmentation, mild to moderate acne flaring, and no reported scarring [81].

Some studies discussed cryotherapy with success in a patient with both EN and inflammatory linear verrucous EN (ILVEN) [76, 82]. A typical cryotherapy regimen consisted of two cycles of an open spray technique, 10–15 seconds each. No scarring was reported, but postinflammatory hypopigmentation occurred in a patient with phototype IV. Postoperative healing time was typically 10–20 days [76]. PDT has also been reported as successful [83].

16.9 Aplasia Cutis

Aplasia cutis congenita (ACC) is a rare congenital disorder, which most commonly involves the scalp, and can affect the galea, the pericranium, the bone, and the dura mater. Although ACC can be located anywhere in the body, in the vast majority (84%) of cases, the defect is found on the scalp [84]. The nonscalp ACC lesions mainly involve the trunk and/or extremities; are usually large, bilateral, and symmetric; and are often associated with epidermolysis bullosa [85]. While a classification of nine different groups of ACC based on the location and presence of other abnormalities [86] exists, this section will focus on scalp management.

The mortality rate of patients with ACC is estimated as high as 20–55%, resulting from associated congenital defects, meningitis, or bleeding from the sagittal sinus secondary to surgical intervention or separation and erosion of desiccated eschar [87]. The presence of a hair collar suggests dysraphism of the skull with the possible presence of ectopic neural tissue [88]. ACC of the scalp should be allowed to heal by secondary intention, when possible, using conservative wound care such as twice daily petrolatum, silver sulfadiazine, or bacitracin application. Petrolatum is considered the best choice because of the low risk of contact allergy or systemic absorption [88]. After healing of the ACC, scar revision may be considered. This might be especially helpful on the scalp due to alopecia over the scar [89]. Silberstein et al. has proposed a new five-level grading classification system subdividing scalp involvement to help direct therapy in a more standardized fashion [90] according to size of defect, layers involved, and involvement of veins. Immediate surgical intervention with allograft, skin substitute, or flap reconstruction was indicated if there was venous involvement with sagittal sinus or brain exposure.

16.10 Dermoid Cysts

Scalp dermoid cysts (DC) are subcutaneous sacs lined with a stratified squamous epithelium. They contain developmentally mature ectodermal tissues, including skin, hair follicles, sweat glands, and sebaceous glands. They are generally benign. Most often they are located on the head, but they can also arise on the neck or trunk [91]. Typically they are limited to an extracranial location and management generally involves simple excision, however, there is a potential for intracranial and/or intradural extension. Preoperative imaging studies are required for lesions on the nose, midline scalp or posterior axis in order to exclude a connection to the CNS [92]. DCs most often remain stable for years, but they may become symptomatic as a result of enlargement and rupture. Rarely, they may extend into surrounding tissues [91].

The periorbital lesion is one of the most commonly approached locations of a dermoid cyst. Traditionally, the surgical approach most commonly used has been incising above the mass. This can lead to a visible scar [93]. A brow technique hiding the incision above, below, or through the brow has also been well documented. However, this may lead to eyebrow follicle damage and subsequent alopecia. Additionally, a scar below the eyebrow would be more evident in females who undergo mechanical hair removal [94]. A superior eyelid incision seems to afford the best esthetic result [95]. Nelson et al. describe 34 patients who underwent a DC removal through this incision, also known as a blepharoplasty incision. They demonstrate great efficacy, with an average surgical time of 30 minutes. Mechanical ptosis was the most commonly encountered problem as it occurred in three patients; however, all cases completely resolved [93]. Endoscopic excision is also an option for surgical excision of any benign dermal tumor of the forehead and cheek [96]. In many cases, the cyst may be adherent to the underlying periosteum. The use of a periosteal elevator can aid in delicately removing these lesions without rupturing the cyst wall [93].

Foam sclerotherapy has been used with success in patients who did not want to undergo excision. One study of four patients reports a technique of aspirating the ectodermal contents with an 18-gauge needle, followed by saline lavage, and intraluminal foam sclerotherapy with STS (30 mg/ml) in a proportion of 10% of the total aspirate volume [97]. At 13 months, there were no recurrences.

16.11 Pilomatricoma

Pilomatricomas frequently occur as a solitary, small tumor on the face or upper extremities of people younger than 20 years old [98]. This lesion is described as a tumor with differentiation toward hair cells [99]. Most commonly, they present as a hard, subcutaneous, slowly growing nodule or mass [100]. Rarely, these lesions can develop to a giant size that resembles a malignant tumor [98, 101]. Occasionally, these tumors can undergo malignant transformation to a pilomatrix carcinoma [102]. Multiple pilomatricomas can also occur [103].

Surgical excision is the treatment of choice but the location of the lesion dictates management [100]. Mohs micrographic surgery (MMS) has also been used in cosmetically sensitive areas [104]. One report of patient with a 5 × 4 × 4 cm pilomatricoma of the earlobe was treated with excision and reconstructed with a posterior-superior pedicled skin flap [99]. When these tumors arise in the brow or forehead, endoscopic excision using brow-lift techniques have been used with success to preserve cosmesis. The procedure can be done with a single small scalp incision 2 cm posterior to the hairline [105].

Recurrence after surgical excision is low. Pilomatrical carcinoma should be considered in the case of local recurrence [106]. In the rare event of a pilomatrix carcinoma, complete excision is prudent to prevent local invasion and metastasis. While no specific guidelines exist, MMS may provide optimal treatment of this neoplasm given the ability to have 100% margin control [107, 108].

16.12 Giant Juvenile Xanthogranuloma

Juvenile Xanthogranuloma (JXG) is a non-Langerhans histiocytosis occurring predominantly in infancy and early childhood. It is usually an asympomatic, red-brown papule which slowly enlarges to a diameter of 1–2 cm. Evolution into a yellow-brown papule, plaque, or nodule often occurs, followed by spontaneous resolution that may leave an atrophic scar, hyperpigmentation, or anetoderma [109, 110].

Giant JXGs have been reported in the literature [111–115]. These tumors are defined as JXGs that are larger than 2 cm. Lesions as large as 10 cm have been reported [114]. This variant can be exophytic or endophytic [116]. With any JXG, extracutaneous involvement occurs in 5% of cases, and the eye represents the most affected site [110]. Surgical excision does not seem to be a viable option as these lesions tend to regress spontaneously. One study discusses the use of CO_2 laser to effectively treat multiple JXG, but with larger lesions this technique should be used with caution [117].

16.13 Epidermolysis Bullosa

Epidermolysis bullosa (EB) comprises a group of genetic blistering disorders of the skin and mucosa following mild mechanical trauma. Some forms of EB are associated with significant morbidity and mortality either directly or indirectly due to EB. Because of the potential for severe blistering, causes of mortality usually occur secondary to infections, organ dysfunction, and squamous cell carcinoma (SCC). The current mainstay of management is based on protection, avoidance of provoking factors, and wound care [118]. The use of tissue-engineered skin (Apligraf; Organogenesis Inc., Canton, Mass) as a wound dressing has been used with success as opposed to conventional dressings to induce rapid healing, with minimal adverse effects [118, 119].

Of note, recessive dystrophic EB (RDEB) and more severe EB classically present with widespread scarring with concomitant formation of SCC. While it is unusual before the second or third decade of life, it has been described in a 6-year-old child [120]. The cumulative risk of developing SCC in RDEB is 90% by age 55. These SCCs tend to be aggressive and multifocal. A high degree of suspicion should be present when tending to the chronic wounds of these patients [120]. These SCCs should be treated as if they were arising in a scar and are, as a result, considered high risk. MMS, surgical excision, radiation therapy, electrodesiccation and curettage, and cryosurgery have been used as primary surgical options for SCCs [121–123]. For surgical excision, margins should be 6 mm for high-risk tumors [121].

16.14 Basal Cell Nevus Syndrome

Basal cell nevus syndrome (BCNS), also known as Gorlin syndrome, is a condition defined by dysregulated hedgehog signaling. This pathway is the pivotal molecular abnormality underlying basal cell carcinomas (BCCs) and thus patients with BCNS develop multiple, aggressive BCCs at a young age [124].

While many treatment options are available for BCCs, this widespread involvement brings forth a conundrum when discussing treatment options for BCNS patients. MMS or wide local excision [125], while the standards of care for many BCCs, may not be feasible in patients with diffuse neoplastic disease. Thus, discussion with the patient and their family about available treatment options are paramount.

PDT with 5-aminolevulinic acid (ALA) has been used in multiple studies with excellent results for patients with BCNS [126–128]. Ultrapulse CO_2 laser may be an option for small BCCs in low-risk areas for patients with BCNS with minimal scarring [129]. For smaller BCCs of the face, pulsed dye laser (PDL), alexandrite, neodymium (Nd), or Nd:YAG laser irradiation have shown to be effective with acceptable cosmetic results [130–132]. CO_2 has also been used for facial BCCs in a patient with BCNS with acceptable cosmesis [133]. Dermabrasion may also be considered an option [134]. Superficial BCCs can be treated with topical imiquimod or 5-fluorouracil (5-FU) [135, 136]. Cryosurgery may be considered for some patients because of the quickness, relative safety and low cost [137, 138]. Combined curettage and excision remains a mainstay of therapy as well for primary BCCs [139].

Vismodegib, a SMO-inhibitor targeting the hedgehog pathway, has been shown to reduce BCC tumor burden and block the growth of new BCCs in patients with BCNS. Near-complete regression of BCNS-associated odontogenic keratocysts are also possible with vismodegib [140]. Most commonly seen adverse events include loss of taste, muscle cramps, hair loss, and weight loss [124]. One can also consider systemic retinoid to prevent new BCCs from appearing [141].

16.15 Dermatofibrosarcoma Protuberans

Dermatofibrosarcoma protuberans (DFSP) is a rare, slow-growing, painless, dermal tumor that typically arises in the third to fifth decade. It characteristically invades local tissue by direct extension and can degenerate into a malignant fibrosarcoma capable of regional and distant metastasis. MMS has the highest cure rates, ranging from 93.4 to 100% [142–146]. Wide local excision (>3 cm margins) and radiation therapy have been used with lower efficacy than MMS [147, 148]. Imatinib therapy has been used in some studies, either as a neoadjuvant therapy or alone in unresectable cases [149, 150].

References

1 Moody, M.N., Landau, J.M., and Goldberg, L.H. (2012). Nevus sebaceous revisited. *Pediatric Dermatology* 29 (1): 15–23.

2 Jaqueti, G., Requena, L., and Sanchez Yus, E. (2000). Trichoblastoma is the most common neoplasm developed in nevus sebaceus of Jadassohn: a clinicopathologic study of a series of 155 cases. *The American Journal of Dermatopathology* 22 (2): 108–118.

3 Alessi, E., Wong, S.N., Advani, H.H. et al. (1988). Nevus sebaceus is associated with unusual neoplasms. An atlas. *The American Journal of Dermatopathology* 10 (2): 116–127.

4 Rosen, H., Schmidt, B., Lam, H.P. et al. (2009). Management of nevus sebaceous and the risk of basal cell carcinoma: an 18-year review. *Pediatric Dermatology* 26 (6): 676–681.

5 Davison, S.P., Khachemoune, A., Yu, D. et al. (2005). Nevus sebaceus of Jadassohn revisited with reconstruction options. *International Journal of Dermatology* 44 (2): 145–150.
6 Donelan, M.B. and Garcia, J.A. (2008). Purse-string closure of scalp defects following tissue expansion: an effective aesthetic alternative. *Journal of Plastic, Reconstructive & Aesthetic Surgery: JPRAS* 61 (4): 419–422.
7 Ashinoff, R. (1993). Linear nevus sebaceus of Jadassohn treated with the carbon dioxide laser. *Pediatric Dermatology* 10 (2): 189–191.
8 Dierickx, C.C., Goldenhersh, M., Dwyer, P. et al. (1999). Photodynamic therapy for nevus sebaceus with topical delta-aminolevulinic acid. *Archives of Dermatology* 135 (6): 637–640.
9 In, S.I., Lee, J.Y., and Kim, Y.C. (2010). Topical photodynamic therapy for nevus sebaceous on the face. *European Journal of Dermatology: EJD* 20 (5): 590–592.
10 Pride, H.B., Tollefson, M., and Silverman, R. (2013). What's new in pediatric dermatology?: part I. Diagnosis and pathogenesis. *Journal of the American Academy of Dermatology* 68 (6): 885. e1–12; quiz 97–8.
11 Alikhan, A., Ibrahimi, O.A., and Eisen, D.B. (2012). Congenital melanocytic nevi: where are we now? Part I. Clinical presentation, epidemiology, pathogenesis, histology, malignant transformation, and neurocutaneous melanosis. *Journal of the American Academy of Dermatology* 67: 495–884. e1–17; quiz 512–4.
12 Mann, J.A. (2014). Update on pediatric dermatologic surgery from tots to teens. *Current Opinion in Pediatrics* 26 (4): 452–459.
13 Arad, E. and Zuker, R.M. (2014). The shifting paradigm in the management of giant congenital melanocytic nevi: review and clinical applications. *Plastic and Reconstructive Surgery* 133 (2): 367–376.
14 Ibrahimi, O.A., Alikhan, A., and Eisen, D.B. (2012). Congenital melanocytic nevi: where are we now? Part II. Treatment options and approach to treatment. *Journal of the American Academy of Dermatology* 67 (4): 515. e1–13; quiz 28–30.
15 Castilla, E.E., da Graca Dutra, M., and Orioli-Parreiras, I.M. (1981). Epidemiology of congenital pigmented naevi: I. Incidence rates and relative frequencies. *The British Journal of Dermatology* 104 (3): 307–315.
16 Ruiz-Maldonado, R. (2004). Measuring congenital melanocytic nevi. *Pediatric Dermatology* 21 (2): 178–179.
17 Tromberg, J., Bauer, B., Benvenuto-Andrade, C. et al. (2005). Congenital melanocytic nevi needing treatment. *Dermatologic Therapy* 18 (2): 136–150.
18 Berg, P. and Lindelöf, B. (2002). Congenital nevocytic nevi: follow-up of a Swedish birth register sample regarding etiologic factors, discomfort, and removal rate. *Pediatric Dermatology* 19 (4): 293–297.
19 Gosain, A.K., Santoro, T.D., Larson, D.L. et al. (2001). Giant congenital nevi: a 20-year experience and an algorithm for their management. *Plastic and Reconstructive Surgery* 108 (3): 622–636.
20 Roldan, F.A., Hernando, A.B., Cuadrado, A. et al. (2009). Small and medium-sized congenital nevi in children: a comparison of the costs of excision and long-term follow-up. *Dermatologic Surgery* 35 (12): 1867–1872.
21 Oh, S.I. and Lee, Y.H. (2013). Multidirectional vector excision leads to better outcomes than traditional elliptical excision of facial congenital melanocytic nevus. *Archives of Plastic Surgery* 40 (5): 570–574.
22 Coyette, M., Elajmi, A., Bayet, B., and Lengele, B. (2014). Hydrosurgery, a new therapeutic perspective in early care of giant congenital nevi: a preliminary series of four cases. *Journal of Plastic, Reconstructive & Aesthetic Surgery* 67 (8): 1063–1069.
23 Al-Hadithy, N., Al-Nakib, K., and Quaba, A. (2012). Outcomes of 52 patients with congenital melanocytic naevi treated with UltraPulse carbon dioxide and frequency-doubled Q-switched Nd-Yag laser. *Journal of Plastic, Reconstructive & Aesthetic Surgery* 65 (8): 1019–1028.

24 Arora, H., Falto-Aizpurua, L., Chacon, A. et al. (2014). Lasers for nevi: a review. *Lasers in Medical Science*.

25 Burns, A.J. and Navarro, J.A. (2009). Role of laser therapy in pediatric patients. *Plastic and Reconstructive Surgery* 124 (1 Suppl): 82e–92e.

26 Funayama, E., Sasaki, S., Furukawa, H. et al. (2012). Effectiveness of combined pulsed dye and Q-switched ruby laser treatment for large to giant congenital melanocytic naevi. *The British Journal of Dermatology* 167 (5): 1085–1091.

27 Zeng, Y. and Zheng, Y.Q. (2014). Successful treatment of congenital melanocytic nevus on tragus with CO_2 laser. *The Journal of Dermatological Treatment* 25 (4): 287–289.

28 English, D.R. and Armstrong, B.K. (1994). Melanocytic nevi in children. I. Anatomic sites and demographic and host factors. *American Journal of Epidemiology* 139 (4): 390–401.

29 Oliveria, S.A., Satagopan, J.M., Geller, A.C. et al. (2009). Study of Nevi in Children (SONIC): baseline findings and predictors of nevus count. *American Journal of Epidemiology* 169 (1): 41–53.

30 Hawryluk, E.B. and Liang, M.G. (2014). Pediatric melanoma, moles, and sun safety. *Pediatric Clinics of North America* 61 (2): 279–291.

31 Tucker, M.A., Halpern, A., Holly, E.A. et al. (1997). Clinically recognized dysplastic nevi. A central risk factor for cutaneous melanoma. *Journal of the American Medical Association* 277 (18): 1439–1444.

32 Tsao, H., Bevona, C., Goggins, W. et al. (2003). The transformation rate of moles (melanocytic nevi) into cutaneous melanoma: a population-based estimate. *Archives of Dermatology* 139 (3): 282–288.

33 Suh, K.Y. and Bolognia, J.L. (2009). Signature nevi. *Journal of the American Academy of Dermatology* 60 (3): 508–514.

34 Westerhof, W. and Gamei, M. (2003). Treatment of acquired junctional melanocytic naevi by Q-switched and normal mode ruby laser. *The British Journal of Dermatology* 148 (1): 80–85.

35 Baba, M. and Bal, N. (2006). Efficacy and safety of the short-pulse erbium: YAG laser in the treatment of acquired melanocytic nevi. *Dermatologic Surgery* 32 (2): 256–260.

36 Spitz, S. (1948). Melanomas of childhood. *The American Journal of Pathology* 24 (3): 591–609.

37 Barnhill, R.L. (2006). The Spitzoid lesion: rethinking Spitz tumors, atypical variants, "Spitzoid melanoma" and risk assessment. *Modern Pathology* 19 (Suppl 2): S21–S33.

38 Spatz, A., Calonje, E., Handfield-Jones, S. et al. (1999). Spitz tumors in children: a grading system for risk stratification. *Archives of Dermatology* 135 (3): 282–285.

39 Joyce, D.P., Prichard, R.S., Gulmann, C. et al. (2013). The surgical management of Spitz naevi and atypical spitzoid neoplasms: a review of the literature. *The Surgeon* 11 (4): 205–209.

40 Metzger, A.T., Kane, A.A., and Bayliss, S.J. (2013). Differences in treatment of Spitz nevi and atypical Spitz tumors in pediatric patients among dermatologists and plastic surgeons. *JAMA Dermatology* 149 (11): 1348–1350.

41 Tlougan, B.E., Orlow, S.J., and Schaffer, J.V. (2013). Spitz nevi: beliefs, behaviors, and experiences of pediatric dermatologists. *JAMA Dermatology* 149 (3): 283–291.

42 Nino, M., Brunetti, B., Delfino, S. et al. (2009). Spitz nevus: follow-up study of 8 cases of childhood starburst type and proposal for management. *Dermatology* 218 (1): 48–51.

43 Lallas, A., Moscarella, E., Longo, C. et al. (2015). Likelihood of finding melanoma when removing a Spitzoid-looking lesion in patients aged 12 years or older. *Journal of the American Academy of Dermatology* 72 (1): 47–53.

44 Massi, D., Tomasini, C., Senetta, R. et al. (2015). Atypical Spitz tumors in patients younger than 18 years. *Journal of the American Academy of Dermatology* 72 (1): 37–46.

45 Kilcline, C. and Frieden, I.J. (2008). Infantile hemangiomas: how common are they? A systematic review of the medical literature. *Pediatric Dermatology* 25 (2): 168–173.

46 North, P.E., Waner, M., Mizeracki, A. et al. (2001). A unique microvascular phenotype shared by juvenile hemangiomas and human placenta. *Archives of Dermatology* 137 (5): 559–570.

47 Hochman, M. (2014). Infantile hemangiomas: current management. *Facial Plastic Surgery Clinics of North America* 22 (4): 509–521.

48 Hochman, M., Adams, D.M., and Reeves, T.D. (2011). Current knowledge and management of vascular anomalies: I. Hemangiomas. *Archives of Facial Plastic Surgery* 13 (3): 145–151.

49 Greene, A.K. (2011). Management of hemangiomas and other vascular tumors. *Clinics in Plastic Surgery* 38 (1): 45–63.

50 Garden, J.M., Bakus, A.D., and Paller, A.S. (1992). Treatment of cutaneous hemangiomas by the flashlamp-pumped pulsed dye laser: prospective analysis. *The Journal of Pediatrics* 120 (4 Pt 1): 555–560.

51 Anderson, R.R. (2006). Infant hemangiomas: a controversy worth solving. *Lasers in Surgery and Medicine* 38 (2): 92–93.

52 Batta, K., Goodyear, H.M., and Moss, C. (2002). Randomised controlled study of early pulsed dye laser treatment of uncomplicated childhood haemangiomas: results of a 1-year analysis. *Lancet* 360 (9332): 521–527.

53 Witman, P.M., Wagner, A.M., and Scherer, K. (2006). Complications following pulsed dye laser treatment of superficial hemangiomas. *Lasers in Surgery and Medicine* 38 (2): 116–123.

54 David, L.R., Malek, M.M., and Argenta, L.C. (2003). Efficacy of pulse dye laser therapy for the treatment of ulcerated haemangiomas: a review of 78 patients. *British Journal of Plastic Surgery* 56 (4): 317–327.

55 Brauer, J.A. and Geronemus, R.G. (2013). Laser treatment in the management of infantile hemangiomas and capillary vascular malformations. *Techniques in Vascular and Interventional Radiology* 16 (1): 51–54.

56 Blei, F. and Guarini, A. (2014). Current workup and therapy of infantile hemangiomas. *Clinics in Dermatology* 32 (4): 459–470.

57 Liang, M.G. and Frieden, I.J. (2014). Infantile and congenital hemangiomas. *Seminars in Pediatric Surgery* 23 (4): 162–167.

58 Mulliken, J.B., Rogers, G.F., and Marler, J.J. (2002). Circular excision of hemangioma and purse-string closure: the smallest possible scar. *Plastic and Reconstructive Surgery* 109 (5): 1544–1554; discussion 55.

59 Chang, C.S., Wong, A., Rohde, C.H. et al. (2012). Management of lip hemangiomas: minimizing peri-oral scars. *Journal of Plastic, Reconstructive & Aesthetic Surgery* 65 (2): 163–168.

60 Mills, S.E., Cooper, P.H., and Fechner, R.E. (1980). Lobular capillary hemangioma: the underlying lesion of pyogenic granuloma. A study of 73 cases from the oral and nasal mucous membranes. *The American Journal of Surgical Pathology* 4 (5): 470–479.

61 Giblin, A.V., Clover, A.J., Athanassopoulos, A. et al. (2007). Pyogenic granuloma – the quest for optimum treatment: audit of treatment of 408 cases. *Journal of Plastic, Reconstructive & Aesthetic Surgery* 60 (9): 1030–1035.

62 Patrice, S.J., Wiss, K., and Mulliken, J.B. (1991). Pyogenic granuloma (lobular capillary hemangioma): a clinicopathologic study of 178 cases. *Pediatric Dermatology* 8 (4): 267–276.

63 Pagliai, K.A. and Cohen, B.A. (2004). Pyogenic granuloma in children. *Pediatric Dermatology* 21 (1): 10–13.

64 Hochman, M. (2012). Management of vascular tumors. *Facial Plastic Surgery* 28 (6): 584–589.

65 Kirschner, R.E. and Low, D.W. (1999). Treatment of pyogenic granuloma by shave excision and laser photocoagulation. *Plastic and Reconstructive Surgery* 104 (5): 1346–1349.

66 Raulin, C., Greve, B., and Hammes, S. (2002). The combined continuous-wave/pulsed carbon dioxide laser for treatment of pyogenic granuloma. *Archives of Dermatology* 138 (1): 33–37.

67 Lee, J., Sinno, H., Tahiri, Y. et al. (2011). Treatment options for cutaneous pyogenic granulomas: a review. *Journal of Plastic, Reconstructive & Aesthetic Surgery* 64 (9): 1216–1220.

68 Mulliken, J.B. and Glowacki, J. (1982). Classification of pediatric vascular lesions. *Plastic and Reconstructive Surgery* 70 (1): 120–121.

69 Mulliken, J.B., Fishman, S.J., and Burrows, P.E. (2000). Vascular anomalies. *Current Problems in Surgery* 37 (8): 517–584.

70 Legiehn, G.M. and Heran, M.K. (2006). Classification, diagnosis, and interventional radiologic management of vascular malformations. *The Orthopedic Clinics of North America* 37 (3): 435–474, vii–viii.

71 Kumar, S., Kumar, V., Kumar, S. et al. (2014). Management strategy for facial venous malformations. *National Journal of Maxillofacial Surgery* 5 (1): 93–96.

72 Berenguer, B., Burrows, P.E., Zurakowski, D. et al. (1999). Sclerotherapy of craniofacial venous malformations: complications and results. *Plastic and Reconstructive Surgery* 104 (1): 1–11; discussion 2–5.

73 Koerper, M.A., Addiego, J.E. Jr., deLorimier, A.A. et al. (1983). Use of aspirin and dipyridamole in children with platelet trapping syndromes. *The Journal of Pediatrics* 102 (2): 311–314.

74 Nguyen, C.M., Yohn, J.J., Huff, C. et al. (1998). Facial port-wine stains in childhood: prediction of the rate of improvement as a function of the age of the patient, size and location of the port-wine stain and the number of treatments with the pulsed dye (585 nm) laser. *The British Journal of Dermatology* 138 (5): 821–825.

75 Huikeshoven, M., Koster, P.H., de Borgie, C.A. et al. (2007). Redarkening of port-wine stains 10 years after pulsed-dye-laser treatment. *The New England Journal of Medicine* 356 (12): 1235–1240.

76 Panagiotopoulos, A., Chasapi, V., Nikolaou, V. et al. (2009). Assessment of cryotherapy for the treatment of verrucous epidermal naevi. *Acta Dermato-Venereologica* 89 (3): 292–294.

77 Dellon, A.L., Luethke, R., Wong, L. et al. (1992). Epidermal nevus: surgical treatment by partial-thickness skin excision. *Annals of Plastic Surgery* 28 (3): 292–296; discussion 6.

78 Hohenleutner, U. and Landthaler, M. (1993). Laser therapy of verrucous epidermal naevi. *Clinical and Experimental Dermatology* 18 (2): 124–127.

79 Paradela, S., Del Pozo, J., Fernandez-Jorge, B. et al. (2007). Epidermal nevi treated by carbon dioxide laser vaporization: a series of 25 patients. *The Journal of Dermatological Treatment* 18 (3): 169–174.

80 Baba, T., Narumi, H., Hanada, K. et al. (1995). Successful treatment of dark-colored epidermal nevus with ruby laser. *The Journal of Dermatology* 22 (8): 567–570.

81 Park, J.H., Hwang, E.S., Kim, S.N. et al. (2004). Er:YAG laser treatment of verrucous epidermal nevi. *Dermatologic Surgery: Official Publication for American Society for Dermatologic Surgery [et al]* 30 (3): 378–381.

82 Fox, B.J. and Lapins, N.A. (1983). Comparison of treatment modalities for epidermal nevus: a case report and review. *The Journal of Dermatologic Surgery and Oncology* 9 (11): 879–885.

83 Sim, J.H., Kang, Y., and Kim, Y.C. (2010). Verrucous epidermal nevus successfully treated with photodynamic therapy. *European Journal of Dermatology: EJD.* 20 (6): 814–815.

84 Demmel, U. (1975). Clinical aspects of congenital skin defects. I. Congenital skin defects on the head of the newborn. *European Journal of Pediatrics* 121 (1): 21–50.

85 Benvenuto, C., Kraemer, C.K., Kruse, R.L. et al. (2003). Familial epidermolysis bullosa with aplasia cutis congenita: Bart's syndrome? *Skinmed* 2 (5): 319–321.

86 Frieden, I.J. (1986). Aplasia cutis congenita: a clinical review and proposal for classification. *Journal of the American Academy of Dermatology* 14 (4): 646–660.

87 Wexler, A., Harris, M., and Lesavoy, M. (1990). Conservative treatment of cutis aplasia. *Plastic and Reconstructive Surgery* 86 (6): 1066–1071.
88 Browning, J.C. (2013). Aplasia cutis congenita: approach to evaluation and management. *Dermatologic Therapy* 26 (6): 439–444.
89 Starcevic, M., Sepec, M.P., and Zah, V. (2010). A case of extensive aplasia cutis congenita: a conservative approach. *Pediatric Dermatology* 27 (5): 540–542.
90 Silberstein, E., Pagkalos, V.A., Landau, D. et al. (2014). Aplasia cutis congenita: clinical management and a new classification system. *Plastic and Reconstructive Surgery* 134 (5): 766e–774e.
91 Orozco-Covarrubias, L., Lara-Carpio, R., Saez-De-Ocariz, M. et al. (2013). Dermoid cysts: a report of 75 pediatric patients. *Pediatric Dermatology* 30 (6): 706–711.
92 Sorenson, E.P., Powel, J.E., Rozzelle, C.J. et al. (2013). Scalp dermoids: a review of their anatomy, diagnosis, and treatment. *Child's Nervous System: ChNS: Official Journal of the International Society for Pediatric Neurosurgery* 29 (3): 375–380.
93 Nelson, K.E., Mishra, A., and Duncan, C. (2011). Upper blepharoplasty approach to frontozygomatic dermoid cysts. *The Journal of Craniofacial Surgery* 22 (6): e41–e44.
94 Park, A.H. and Siddiqi, F. (2006). An approach to pediatric brow dermoids: an upper eyelid crease incision. *International Journal of Pediatric Otorhinolaryngology* 70 (2): 349–351.
95 Hachach-Haram, N., Benyon, S., Shanmugarajah, K. et al. (2013). Back to basics: a case series of angular dermoid cyst excision. *Journal of Plastic, Reconstructive & Aesthetic Surgery: JPRAS* 66 (1): 57–60.
96 Im, J.T., Park, B.Y., Lim, S.Y. et al. (2014). Endoscopic excision of benign facial tumors: a decade of experience with 152 patients. *Annals of Plastic Surgery* 72 (5): 556–559.
97 Naik, M.N., Batra, J., Nair, A.G. et al. (2014). Foam sclerotherapy for periorbital dermoid cysts. *Ophthalmic Plastic and Reconstructive Surgery* 30 (3): 267–270.
98 Yamauchi, M., Yotsuyanagi, T., Saito, T. et al. (2010). Three cases of giant pilomatrixoma – considerations for diagnosis and treatment of giant skin tumours with abundant inner calcification present on the upper body. *Journal of Plastic, Reconstructive & Aesthetic Surgery: JPRAS* 63 (6): e519–e524.
99 Sevin, K., Can, Z., Yilmaz, S. et al. (1995). Pilomatrixoma of the earlobe. *Dermatologic Surgery: Official Publication for American Society for Dermatologic Surgery [et al]* 21 (3): 245–246.
100 Pirouzmanesh, A., Reinisch, J.F., Gonzalez-Gomez, I. et al. (2003). Pilomatrixoma: a review of 346 cases. *Plastic and Reconstructive Surgery* 112 (7): 1784–1789.
101 Kovacic, M., Rudic, M., Nekic, I. et al. (2007). Giant pilomatrixoma (benign calcifying epithelioma of Malherbe) of the neck and face. *Dermatologic Surgery: Official Publication for American Society for Dermatologic Surgery [et al]* 33 (3): 340–343.
102 Sassmannshausen, J. and Chaffins, M. (2001). Pilomatrix carcinoma: a report of a case arising from a previously excised pilomatrixoma and a review of the literature. *Journal of the American Academy of Dermatology* 44 (2 Suppl): 358–361.
103 Reddy, S.S., Gadre, S.A., Adegboyega, P. et al. (2008). Multiple pilomatrixomas: case report and literature review. *Ear, Nose, & Throat Journal* 87 (4): 230–233.
104 Behroozan, D.S., Goldberg, L.H., Glaich, A.S. et al. (2006). Mohs micrographic surgery for deeply penetrating, expanding benign cutaneous neoplasms. *Dermatologic Surgery: Official publication for American Society for Dermatologic Surgery [et al]* 32 (7): 958–965.
105 Dutta, S., Lorenz, H.P., and Albanese, C.T. (2006). Endoscopic excision of benign forehead masses: a novel approach for

pediatric general surgeons. *Journal of Pediatric Surgery* 41 (11): 1874–1878.

106 Chan, J.J. and Tey, H.L. (2010). Multiple pilomatricomas: case presentation and review of the literature. *Dermatology Online Journal* 16 (4): 2.

107 Sable, D. and Snow, S.N. (2004). Pilomatrix carcinoma of the back treated by mohs micrographic surgery. *Dermatologic Surgery: Official Publication for American Society for Dermatologic Surgery [et al]* 30 (8): 1174–1176.

108 Melancon, J.M., Tom, W.L., Lee, R.A. et al. (2011). Management of pilomatrix carcinoma: a case report of successful treatment with Mohs micrographic surgery and review of the literature. *Dermatologic Surgery: Official Publication for American Society for Dermatologic Surgery [et al]* 37 (12): 1798–1805.

109 Gunson, T.H. and Birchall, N.M. (2008). Symmetrical giant facial plaque-type juvenile xanthogranuloma. *Journal of the American Academy of Dermatology* 59 (2 Suppl 1): S56–S57.

110 Pinto, C., Lechuga, M., Bellolio, E. et al. (2014). Giant congenital juvenile xanthogranuloma presenting as a yellowish atrophic plaque. *The Journal of Dermatology* 41 (7): 646–647.

111 Bazan, A., Lasso, J.M., Elejabeitia, J. et al. (1998). Giant juvenile xanthogranuloma present since birth. *Annals of Plastic Surgery* 41 (3): 335–337.

112 Behne, K. and Casey, T. (2003). Ulcerated juvenile xanthogranuloma of the scalp. *The Australasian Journal of Dermatology* 44 (1): 74–75.

113 Campbell, L., McTigue, M.K., Esterly, N.B. et al. (1988). Giant juvenile xanthogranuloma. *Archives of Dermatology* 124 (11): 1723–1724.

114 Imiela, A., Carpentier, O., Segard-Drouard, M. et al. (2004). Juvenile xanthogranuloma: a congenital giant form leading to a wide atrophic sequela. *Pediatric Dermatology* 21 (2): 121–123.

115 Magana, M., Vazquez, R., Fernandez-Diez, J. et al. (1994). Giant congenital juvenile xanthogranuloma. *Pediatric Dermatology* 11 (3): 227–230.

116 Resnick, S.D., Woosley, J., and Azizkhan, R.G. (1990). Giant juvenile xanthogranuloma: exophytic and endophytic variants. *Pediatric Dermatology* 7 (3): 185–188.

117 Klemke, C.D., Held, B., Dippel, E. et al. (2007). Multiple juvenile xanthogranulomas successfully treated with CO laser. *Journal der Deutschen Dermatologischen Gesellschaft = Journal of the German Society of Dermatology: JDDG* 5 (1): 30–33.

118 Falabella, A.F., Valencia, I.C., Eaglstein, W.H. et al. (2000). Tissue-engineered skin (Apligraf) in the healing of patients with epidermolysis bullosa wounds. *Archives of Dermatology* 136 (10): 1225–1230.

119 Fivenson, D.P., Scherschun, L. et al. (2003). Apligraf in the treatment of severe mitten deformity associated with recessive dystrophic epidermolysis bullosa. *Plastic and Reconstructive Surgery* 112 (2): 584–588.

120 Pope, E., Lara-Corrales, I., Mellerio, J. et al. (2012). A consensus approach to wound care in epidermolysis bullosa. *Journal of the American Academy of Dermatology* 67 (5): 904–917.

121 Brodland, D.G. and Zitelli, J.A. (1992). Surgical margins for excision of primary cutaneous squamous cell carcinoma. *Journal of the American Academy of Dermatology* 27 (2 Pt 1): 241–248.

122 Hernandez-Machin, B., Borrego, L., Gil-Garcia, M. et al. (2007). Office-based radiation therapy for cutaneous carcinoma: evaluation of 710 treatments. *International Journal of Dermatology* 46 (5): 453–459.

123 Leibovitch, I., Huilgol, S.C., Selva, D. et al. (2005). Cutaneous squamous cell carcinoma treated with Mohs micrographic surgery in Australia I. Experience over 10 years. *Journal of the American Academy of Dermatology* 53 (2): 253–260.

124 Tang, J.Y., Mackay-Wiggan, J.M., Aszterbaum, M. et al. (2012). Inhibiting the hedgehog pathway in patients with the basal-cell nevus syndrome. *The New England Journal of Medicine* 366 (23): 2180–2188.
125 Krunic, A.L., Viehman, G.E., Madani, S. et al. (1998). Microscopically controlled surgical excision combined with ultrapulse CO_2 vaporization in the management of a patient with the nevoid basal cell carcinoma syndrome. *The Journal of Dermatology* 25 (1): 10–12.
126 Oseroff, A.R., Shieh, S., Frawley, N.P. et al. (2005). Treatment of diffuse basal cell carcinomas and basaloid follicular hamartomas in nevoid basal cell carcinoma syndrome by wide-area 5-aminolevulinic acid photodynamic therapy. *Archives of Dermatology* 141 (1): 60–67.
127 Loncaster, J., Swindell, R., Slevin, F. et al. (2009). Efficacy of photodynamic therapy as a treatment for Gorlin syndrome-related basal cell carcinomas. *Clinical Oncology (Royal College of Radiologists (Great Britain))* 21 (6): 502–508.
128 Girard, C., Debu, A., Bessis, D. et al. (2013). Treatment of Gorlin syndrome (nevoid basal cell carcinoma syndrome) with methylaminolevulinate photodynamic therapy in seven patients, including two children: interest of tumescent anesthesia for pain control in children. *Journal of the European Academy of Dermatology and Venereology: JEADV* 27 (2): e171–e175.
129 Nouri, K., Chang, A., Trent, J.T. et al. (2002). Ultrapulse CO_2 used for the successful treatment of basal cell carcinomas found in patients with basal cell nevus syndrome. *Dermatologic Surgery: Official Publication for American Society for Dermatologic Surgery [et al]* 28 (3): 287–290.
130 Moskalik, K., Kozlov, A., Demin, E. et al. (2009). The efficacy of facial skin cancer treatment with high-energy pulsed neodymium and Nd:YAG lasers. *Photomedicine and Laser Surgery* 27 (2): 345–349.
131 Konnikov, N., Avram, M., Jarell, A. et al. (2011). Pulsed dye laser as a novel non-surgical treatment for basal cell carcinomas: response and follow up 12–21 months after treatment. *Lasers in Surgery and Medicine* 43 (2): 72–78.
132 Ibrahimi, O.A., Sakamoto, F.H., Tannous, Z. et al. (2011). 755 nm alexandrite laser for the reduction of tumor burden in basal cell nevus syndrome. *Lasers in Surgery and Medicine* 43 (2): 68–71.
133 Doctoroff, A., Oberlender, S.A., and Purcell, S.M. (2003). Full-face carbon dioxide laser resurfacing in the management of a patient with the nevoid basal cell carcinoma syndrome. *Dermatologic Surgery: Official Publication for American Society for Dermatologic Surgery [et al]* 29 (12): 1236–1240.
134 Melandri, D. and Carruthers, A. (1992). Widespread basal cell carcinoma of the scalp treated by dermabrasion. *Journal of the American Academy of Dermatology* 26 (2 Pt 1): 270–271.
135 Love, W.E., Bernhard, J.D., and Bordeaux, J.S. (2009). Topical imiquimod or fluorouracil therapy for basal and squamous cell carcinoma: a systematic review. *Archives of Dermatology* 145 (12): 1431–1438.
136 Geisse, J., Caro, I., Lindholm, J. et al. (2004). Imiquimod 5% cream for the treatment of superficial basal cell carcinoma: results from two phase III, randomized, vehicle-controlled studies. *Journal of the American Academy of Dermatology* 50 (5): 722–733.
137 Kuflik, E.G. (1997). Cryosurgery for cutaneous malignancy. An update. *Dermatologic Surgery: Official Publication for American Society for Dermatologic Surgery [et al]* 23 (11): 1081–1087.
138 Tsuji, T., Otake, N., and Nishimura, M. (1993). Cryosurgery and topical fluorouracil: a treatment method for widespread basal cell epithelioma in basal cell nevus syndrome. *The Journal of Dermatology* 20 (8): 507–513.

139 Johnson, T.M., Tromovitch, T.A., and Swanson, N.A. (1991). Combined curettage and excision: a treatment method for primary basal cell carcinoma. *Journal of the American Academy of Dermatology* 24 (4): 613–617.

140 Goldberg, L.H., Landau, J.M., Moody, M.N. et al. (2011). Resolution of odontogenic keratocysts of the jaw in basal cell nevus syndrome with GDC-0449. *Archives of Dermatology* 147 (7): 839–841.

141 Campbell, R.M. and DiGiovanna, J.J. (2006). Skin cancer chemoprevention with systemic retinoids: an adjunct in the management of selected high-risk patients. *Dermatologic Therapy* 19 (5): 306–314.

142 Galimberti, G., Montano, A.P., Kowalczuk, A. et al. (2012). Outcomes in 11 patients with dermatofibrosarcoma protuberans treated with Mohs micrographic surgery. *International Journal of Dermatology* 51 (1): 89–93.

143 Hobbs, E.R., Wheeland, R.G., Bailin, P.L. et al. (1988). Treatment of dermatofibrosarcoma protuberans with Mohs micrographic surgery. *Annals of Surgery* 207 (1): 102–107.

144 Paradisi, A., Abeni, D., Rusciani, A. et al. (2008). Dermatofibrosarcoma protuberans: wide local excision vs. Mohs Micrographic Surgery. *Cancer Treatment Reviews* 34 (8): 728–736.

145 Snow, S.N., Gordon, E.M., Larson, P.O. et al. (2004). Dermatofibrosarcoma protuberans: a report on 29 patients treated by Mohs micrographic surgery with long-term follow-up and review of the literature. *Cancer* 101 (1): 28–38.

146 Tan, W.P., Barlow, R.J., Robson, A. et al. (2011). Dermatofibrosarcoma protuberans: 35 patients treated with Mohs micrographic surgery using paraffin sections. *The British Journal of Dermatology* 164 (2): 363–366.

147 Suit, H., Spiro, I., Mankin, H.J. et al. (1996). Radiation in management of patients with dermatofibrosarcoma protuberans. *Journal of Clinical Oncology: Official Journal of the American Society of Clinical Oncology* 14 (8): 2365–2369

148 Sun, L.M., Wang, C.J., Huang, C.C. et al. (2000). Dermatofibrosarcoma protuberans: treatment results of 35 cases. *Radiotherapy and Oncology: Journal of the European Society for Therapeutic Radiology and Oncology* 57 (2): 175–181.

149 Kerob, D., Porcher, R., Verola, O. et al. (2010). Imatinib mesylate as a preoperative therapy in dermatofibrosarcoma: results of a multicenter phase II study on 25 patients. *Clinical Cancer Research: An Official Journal of the American Association for Cancer Research* 16 (12): 3288–3295.

150 Rutkowski, P., Debiec-Rychter, M., Nowecki, Z. et al. (2011). Treatment of advanced dermatofibrosarcoma protuberans with imatinib mesylate with or without surgical resection. *Journal of the European Academy of Dermatology and Venereology: JEADV* 25 (3): 264–270.

17

Lasers for Vascular Lesions

Nawaf Almutairi[1] and Jasem Alshaiji[2]

[1] *Faculty of Medicine, Department of Medicine, Dermatology Unit, Kuwait University, Kuwait City, Kuwait*
[2] *Department of Dermatology, Amiri Hospital, Kuwait City, Kuwait*

17.1 Introduction

"LASER" stands for **L**ight **A**mplification by the **S**timulated **E**mission of **R**adiation.

Lasers are sources of high-intensity light with the following properties:

- monochromatic, i.e. the light is of a single wavelength
- coherent, i.e. the light beam waves are in phase
- collimated, i.e. the light beams travel in parallel.

Laser light can be accurately focused into small spots with very high energy. The light is produced within an optical cavity containing a medium, which may be a gas (e.g. argon, krypton, carbon dioxide), liquid (e.g. dye) or solid (e.g. ruby, neodymium:yttrium-aluminum-garnet, alexandrite). The process involves excitation of the molecules of the laser medium, which results in the release of a photon of light as it returns to a stable state. Each medium produces a specific wavelength of light, which may be within the visible spectrum (violet 400 nm through to red 700 nm) or infrared spectrum (more than 700 nm). Laser irradiation can selectively destroy specific targets (chromophores) within the skin by using an appropriate wavelength, pulse duration, and energy setting. To limit damage to surrounding structures, pulse duration must always be less than or equal to the targeted thermal relaxation time of the chromophore, i.e. the time necessary for the target to cool by half of its peak temperature after laser irradiation

17.2 Vascular Lasers

The use of lasers to treat vascular skin lesions started over 40 years ago. During that time, argon and carbon dioxide (CO_2) lasers in a continuous wave mode (CW) were commonly used to treat benign vascular birthmarks such as port-wine stains and hemangiomas. Although significant lightening of these birthmarks could be achieved, a common side effect of scar formation, with an unacceptably high rate, was noticed in many patients. However, in the last two decades several major advances in laser technology have taken place, which has revolutionized their use in the treatment of vascular lesions, with minimal side effects.

Vascular skin lesions contain oxygenated hemoglobin, which strongly absorbs visible light at 418, 542, and 577 nm. Pulsed-laser systems; such as the 585 or 595 nm pulsed dye laser (PDL), have now become the mainstay of therapy for both congenital and acquired vascular lesions [7]. These lasers act on intravascular oxyhemoglobin (targeted chromophore)

Pediatric Dermatologic Surgery, First Edition. Edited by Keyvan Nouri, Latanya Benjamin, Jasem Alshaiji, and Jan Izakovic.

in vascular lesions; thus, thermal damage is largely restricted to cutaneous blood vessels. Current technological improvements include dynamic surface cooling and extended pulse duration, which enhance clinical results and minimize adverse effects.

There are many different types and combinations of lasers that can be used to treat vascular lesions and are broadly classified as follows:

A) Continuous or quasi continuous wave lasers:
   - Argon laser
   - Argon pumped tuneable dye laser
   - Krypton laser
   - Copper vapor and copper bromide laser (now rarely used)
   - Potassium Titanyl Phosphate (KTP) laser

B) Pulsed lasers:
   1) PDL
   2) Long-pulse dye lasers
   3) Frequency-doubled Q-switched Nd:YAG laser

C) IPL

IPL stands for intense pulsed light, which is not a true laser but can be used to treat vascular lesions by using filters to deliver an appropriate wavelength of light.

The aim is to destroy the target cells, and not to harm the surrounding tissue. Short pulses reduce the amount that the damaged cells heat up, thereby reducing thermal injury that could result in scarring. Automated scanners aim to reduce the chance of overlapping treatment areas.

Following types of skin lesions can be treated with vascular lasers

- Port-wine stain birthmarks
- Broken capillaries or telangiectasias
- Redness of the face and neck
- Rosacea
- Spider nevi
- Cherry angiomas
- Infantile hemangiomas
- Venous lakes
- Some leg veins
- Early scars
- Red stretch marks
- Warts

17.3 Types of Vascular Lesions

Cutaneous vascular lesions can be classified according to histopathology and age of onset [1–5]. Congenital lesions begin in infancy and include port-wine stains, hemangiomas, venous malformations, and lymphangiomas. Congenital lesions are found most commonly on the head or neck and may be isolated or found as part of a congenital syndrome such as Sturge–Weber syndrome. Acquired lesions develop in persons of any age and include telangiectasias, cherry angiomas, pyogenic granulomas, venous lakes, poikiloderma, and Kaposi sarcoma. Acquired lesions may occur spontaneously, or they may occur in response to trauma, ultraviolet exposure, or hormonal changes. According to the classification proposed by International Society for the Study of Vascular Anomalies (ISSVA) in 1996, these can be classified as follows:

A) Vascular malformations:
   a) Simple:
      - Capillary
      - Lymphatic
      - Venous
      - Arterial
      - Arteriovenous malformation
      - Arteriovenous fistula
   b) Combined
   c) Of major named vessels
   d) Associated with other anomalies

B) Vascular tumors:
   a) Benign:
      - Infantile hemangioma (IH)/hemangioma of infancy (HOI)
      - Congenital hemangioma (CH)
        – Rapidly involuting CH (RICH)
        – Non-involuting CH (NICH)
        – Partially involuting CH (PICH)

- Tufted angioma
- Spindle cell hemangioma
- Epithelioid hemangioma
- Pyogenic granuloma (or lobular capillary hemangioma)
- Others

b) locally aggressive
- Kaposiform hemangioendothelioma
- Retiform hemangioendothelioma
- Papillary intralymphatic angioendothelioma
  - Dabska tumor
- Composite hemangioendothelioma
- Kaposi sarcoma
- Others

c) Malignant tumors
- Angiosarcoma
- Epithelioid hemangioendothelioma
- Others

17.4 Common Vascular Lesions

17.4.1 Port-Wine Stains

Also known as nevus flammeus or capillary malformations, port-wine stains are usually present at birth and affect both sexes equally. The prevalence rate in the general population is estimated to be around 0.3–0.5%. They are usually located on the face, with V2 dermatome being most commonly affected. They begin as light-pink macules, and can darken and become hypertrophy over time. Overlying soft tissue or bony hypertrophy may sometimes be associated with these lesions. These lesions tend to grow with the patient, without a tendency toward regression. Numerous epidemiologic studies have demonstrated that patients treated earlier in the natural history (e.g. < 1 year of age) have the most effective lightening, require fewer treatments than older individuals and have decreased likelihood of recurrence.

PDL is the gold standard for the treatment of port-wine stains and it is highly effective and safe, especially for small facial PWS in infants <6 months of age under local anesthesia, with clearance rate of 88.6%. PWS located on the periorbital area, lateral facial cheeks, chest, and proximal aspect of the arms respond best to treatment, whereas the malar areas of the face and distal limbs do not respond well, even with many treatment sessions.

The typical parameters used are fluency 6–12 j/cm^2, spot size of 7–10 mm, and pulse duration of 0.45–1.5 ms. The session can be repeated at four to eight weeks interval. In general, 6–12 sessions are required to achieve significant clearing

For those PWSs that are resistant to PDL (due to their sizes, anatomic locations, age of the patients, vessel depth and diameter), long-pulsed (600 nm), Nd:YAG (1064 nm), and alexandrite (755 nm) lasers can be utilized, but there is a risk of complications (e.g. purpura, and pigmentary alterations).

17.4.2 Hemangiomas

These are benign proliferations of blood vessels seen in 1–2% of newborns and 10% of infants. Only one third of these lesions are present at birth. They most commonly are seen as solitary lesions on the head (40%) or neck (20%), and typically undergo a rapid growth phase before involuting after an undetermined amount of time, although involution usually starts by the end of the first year and continues for several years (3–7 years).

A total of 92% of hemangiomas are expected to disappear by four years of age. Some of the common complications associated with these lesions include ulceration, bleeding, infection, and scarring. Rapidly proliferating hemangiomas located on the face are particularly concerning because they may compromise vital structures or obscure vision. Larger lesions may be associated with Kasabach–Merritt syndrome, which has a constellation of findings that includes platelet destruction, hemolytic anemia, and coagulopathy. Treatment of IH remains extremely controversial, due to wide ranges of outcomes, from fully resolved to disfiguring scars to life-threatening obstructions. One argument dictates an aggressive approach, using early intervention to lessen the impact of a potentially threatening lesion, whereas the contrasting argument advises a wait-and-see approach, in the belief that most IH resolve with a more cosmetically adequate outcome without treatment. Some authors recommend using PDL for early initially flat IH to prevent further progression and complications, or superficial IH during proliferative phase utilizing frequent treatments at two- to three-week intervals at higher energies (11–12 J/cm^2, 7 mm spot size), while others advocate the use of PDL to treat superficial involuting and ulcerating IH.

The treatment is indicated for lesions with life/function-threatening complications, treating ulceration, pain, and bleeding, preventing permanent disfigurement and minimizing psychosocial distress to the patient/families.

Current first-line therapy for IH is beta-blockers, mainly oral propranolol. Other treatment modalities that have also been successfully used to treat these lesions include systemic corticosteroids, interferon alfa-2a and 2b, vincristine, topical timolol, imiquimod, topical/intralesional corticosteroids, PDL, excisional surgery, and cryosurgery. Although laser treatment of hemangiomas remains debatable, PDL has shown the best-documented safety record. Typical parameter used are fluency 5–8 J/cm^2, spot size of 7–10 mm and pulse duration 1.5 ms. The main limitation of the PDL is the depth of the lesion, with lesions thicker than 3 mm usually not responding well. In these lesions, KTP or CW/long-pulsed Nd:YAG laser can be used although there is a risk of scarring, blistering, crusting, dyschromias and textural abnormalities.

Currently, PDL is used for thin superficial lesions, residual erythema, and telangiectasia. It has also been used to treat ulcerated lesions, for reducing the pain, infection, and bleeding by assisting with the epithelialization of the ulcer.

Complications of PDL treatment include atrophic scarring, ulceration, hemorrhage, and pain. Long-pulsed PDL has been reported to be a safe and effective therapy for treating childhood hemangioma when compared with PDL.

17.4.3 Spider Angiomas

Also known as nevus araneus or spider nevus, this is a common benign vascular lesion present in 10–15% of healthy adults and young children. The name originates from its characteristic physical appearance, of central red arteriole, or punctum, resembling the body of the spider, surrounded by a radial pattern of thin-walled capillaries, resembling the legs of the spider. The lesions range in size from 1 to 10 mm in diameter. Compression of the central vessel with a slide/pin head results in blanching and temporary obliteration of the lesion, followed by rapid return of blood flow upon release. Occasionally, pulsations may be felt upon compression of the punctum. In children, the backs of the hands and fingers are commonly affected, whereas in adults these lesions are most frequent on exposed areas of the body, such as the face, neck, chest, and upper extremities. They may appear as a solitary lesion or as multiple lesions. In cases with multiple lesions, an association with liver disease, estrogen therapy, and thyrotoxicosis should be investigated. They occur as a result of the dilation of preexisting vessels. The exact etiology of the spider nevus is not clear. However, estrogen-excess states such as pregnancy and liver disease have been commonly associated with these lesions. Additionally, other biologic substances, including vascular endothelial growth factor (VEGF), basic fibroblastic growth factor (bFGF), substance P, and endogenous vasodilators, have also been implicated in the pathogenesis of spider angioma. Their treatment in children is usually not necessary, and the lesions may resolve spontaneously over the course of several years, whereas in young women these lesions often resolve spontaneously within six weeks to nine months after the birth of a child or after discontinuing oral contraceptives.

In addition, multiple lesions associated with liver disease may improve upon treatment of the underlying condition. Surgical therapy, including electrodesiccation and laser treatment, can both be effective for bothersome facial lesions. They respond well to pulsed dye lasers, and usually require one to two sessions to clear completely.

Typical parameters used are fluency 9–12 J/cm^2, spot size 7 mm, and pulse duration of 1.5–6 ms. Although there is a risk of a scar formation, good results are generally achieved with either mode. The risk of scarring is slightly higher with electrodesiccation.

17.4.4 Pyogenic Granuloma

It is an acquired, benign, vascular cutaneous tumor that can also affect mucous membranes. These are commonly found in infants and children, accounting for approximately 0.5% of all skin nodules in children. Clinically, they usually manifest as rapidly enlarging soft to firm red papules commonly located on the head and neck region. These lesions frequently bleed or ulcerate, and can be treated with various options that include complete excision, shave excision with electrodesiccation of the base, electrocautery alone, and lasers (PDLs, Nd:YAG, and carbon dioxide lasers). It has been demonstrated that PDL is safe and effective for small pyogenic granulomas in children. Typical parameters used are fluency 10–12 J/cm^2, spot size 7 mm, and pulse duration of 1.5–6 ms. The continuous-wave carbon dioxide laser has proved to be effective, but nonspecific coagulation may lead to scars. Other lasers that have been used to treat pyogenic granulomas are Nd:YAG and intense pulsed light, requiring multiple sessions.

17.4.5 Lymphatic Malformations

Also known as lymphangiomas, these are slow-growing lymphatic malformations that mostly are congenital, and likely arise from a combination of abnormal budding of lymphatic structures, failure of venous vasculature to unite with the lymphatics, and atypical lymphatic tissue sequestration during embryogenic development. Most of these lesions are diagnosed by age two years, with nearly half diagnosed at birth, though these lesions can be acquired after lymphatic drainage obstruction, chronic inflammation, infections, trauma, or surgical procedures. These are typically seen as soft tissue masses in the axillae or neck regions, but they can occur in other locations such as the tongue, esophagus, and upper airways. These lesions can be classified as either superficial (e.g. lymphangioma circumscriptum) or deep (e.g. cystic hygroma).

In asymptomatic patients they may not require treatment, and up to 15% of cystic hygromas may spontaneously regress. However, complete surgical excision is typically the preferred treatment modality.

However, because of the location and possible involvement of vital structures, complete excision may not always be possible. Other options include sclerosing agents and laser therapy.

Successful treatment with lasers (i.e. Nd:YAG, PDL, carbon dioxide) has been reportedly used for ablation, debulking, and complete excision. However, scarring after laser treatment, recurrence, and multiple treatment sessions are a matter of concern.

17.4.6 Laser Therapy

Anesthesia is an important component of the laser therapy when treating infants and children. Local anesthesia prior to therapy is advisable in children. Intradermal injection of 0.1–0.2 ml physiological saline solution injected using 30G needle produces brief complete anesthesia of the site and does not sting on injection. This represents a viable alternative to lidocaine. Alternatively, EMLA cream can be applied under occlusion for one hour before the procedure. However, smaller but significant methemoglobinemia risk in neonates and young infants has been reported because of the prilocaine component in the cream. Because of the significant risk associated, general anesthesia should be avoided in infants as far as possible.

Standard protective goggles are too large for infants and children, and two to three layers of moist white gauzes can be used safely to protect the eyes. Also, pediatric metal corneal should be used while treating periorbital area [6, 7].

17.4.7 Pulsed Dye Laser

The pulsed dye laser or PDL is considered the gold standard treatment for port-wine stains, and it can be used to treat infants aged only a few weeks. A newer 595-nm ultralong-PDL can be adjusted for pulse durations from 1.5 to 40 milliseconds. It has a cryogen-cooling device to decrease pain and adverse effects (e.g. purpura). The long-pulsed dye laser has deeper penetration than the 585-nm laser, and may be preferred for treating certain telangiectasias. Typically, larger-caliber vessels require longer pulse durations to be effective, and the 595-nm PDL can be adjusted to correspond to the different-sized vessels being treated. The PDL is useful in the treatment of superficial hemangiomas and in a variety of acquired cutaneous vascular lesions, including telangiectasias, cherry angiomas, pyogenic granulomas, and poikiloderma of Civatte.

Pyogenic granulomas have also been successfully treated with the 585-nm PDL. However, some thicker lesions may not respond to therapy because of the greater depth. Some physicians prefer multiple, overlapping pulses to treat these lesions. However, some others compress the superficial vessels with a glass slide and then administer the laser.

After the deeper portion has been treated, the slide is removed and the superficial portion is treated. PDL treatment is especially effective for reducing diffuse erythema and matted telangiectasias associated with acne rosacea, actinic damage, and long-term corticosteroid use. Laser treatment parameters depend on several factors, including age of the patient, location of lesion, morphology, and patient skin type. Spot sizes ranging from 2 to 10 mm are used to deliver a fluence averaging 5–10 J/cm^2.

The use of larger spot sizes and a higher fluence permit deeper dermal penetration and destruction of larger-caliber vessels. Lower energy densities are necessary in anatomic locations, with an increased risk of scarring, such as the anterior chest, neck, and periorbital area. The physician should also apply laser pulses in a non-overlapping manner to prevent excessive thermal damage that could result in vesiculation and fibrosis. In general, port-wine stains are expected to fade by 80% after about 8–10 treatments. Lesions on the face or neck tend to respond more quickly than those on the lower extremities. Superficial and ulcerated hemangiomas also respond favorably to the PDL. However, hemangiomas with a deeper component tend to be more resistant to laser therapy, often requiring concomitant beta-blockers or corticosteroids.

17.4.8 Long-Pulsed Nd:YAG Laser

The long-pulsed 1064-nm Nd:YAG laser has gained popularity for the treatment of telangiectasia, small-to-medium vessels of leg veins (up to 4 mm in diameter), and reticular veins below lower eyelids.

It has also been used to treat rosacea, poikiloderma, hemangiomas, and port-wine stains. The main advantage of the 1064-nm Nd:YAG laser over other shorter-wavelength lasers is that with equivalent absorption of blood, the 1064-nm laser has lower melanin absorption and deeper penetration. It also has a high absorption coefficient of methemoglobin and deoxyhemoglobin, which are the main components of blue veins. With the long-pulsed duration setting, this laser is more likely to heat the vessels slowly and uniformly, which allows sufficient vessel damage to cause coagulation, but avoids vessel rupture, subsequent purpura, and possible post-laser hyperpigmentation.

When used with the appropriate setting (spot size, fluence, and pulse duration) and adequate cooling (re-parallel-post-cooling), adverse effects seen with it are minimal and include crusting that lasts two to three weeks, with or without transient pigmentary alteration.

17.4.9 Post-Operative Care

Cooling the treated skin with a damp cloth soaked in cold water provides immediate relief. Photoprotection and strict use of sunscreen are very important to decrease the incidence of post-inflammatory hyperpigmentation. Also, the patient is advised to gently cleanse and moisturize the treated area.

17.4.10 Complications of Lasers

The most common adverse effects include transient edema and purpura, which may last up to 7–14 days. Patients or the parents have to be warned of postoperative purpura to avoid unnecessary panic.

As a consequence, patients may prefer treatment with a 532-nm KTP laser despite the superior efficacy of the PDL in eradicating telangiectasias with fewer treatments. Although the use of smaller spot sizes and lower energy densities reduces the degree of purpura, these measures also compromises the clinical efficacy. Other potential post-treatment adverse effects include transient hypopigmentation or hyperpigmentation, particularly in dark-skinned or tanned individuals. Blistering and scabbing may occur if there has been inadequate peri-operative skin cooling or higher fluences are used. The use of a dynamic cooling device, which serves to cool the epidermis during laser irradiation, permits safe application of a higher fluence, even in patients with dark skin tones helps to minimize this. The cooling device also reduces the intensity and duration of postoperative purpura. Importantly, the patients should avoid unnecessary sun exposure before, during, and after laser treatment because sun exposure may decrease the efficacy of the procedure and may contribute to adverse events such as postoperative pigmentary changes.

17.4.11 Future Directions

As research in the field continues, lasers capable of removing ectatic vascular growths, regardless of size or location, with minimal risk and low morbidity, will likely become available. Improvement of cooling systems seems to minimize scarring, reduce patient discomfort, and enhance overall results. Further research is needed to optimize these treatments.

References

1 Garzon, M.C., Huang, J.T., Enjolras, O., and Frieden, I.J. (2007). Vascular malformations. Part II: associated syndromes. *J. Am. Acad. Dermatol.* 56 (4): 541–564.

2 Requena, L. and Sangueza, O.P. (1997). Cutaneous vascular proliferation. Part II. Hyperplasias and benign neoplasms. *J. Am. Acad. Dermatol.* 37 (6): 887–919.

3 Garzon, M.C., Enjolras, O., and Frieden, I.J. (2000). Vascular tumors and vascular malformations: evidence for an association. *J. Am. Acad. Dermatol.* 42 (2 Pt 1): 275–279.

4 Wassef, M., Blei, F., Denise, A. et al. (2015). Vascular anomalies classification: recommendations from the International Society for the Study of vascular anomalies. *Pediatrics* 136 (1): 1–12.

5 Requena, L. and Sangueza, O.P. (1998). Cutaneous vascular proliferations. Part III. Malignant neoplasms, other cutaneous neoplasms with significant vascular component, and disorders erroneously considered as vascular neoplasms. *J. Am. Acad. Dermatol.* 38 (2): 541–564.

6 Adamic, M., Troilius, A., Adatto, M. et al. (2007). Vascular lasers and IPLS: guidelines for care from the European Society for Laser Dermatology (ESLD). *J. Cosmet. Laser. Ther.* 9 (2): 113–124.

7 Alshaiji, J. (2016). Laser therapy: when, where, and why. In: *Practical Pediatric Dermatology: Controversies in Diagnosis and Treatment* (ed. A.P. Oranje, N. Al-Mutairi and T. Shwayder), 251–258. New York: Springer.

18

Lasers for Scars and Striae

Sebastian Verne[1], Robert Magno[1], Ariel Eber[1], Marina Perper[1], Ibrahim Alomair[2], Abdulkareem Alfuraih[2], Mana Alharbi[2], and Keyvan Nouri[3]

[1] Department of Dermatology & Cutaneous Surgery, University of Miami Miller School of Medicine, Miami, FL, USA
[2] Al-Imam Mohammad Ibn Saud Islamic University (IMSIU), Riyadh, Saudi Arabia
[3] Department of Dermatology, Ophthalmology, Otolaryngology & Surgery, University of Miami Leonard M. Miller School of Medicine, Miami, FL, USA

18.1 Introduction

Wound healing occurs in almost all tissues and progresses through three sequential phases: inflammation, new tissue formation, and remodeling. Stage one, inflammation, begins immediately after tissue damage and serves to prevent blood and fluid loss, remove dead tissue, and prevent infection. A platelet plug is formed, followed by a fibrin matrix. Neutrophils and macrophages are then recruited to the wound, whose importance in repair is incompletely understood, although thought to be crucial. Stage two, new tissue formation, occurs 2–10 days after initial injury and is illustrated by cellular migration and proliferation. Keratinocyte migration, proliferation, and maturation results in skin barrier restoration. Fibroblasts, some differentiating into myofibroblasts, migrate to the wound and produce extracellular matrix, primarily in the form of collagen. Angiogenesis also develops due to multiple growth factors during this stage. Stage three, remodeling, begins two to three weeks after initial injury and is the final stage of wound healing, lasting a year or more. Cell apoptosis and migration out of the wound results in tissue composed primarily of collagen and extracellular matrix proteins with few cells. Matrix metalloproteinases remodel the skin components from primarily type III collagen to mainly type I collagen. The tissue strengthens, but does not reach the properties of undamaged skin [1].

The wound healing process described results in scar formation and occurs after most injuries. Clinical scar formation may arise from any significant injury to the dermis, including trauma, inflammation, and surgery. For the pediatric population, scars can be not only physically symptomatic, but may also come with cosmetic and psychosocial sequelae that must be taken into account when evaluating this patient population. In children, the prevalence of keloids and hypertrophic scars is estimated at 11 million and the prevalence of striae distensae ranges from 6 to 80% [2, 3]. Acne scarring, an important entity in the pediatric population, has been described as complicating 95% of acne patients to some degree, with acne afflicting 83–100% of adolescents [4, 5]. Specific guidelines for the management of scars in the pediatric population do not exist and thus much information is based on adult studies.

Pediatric Dermatologic Surgery, First Edition. Edited by Keyvan Nouri, Latanya Benjamin, Jasem Alshaiji, and Jan Izakovic.

18.1.1 Summary

- Wound healing progresses through three stages: inflammation, new tissue formation, and remodeling.
- Wound healing leads to the formation of a scar.

18.2 Types of Scars

18.2.1 Keloids

A keloid forms due to a dysregulation of wound healing that results in a raised scar that extends beyond the borders of the initial wound and can appear many years after injury. Keloids along with adjacent skin may be red with symptomatic burning, stinging, and itching [6, 7]. Histologically, scars have a reduced amount of elastic fibers with an increase of mucin [8]. Distinctly, keloids show thick hyalinized collagen nodules and whirls with mucinous ground substance and reduced fibroblasts. There is a tongue-like protruding front at the active edge and the overlying epidermis and papillary dermis remain uninvolved [9].

Keloids have a tendency to occur in usual locations including the anterior chest, shoulder, scapular, and suprapubic regions [10]. After formation, they rarely progress and are associated with recurrence after excisional procedures. Studying keloid formation in animal models is difficult as they only occur naturally in humans [7]. Although mostly sporadic, the presence of familial cases of keloids and the higher occurrence in darker-skinned races may indicate an inheritable predisposition that is triggered by environmental factors [11].

18.2.2 Hypertrophic Scars

Hypertrophic scars form due to a dysregulation of wound healing that results in a raised scar that is within the bounds of the initial wound and usually develops within one to two months of injury. They are rarely symptomatic, less so than keloids and without adjacent skin redness [6, 7]. Histologically, the epidermis is flattened and the dermis is replaced by scar tissue. The upper dermis shows horizontal fibrous collections while the deep dermis shows whirled fibrous collections. The dermal blood vessels are oriented vertically. Hypertrophic scars and keloids both have inflammatory infiltrates with variable presentation and lack adnexal structures [9].

There is no predilection for formation at any particular body location and also unlike keloids, hypertrophic scars progress to mature scars and regress over time [10]. Less evidence exists to support the genetic predisposition for hypertrophic scar formation.

18.2.3 Atrophic Scars

Atrophic scars appear as depressions below the surrounding skin. Histologically, this scar shows a thin epidermis with few cell layers, a lack of epidermal crests, and the dermis with fibers that are parallel and interlaced with broad interfibrillar spaces [12]. The main causes for the development of atrophic scars include acne, varicella, surgery, burns, and other injuries [13]. Atrophic scars due to acne are a common complication in the adolescent population and have been thoroughly studied.

Acne scars form when there is a severe inflammatory response to the acne. The type and depth of scarring is determined by the depth and extent of initial inflammation [5]. Many terms have been used to classify the different types of acne scars. They can be simply classified into three commonly clinically distinguishable types: icepick, rolling, and boxcar scars. Icepick scars are narrow, sharply demarcated tracts extending to the deep dermis or subcutaneous tissue. Measuring approximately 2 mm at the surface, they taper in width as depth increases. Rolling scars are usually the widest acne scars (4–5 mm), with shallow depressions giving an undulating appearance to the skin. They consist of dermal tethering to the subcutaneous tissue. Boxcar scars are sharply demarcated round depressions and can be shallow or deep. They tend to be wider (1.5–4 mm) than icepick scars and do not have tapering at increasing depth [14].

18.2.4 Striae

Striae distensae, often called striae, stretch marks, striae atrophicans, and striae gravidarum, can be divided into striae rubrae and striae albae. Striae rubrae are initial violet to red-colored lesions. Striae albae are the permanent form that develop from striae rubrae and present as hypopigmented, atrophic lesions similar to scars [2]. Histologically, features of striae include a flattened and atrophic dermis, reduction of dermal elastin with fragmentation, alignment and layering of dermal collagen in the direction of stress, and parallel orientation of dermal blood vessels with collagen [15].

In both male and female adolescents, the most common location is the buttocks followed by the lower back and knees in males and the thighs and calves in females. Striae have been described as forming in pregnancy, adolescence, obesity, weight training, corticosteroid use, and many other associations. Among adolescents, proposed mechanisms are stretching of the skin and adrenocortical hyperactivity, with BMI and childhood obesity as important risk factors along with a genetic predisposition [2].

18.2.5 Summary

- Keloids: symptomatic raised scar that extends beyond the borders of the initial injury.
- Hypertrophic scars: asymptomatic raised scar that remains within the bounds of the initial injury.
- Atrophic scars: depressed scars commonly a result of acne.
- Striae: hypo- or hyperpigmented atrophic skin lesions with many causes.

18.3 Types of Laser

18.3.1 Ablative Lasers

18.3.1.1 CO_2 Lasers

CO_2 lasers, like all ablative lasers, function by emitting beams of light that are absorbed by intracellular water within the skin resulting in local tissue destruction. CO_2 lasers have been shown to be ineffective when treating keloid scars and are associated with high levels of recurrence. Some authors believe that CO_2 treatment by itself can actually worsen keloids; however, it has been shown that combinatorial CO_2 treatments can lessen rates of recurrence [16].

The CO_2 laser for treatment of hypertrophic scars has proven itself to be an effective treatment modality. The fractional, ablative laser works by inducing a wound healing response within the scar, involving heat shock proteins, myofibroblasts, and an increase in collagen III production that can lead to remodeling of scar tissue [17].

Atrophic scars, particularly acne scars, have been successfully treated using CO_2 lasers. Research conducted by Majid et al. showed that CO_2 lasers were effective in treating rolling and boxcar scars while they were less effective at resolving icepick scars [18].

CO_2 lasers have shown little effect on striae, but there are studies indicating successful treatment of different types of striae disease. Recent research conducted by El Taieb et al. compared the efficacy of CO_2 lasers vs. intense pulsed light (IPL) for the treatment of striae distensae. The study showed that both modalities successfully treated the striae, with the CO_2 being more effective since it could provide a therapeutic effect in the same time frame with fewer treatments [19]. Additional research conducted by Naeini et al. compared the use of CO_2 lasers singularly against a combination treatment of CO_2 laser and pulsed dye laser for the treatment of striae alba. Their findings showed that CO_2 lasers were successful at treating striae alba; however, they saw better results in the CO_2 with PDL treatment group [20].

Overall, CO_2 lasers can be seen as effective treatment modalities for different types of scars, and less so with striae, when used solely or in conjunction with other treatment modalities.

18.3.1.2 Erbium-Doped: Yttrium, Aluminum, and Garnet Laser (Er:YAG)

Erbium-doped yttrium, aluminum, and garnet lasers (Er:YAG) were designed to be a less aggressive alternative to CO_2 lasers. Er:YAG lasers are ablative lasers that use the 2940 nm wavelength to target intracellular water which superheats the surrounding cells resulting in localized tissue damage.

Er:YAG lasers are not as extensively researched as CO_2 lasers; however, there has been one study that demonstrated their effectiveness for treating keloids. The study successfully treated 21 patients using the Er:YAG laser in an ablative manner. The laser heated the skin to supraphysiologic temperatures causing a metabolic response and upregulation of heat shock proteins. The complete mechanism is believed to decrease the clumping of collagen bundles and increase thin, oriented collagen fibers within the keloid [21].

Hypertrophic scars can also be treated with Er:YAG lasers. A study by Tidwell et al. took hypertrophic scars and divided the scars in half and treated each half with either fractioned or fully ablative Er:YAG lasers. The study showed a statistically significant outcome concluding that fractioned Er:YAG resulted in better patient outcome and satisfaction when compared to patients treated with fully ablative Er:YAG [22].

Various studies have been performed looking at the efficacy of Er:YAG lasers for the treatment of atrophic scars, particularly acne scars. However, there are very few published studies that include large sample sizes. Er:YAG treatment has been shown to be a successful treatment modality and is associated with shorter social downtime and fewer adverse effects when compared with CO_2 lasers [23].

Research conducted by Gungor et al. showed that Er:YAG lasers were not an effective treatment modality for treating striae distensae of the albae type. However, they were moderately helpful in treating striae distensae of the rubrae type [24].

In conclusion, ablative lasers have shown promise in treating keloids, certain types of scars, and striae. Research suggests that certain lasers may be more effective given a particular diagnosis. However, more studies with bigger sample sizes will be needed in order to provide accurate predictions as to which laser will be the most effective for a particular diagnosis.

18.3.2 Non-Ablative Lasers

18.3.2.1 Pulsed-Dye Lasers (PDL)

Pulsed-dye lasers (PDL) function by targeting hemoglobin, melanin, or other chromophores within the skin. PDL treatment is hypothesized to contribute to the treatment of keloids by selectively damaging blood supply to the scar. In addition to selectively damaging blood supply, PDL lasers have been experimentally shown to alter the expression of growth factors and enzymes related to keloid metabolism [25, 26].

Hypertrophic scars have also been successfully treated with pulsed dye lasers by reducing scar volume and increasing scar softness. Various studies have looked at the effect of PDL for the treatment of hypertrophic scars and the general consensus in the literature is that 595 nm wavelength is more effective than 585 nm [27, 28].

Additionally, pulsed dye lasers have been shown to be an effective treatment modality for atrophic and acne scars. One study conducted by Patel et al. found the application of the pulsed dye laser contributed to a 47.8% reduction in scar depth [29]. Another such study treated acne scars with PDL and Nd:YAG lasers, with their results showing both lasers were effective treatment modalities for acne scars. The authors hypothesized that specific lasers may be more effective for treating different types of acne scars but their results did not support a statistically significant conclusion [30].

Research conducted by Shokeir et al. determined that pulsed dye lasers were effective in treating striae rubrae while they were less effective in treating striae albae [31].

An additional study confirmed that PDL has a beneficial impact on striae rubrae, by reducing erythema [32]. This same study supported earlier results showing that PDL is not effective for treating striae of the albae type.

Overall, pulsed dye lasers are a good alternative for treating these different forms of scars and striae. They achieve a therapeutic effect while avoiding some of the negative side effects that are seen in ablative lasers.

18.3.2.2 Neodymium-Doped: Yttrium, Aluminum, and Garnet Laser (Nd:YAG)

Neodymium-doped yttrium, aluminum and garnet lasers (Nd:YAG) have a wavelength of 1064 nm. There are various studies showing the effectiveness of the Nd:YAG laser to treat keloids, with the consensus being that efficacy decreases as the size of the keloid increases [33, 34]. Koike et al. have demonstrated that Nd:YAG lasers are more applicable to treating hypertrophic scars than keloids. In their analysis of 102 cases where keloids and hypertrophic scars were treated with the Nd:YAG laser, they saw significant beneficial outcomes for the hypertrophic scar group that resulted in very few cases of recurrence (4%). This was in comparison to the keloid treatment group, which had recurrence levels ranging from 25 to 52.9% based on the location of the keloid [34].

Nd:YAG lasers have been used for the treatment of atrophic and acne scars but the extent of their effectiveness needs to be assessed with further research. Asilian et al. demonstrated that the Nd:YAG laser produced beneficial results for treating atrophic and acne scars however it was not as effective as the CO_2 laser [35].

Striae albae and rubrae can both be treated effectively with the Nd:YAG laser. A recent study compared two difference fluences of the Nd:YAG laser for the treatment of striae. The study concluded that 100 J/cm^2 was more effective at treating striae albae while 75 J/cm^2 was more effective for striae rubrae. Overall, the researchers recommend the Nd:YAG laser for the treatment of striae since it is a safe and effective modality [36].

In conclusion, the Nd:YAG laser provides another treatment modality for many different scars or striae and while it tends to be effective, sometimes other lasers are better suited for handling a particular treatment.

18.3.3 Summary

- CO_2 laser: Ablative laser causing local tissue destruction, demonstrating effectiveness for atrophic acne scars and less so for striae.
- Er:Yag laser: Ablative laser causing local tissue destruction, demonstrating varied effectiveness for scars and striae requiring more evidence.
- PDL: Non-ablative laser with selective targets, demonstrating effectiveness for scars and striae with a better side effect profile than ablative lasers.
- Nd:YAG laser: Non-ablative laser, demonstrating effectiveness for hypertrophic scars, atrophic scars, and striae although other lasers may prove more beneficial.

18.4 Techniques

Treating scars with lasers requires the doctor to first follow the proper ANSI guidelines regarding the safe use of lasers within health care facilities. For pre-operative care the treatment area should be cleaned thoroughly, making sure to also remove all make-up. Additionally, an anesthetic can be applied to the treatment site to aid in patient comfort. Proper laser therapy involves adjusting parameters to therapeutic treatment levels. Although there is yet to be a defined range of values that provides therapeutic effect while at the same time limiting complications, Tables 18.1–18.4 show a wide range of power outputs, fluences, spot sizes, and pulse durations used by several studies for the application of lasers in treating scars and striae. Many more studies will need to be conducted in order to better define a therapeutic range of laser parameters. Post-operative care involves keeping the treatment area covered and out of direct sunlight.

Table 18.1 Lasers for keloids.

	Keloids		
Laser Type	Power/Fluence	Spot Size	Pulse Speed/Duration
Carbon dioxide [16]	0.5–15 W	—	200–400 ms
Carbon dioxide [17]	30 W	—	1000 μs
Er:YAG [21]	3–4 J/cm^2	5 mm	—
Pulsed dye laser [26]	10–18 J/cm^2	5 mm	450 μs
Pulsed dye laser [27]	7 J/cm^2	—	0.45 or 40 ms
Nd:YAG [34]	14 J/cm^2	5 mm	0.3 ms

Table 18.2 Lasers for hypertrophic scars.

	Hypertrophic Scars		
Laser Type	Power/Fluence	Spot Size	Pulse Speed/Duration
Carbon dioxide [17]	25 W	—	600–800 μs
Er:YAG [21]	3–4 J/cm^2	5 mm	—
Er:YAG [22]	25–50 J/cm^2	—	—
Pulsed dye laser [37]	9–10 J/cm^2	7 mm	1.5–10 ms
Pulsed dye laser [38]	6.5–7.25 J/cm^2	—	0.45 ms
Pulsed dye laser [39]	7–8 J/cm^2	5 mm	2.5 ms
Nd:YAG [33]	14 J/cm^2	5 mm	0.3 ms

Table 18.3 Lasers for atrophic scars.

	Atrophic Scars		
Laser Type	Power/Fluence	Spot Size	Pulse Speed/Duration
Carbon dioxide [18]	15–25 J/cm^2	—	—
Pulse dye lasers [29]	1.9–2.4 J/cm^2	5 mm	350 μs
Pulse dye lasers [30]	10–11 J/cm^2	7 mm	40 ms
Nd:YAG [30]	50–70 J/cm^2	7 mm	50–100 ms
Nd:YAG [35]	2.5 J/cm^2	7 mm	—

18.5 Complications

The use of lasers for the treatment of scars is not without side effects. Ablative lasers and, although to a lesser extent, non-ablative lasers have similar side effects when used for the treatment of scars. Ablative lasers, CO_2 and Er:YAG, have been associated with erythema, pain, burning sensation, pruritus, bleeding, oozing, and post-inflammatory

Table 18.4 Lasers for striae.

	Striae		
Laser Type	Power/Fluence	Spot Size	Pulse Speed/Duration
Carbon dioxide [19]	40 mJ	0.1 cm^2	—
Er:YAG [24]	1–3.2 J	7 mm	250 ms
Pulsed dye laser [31]	2.5 J/cm^2	10 mm	0.5 ms
Pulsed dye laser [32]	3 J/cm^2	10 mm	450 μs
Pulsed dye laser [20]	16 ± 2 J/cm^2	7 mm	0.5 ms
Nd:YAG [36]	75–100 J/cm^2	5 mm	15 ms
Nd:YAG [24]	50 J/cm^2	6 mm	0.3 ms

hyperpigmentation [18–20, 22, 23, 35]. The non-ablative lasers, PDL and Nd:YAG, have been associated with erythema, pain, burning sensation, pruritus, post-inflammatory hyperpigmentation and transient purpura as well, with one study identifying no adverse events [27, 29–32, 36].

18.6 Future Directions

There are a multitude of non-laser treatment modalities available for scar and striae therapy. While cryotherapy, pressure therapy, fluorouracil (5-FU) injections, silicone gel sheeting, corticosteroids, surgical excision, and radiation therapy have all been successfully tested, combination of these therapies has been advocated by extensive clinical use [40]. There is a dearth of literature adequately testing these combination therapies; however, some multimodal options are more prominently represented. A combination of corticosteroid, 5-FU injection and PDL laser therapy is a common treatment [40, 41]. In one study, corticosteroid, 5-FU injection and PDL laser therapy was compared to corticosteroid and 5-FU treatment in a study with 60 patients. Patients preferred treatment that included PDL laser, although efficacy of both treatments were comparable [42]. Surgical excision combined with cryotherapy and corticosteroid injection is another of the most commonly used combination therapies in treatment of hypertrophic and keloid scars [40, 43]. New combinations incorporating the latest treatments such as photodynamic therapy (PDT) and imiquimod cream promise to offer advancements in treatment of scars and striae going forward. Imiquimod is a topical cream that increases collagen breakdown and PDT is being considered for use in keloids for its ability to reduce type I collagen synthesis [40]. These therapies are also favorable options for children as they are painless.

Researchers' developing understanding of the wound healing process has also made growth factors a focus for research concerning the next generation of wound healing therapies [41]. Growth factors play an important role in the pathogenesis of wound healing and scar formation. The transforming growth factor-β (TGF-β) family has been specifically studied in hypertrophic scars for its importance in the wound healing β-pathway [44]. Treatment with TGF-β3 reduced dermal scarring and resulted in the regeneration of normal skin structure [45]. Additionally, neutralizing TGF-β1 and TGF-β2 has been shown to reduce post-operative scarring and collagen synthesis in animals [46]. Other growth factor regulation studies focus on pathways that include the platelet-derived growth factor, connective tissue growth factor, epidermal growth factor, and the vascular endothelial growth factor [44]. As growth factor pathways are increasingly understood, growth factor regulation will contribute to innovative treatments.

18.7 Conclusion

Skin scarring and striae can be a burden to any patient, especially in young patients. The high prevalence of acne scarring and striae in the adolescent population indicate the importance of appropriate treatment, and yet specific guidelines for pediatric patients do not exist. Though treatment varies based on location, type of scar, and color; laser therapy can be a useful tool for functional, symptomatic, and cosmetic improvement. Developing technologies and techniques in laser, medical, and combination therapy are promising for the treatment of scars now and in the future.

References

1 Gurtner, G.C., Werner, S., Barrandon, Y. et al. (2008). Wound repair and regeneration. *Nature* 453: 314–321.
2 Al-Himdani, S., Ud-Din, S., Gilmore, S. et al. (2014). Striae distensae: a comprehensive review and evidence-based evaluation of prophylaxis and treatment. *Br. J. Dermatol.* 170: 527–547.
3 Krakowski, A.C., Totri, C.R., Donelan, M.B. et al. (2016). Scar management in the pediatric and adolescent populations. *Pediatrics* 137: e20142065.
4 Layton, A.M., Henderson, C.A., and Cunliffe, W.J. (1994). A clinical evaluation of acne scarring and its incidence. *Clin. Exp. Dermatol.* 19: 303–308.
5 Goodman, G.J. (2001). Post-acne scarring: a short review of its pathophysiology. *Austr. J. Dermatol.* 42: 84–90.
6 Akaishi, S., Ogawa, R., and Hyakusoku, H. (2008). Keloid and hypertrophic scar: neurogenic inflammation hypotheses. *Med. Hypotheses* 71: 32–38.
7 Berman, B., Maderal, A., and Raphael, B. (2017). Keloids and hypertrophic scars: pathophysiology, classification, and treatment. *Dermatol. Surg.* 43: S3–S18.
8 Kamath, N.V., Ormsby, A., Bergfeld, W.F. et al. (2002). A light microscopic and immunohistochemical evaluation of scars. *J. Cutan. Pathol.* 29: 27–32.
9 Lee, J.Y., Yang, C.C., Chao, S.C. et al. (2004). Histopathological differential diagnosis of keloid and hypertrophic scar. *Am. J. Dermatopathol.* 26: 379–384.
10 Ogawa, R. (2011). Mechanobiology of scarring. *Wound Repair Regen.* 19 (Suppl 1): s2–s9.
11 Halim, A.S., Emami, A., Salahshourifar, I. et al. (2012). Keloid scarring: understanding the genetic basis, advances, and prospects. *Arch. Plast. Surg.* 39: 184–189.
12 Trelles, M.A. and Martinez-Carpio, P.A. (2016). Clinical and histological results in the treatment of atrophic and hypertrophic scars using a combined method of radiofrequency, ultrasound, and transepidermal drug delivery. *Int. J. Dermatol.* 55: 926–933.
13 Patel, L., McGrouther, D., and Chakrabarty, K. (2014). Evaluating evidence for atrophic scarring treatment modalities. *JRSM Open* 5: 2054270414540139.
14 Jacob, C.I., Dover, J.S., and Kaminer, M.S. (2001). Acne scarring: a classification system and review of treatment options. *J. Am. Acad. Dermatol.* 45: 109–117.
15 Arem, A.J. and Kischer, C.W. (1980). Analysis of striae. *Plast. Reconstr. Surg.* 65: 22–29.
16 Garg, G.A., Sao, P.P., and Khopkar, U.S. (2011). Effect of carbon dioxide laser ablation followed by intralesional steroids on keloids. *J. Cutan. Aesthet. Surg.* 4: 2–6.
17 Azzam, O.A., Bassiouny, D.A., El-Hawary, M.S. et al. (2016). Treatment of hypertrophic scars and keloids by fractional carbon dioxide laser: a clinical, histological,

and immunohistochemical study. *Lasers Med. Sci.* 31: 9–18.

18 Majid, I. and Imran, S. (2014). Fractional CO_2 laser resurfacing as monotherapy in the treatment of atrophic facial acne scars. *J. Cutan. Aesthet. Surg.* 7: 87–92.

19 El Taieb, M.A. and Ibrahim, A.K. (2016). Fractional CO_2 laser versus intense pulsed light in treating striae distensae. *Ind. J. Dermatol.* 61: 174–180.

20 Naeini, F.F., Nikyar, Z., Mokhtari, F. et al. (2014). Comparison of the fractional CO_2 laser and the combined use of a pulsed dye laser with fractional CO_2 laser in striae alba treatment. *Adv. Biomed. Res.* 3: 184.

21 Wagner, J.A., Paasch, U., Bodendorf, M.O. et al. (2011). Treatment of keloids and hypertrophic scars with the triple-mode Er:YAG laser: a pilot study. *Med. Laser Appl.* 26: 10–15.

22 Tidwell, W.J., Owen, C.E., Kulp-Shorten, C. et al. (2016). Fractionated Er:YAG laser versus fully ablative Er:YAG laser for scar revision: results of a split scar, double blinded, prospective trial. Lasers Surg. Med.

23 You, H.J., Kim, D.W., Yoon, E.S. et al. (2016). Comparison of four different lasers for acne scars: resurfacing and fractional lasers. *J. Plast. Reconstr. Aesthet. Surg.* 69: e87–e95.

24 Gungor, S., Sayilgan, T., Gokdemir, G. et al. (2014). Evaluation of an ablative and non-ablative laser procedure in the treatment of striae distensae. *Ind. J. Dermatol. Venereol. Leprol.* 80: 409–412.

25 Wolfram, D., Tzankov, A., Pulzl, P. et al. (2009). Hypertrophic scars and keloids – a review of their pathophysiology, risk factors, and therapeutic management. *Dermatol. Surg.* 35: 171–181.

26 Kuo, Y.R., Jeng, S.F., Wang, F.S. et al. (2004). Flashlamp pulsed dye laser (PDL) suppression of keloid proliferation through down-regulation of TGF-beta1 expression and extracellular matrix expression. *Lasers Surg. Med.* 34: 104–108.

27 Manuskiatti, W., Wanitphakdeedecha, R., and Fitzpatrick, R.E. (2007). Effect of pulse width of a 595-nm flashlamp-pumped pulsed dye laser on the treatment response of keloidal and hypertrophic sternotomy scars. *Dermatol. Surg.* 33: 152–161.

28 Brewin, M.P. and Lister, T.S. (2014). Prevention or treatment of hypertrophic burn scarring: a review of when and how to treat with the pulsed dye laser. *Burns* 40: 797–804.

29 Patel, N. and Clement, M. (2002). Selective nonablative treatment of acne scarring with 585 nm flashlamp pulsed dye laser. *Dermatol. Surg.* 28: 942–945; discussion 5.

30 Lee, D.H., Choi, Y.S., Min, S.U. et al. (2009). Comparison of a 585-nm pulsed dye laser and a 1064-nm Nd:YAG laser for the treatment of acne scars: a randomized split-face clinical study. *J. Am. Acad. Dermatol.* 60: 801–807.

31 Shokeir, H., El Bedewi, A., Sayed, S. et al. (2014). Efficacy of pulsed dye laser versus intense pulsed light in the treatment of striae distensae. *Dermatol. Surg.* 40: 632–640.

32 Jimenez, G.P., Flores, F., Berman, B. et al. (2003). Treatment of striae rubra and striae alba with the 585-nm pulsed-dye laser. *Dermatol. Surg.* 29: 362–365.

33 Akaishi, S., Koike, S., Dohi, T. et al. (2012). Nd:YAG laser treatment of keloids and hypertrophic scars. *Eplasty* 12: e1.

34 Koike, S., Akaishi, S., Nagashima, Y. et al. (2014). Nd:YAG laser treatment for keloids and hypertrophic scars: an analysis of 102 cases. *Plast. Reconstr. Surg. Glob. Open* 2: e272.

35 Asilian, A., Salimi, E., Faghihi, G. et al. (2011). Comparison of Q-switched 1064-nm Nd:YAG laser and fractional CO_2 laser efficacies on improvement of atrophic facial acne scar. *J. Res. Med. Sci.* 16: 1189–1195.

36 Elsaie, M.L., Hussein, M.S., Tawfik, A.A. et al. (2016). Comparison of the effectiveness of two fluences using long-pulsed Nd:YAG laser in the treatment of striae distensae. Histological and morphometric evaluation. *Lasers Med. Sci.* 31 (9): 1845–1853.

37 Kono, T., Ercocen, A.R., Nakazawa, H. et al. (2005). Treatment of hypertrophic scars using a long-pulsed dye laser with cryogen-spray cooling. *Ann. Plast. Surg.* 54: 487–493.
38 Kuo, Y.R., Wu, W.S., Jeng, S.F. et al. (2005). Activation of ERK and p38 kinase mediated keloid fibroblast apoptosis after flashlamp pulsed-dye laser treatment. *Lasers Surg. Med.* 36: 31–37.
39 Chan, H.H., Wong, D.S., Ho, W.S. et al. (2004). The use of pulsed dye laser for the prevention and treatment of hypertrophic scars in Chinese persons. *Dermatol. Surg.* 30: 987–994; discussion 94.
40 Gauglitz, G.G. (2013). Management of keloids and hypertrophic scars: current and emerging options. *Clin. Cosmet. Investig. Dermatol.* 6: 103–114.
41 Tziotzios, C., Profyris, C., and Sterling, J. (2012). Cutaneous scarring: pathophysiology, molecular mechanisms, and scar reduction therapeutics part II. Strategies to reduce scar formation after dermatologic procedures. *J. Am. Acad. Dermatol.* 66: 13–24; quiz 5–6.
42 Asilian, A., Darougheh, A., and Shariati, F. (2006). New combination of triamcinolone, 5-fluorouracil, and pulsed-dye laser for treatment of keloid and hypertrophic scars. *Dermatol. Surg.* 32: 907–915.
43 Lawrence, W.T. (1991). In search of the optimal treatment of keloids: report of a series and a review of the literature. *Ann. Plast. Surg.* 27: 164–178.
44 Lian, N. and Li, T. (2016). Growth factor pathways in hypertrophic scars: molecular pathogenesis and therapeutic implications. *Biomed. Pharmacother.* 84: 42–50.
45 Occleston, N.L., Laverty, H.G., O'Kane, S. et al. (2008). Prevention and reduction of scarring in the skin by transforming growth factor beta 3 (TGFbeta3): from laboratory discovery to clinical pharmaceutical. *J. Biomater. Sci. Polym. Ed.* 19: 1047–1063.
46 Gauglitz, G.G., Korting, H.C., Pavicic, T. et al. (2011). Hypertrophic scarring and keloids: pathomechanisms and current and emerging treatment strategies. *Mol. Med.* 17: 113–125.

19

Lasers for Acne

Mohammad-Ali Yazdani Abyaneh[1], *Robert D. Griffith*[1], *Leyre Falto-Aizpurua*[1], *Harleen Arora*[2], *and Keyvan Nouri*[3]

[1] Department of Dermatology & Cutaneous Surgery, University of Miami Miller School of Medicine, Miami, FL, USA
[2] University of Miami, Coral Gables, FL, USA
[3] Department of Dermatology, Ophthalmology, Otolaryngology & Surgery, University of Miami Leonard M. Miller School of Medicine, Miami, FL, USA

19.1 Introduction

- Acne vulgaris the most common disease of the skin and primarily affects adolescents.
- Laser and light therapies target *Propionibacterium acnes* and the sebaceous gland.
- Preliminary studies suggest efficacy and a good side effect profile for treatment of inflammatory acne with narrowband light, infrared lasers, and photodynamic therapy.

Acne vulgaris is the most common disease of the skin. Its prevalence is estimated to be somewhere between 70 and 87% among adolescents, who are classically affected by the disease [1]. The mean age of onset of disease is between 11 and 12 years of age, with girls inclined toward an earlier onset. The frequency of acne increases drastically into the late teens [2]. The pediatric population is therefore significantly affected by the disease and stands to benefit from breakthroughs in safe and effective treatment options.

The diagnosis and early treatment of acne is important to address its social and psychological burden as well as to prevent the potential development of scars [3]. The first-line treatment for acne is usually a combination of topical and oral retinoids, antibiotics, and benzoyl peroxide [4]. But recalcitrant and recurrent acne, side effects from standard treatments, and concerns over antibiotic resistance have impelled research into further treatment modalities. The use of lights and lasers both for the treatment of active acne lesions and for acne scars has been the subject of ample research in recent years.

For active acne lesions, intense narrowband blue light, mid-infrared 1450 nm diode laser, and photodynamic therapy have shown promise in efficacy and safety in a multitude of studies. A narrowband blue light device (ClearLight, Lumenis, Inc. Santa Clara, CA) and a 1450 nm diode laser device (Smoothbeam, Candela Corp., Wayland, MA) have Food and Drug Administration (FDA) approvals for the treatment of mild to moderate inflammatory acne [5, 6]. These therapies target *P. acnes* and sebaceous gland function [7].

P. acnes produces porphyrins as part of its natural metabolism. These porphyrins absorb light maximally at certain absorption peaks within the electromagnetic spectrum (Figure 19.1). The highest of these peaks is the Soret Band between 400 and 420 nm, with other smaller peaks, or Q Bands, falling in the range of 500–700 nm. Absorption of light at these peaks by porphyrins generates

Pediatric Dermatologic Surgery, First Edition. Edited by Keyvan Nouri, Latanya Benjamin, Jasem Alshaiji, and Jan Izakovic.

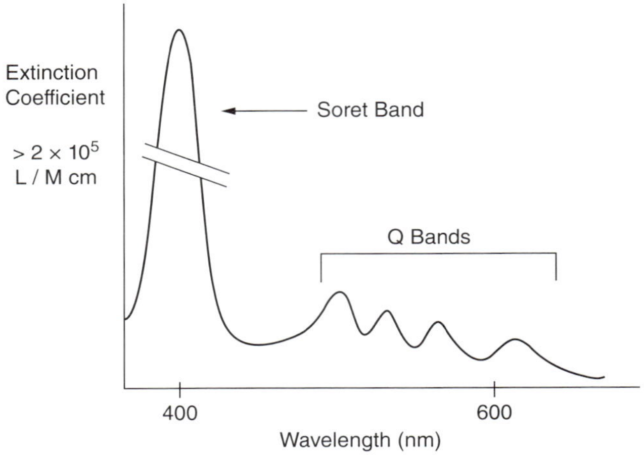

Figure 19.1 Porphyrin light absorption peaks on the electromagnetic spectrum. Note that the peak designated as the Soret Band corresponds to the wavelengths emitted by narrowband blue light. *Source:* Mariwalla and Rohrer [7]. Reprinted with permission of John Wiley & Sons, Inc.

singlet oxygen molecules which are believed to damage the cell walls of *P. acnes*, thereby destroying the bacteria [8]. Narrowband light (i.e. blue and red light), broadband light (i.e. intense pulsed light [IPL]), pulsed dye laser (PDL) (585 nm, 595 nm), and potassium titanyl phosphate (KTP) laser (532 nm) all have wavelengths which correspond to a porphyrin absorption peak [4].

Infrared lasers, owing to their higher wavelength, penetrate deeper into the skin and are believed to damage the sebaceous gland and decrease sebum output as well as glandular size [9, 10]. A similar mechanism is suspected in photodynamic therapy (PDT), where the application of photosensitizers (which are porphyrin precursors) and subsequent irradiation of the skin is believed to produce free radicals damaging the sebaceous gland [11].

The published data for light and laser therapies presents an exciting and promising new approach to the treatment of acne, with need for further study.

19.2 Indications

- Physicians may consider treatment on an individual basis for patients unresponsive to standard therapy, those who suffer significant adverse effects or recurrence on standard therapy, and those with contraindications to standard therapy.
- Most studies on light and laser therapies have focused on mild to moderate inflammatory acne.
- Use of laser treatment in patients under 18 years of age is limited in the literature.

The proper place for laser therapy in the arsenal of acne treatments remains to be determined. The use of lasers in acne is not recommended as a first-line treatment or as monotherapy [4]. Instead, it is reserved for patients who do not respond to standard therapy or show only partial response, those who suffer significant adverse effects or recurrences on standard therapy, and those with contraindications to standard therapy [12].

Laser therapy has been most effective in patients with mild to moderate inflammatory acne, and should therefore be considered as an option primarily in this group of patients. One potential approach is to administer laser and light-based therapies as an adjunct to oral and topical therapies that have failed on their own. The use of standard treatments for maintenance of results is important because light and laser therapies that target *P. acnes* can be short-lived [7].

The indications for using lasers in treating pediatric acne are less clear. Of the small number of subjects studied in trials of lights and lasers for acne, an even smaller proportion have constituted patients under 18 years of age (Tables 19.1 and 19.2). Therefore, any decision to treat pediatric patients should be made more cautiously and only after a thorough discussion with the patient and the patient's guardian(s).

19.3 Types of Lasers

- Intense narrowband blue light and 1450 nm diode laser have demonstrated safety and efficacy in multiple studies and have FDA approvals for treating inflammatory acne.
- PDT has shown a lot of promise in treating inflammatory acne, but treatment protocols in different studies have varied widely.
- Other lasers have been studied to a lesser extent.

In recent years, various types of lights and lasers have been studied for the treatment of acne. Among the treatments studied are narrowband light sources (blue and red light), infrared lasers, PDT, IPL, PDL, and the KTP laser. The FDA has approved the use of intense narrowband blue light and the mid-infrared 1450 nm diode laser for the treatment of inflammatory acne based on the preliminary evidence supporting their safety and efficacy [5, 6]. The FDA has also approved PDL and another infrared device exclusively for back acne [13, 14]. It is important to note that FDA approval for devices entails a much less rigorous process than it does for drugs [4].

19.3.1 Narrowband Light

In 2001, Shalita et al. published the results of an uncontrolled trial of twice weekly treatments for four weeks with a blue metal halide lamp (ClearLight) in 35 patients with facial and back acne [15]. They reported a 68% decline in inflammatory lesions. This study was followed by a number of controlled trials to assess narrowband light therapy for mild to moderate inflammatory facial acne (Table 19.1, Figure 19.2). A number of these studies have demonstrated statistically significant better results with light treatment vs. no treatment (or a mixture of blue and red light vs benzoyl peroxide alone [16]), but no studies have yet compared light therapy to a standard combination of topical and/or oral medications for acne.

These studies show that narrowband blue light, especially in combination with red light, can have efficacy and a favorable adverse effect profile in treating inflammatory facial acne. A few of the studies enrolled subjects under 18 years of age [16–18]. However, the number of pediatric patients studied was small and not explicitly specified.

19.3.2 Infrared Lasers

Infrared lasers penetrate deeper into the dermis and target water, which constitutes the major chromophore in sebaceous glands [9]. By inducing thermal injury to the glands, infrared lasers reduce glandular size and sebum production and help in clearing inflammatory lesions. A dynamic cooling device is used concurrently to protect the epidermis from injury.

To date, the most studied of infrared lasers for the treatment of acne is the 1450 nm diode laser. In the first major study of this laser, Paithankar et al. conducted a three-part experiment with the 1450 nm diode laser [9]. First, they demonstrated that thermal injury in the upper dermis with preservation of the epidermis was possible in *ex-vivo* human skin. Then they demonstrated similar results (with histologic evidence of damaged sebaceous glands) *in vivo* in rabbit ears. Finally, the trial compared four treatments, separated by three-week intervals, with 1450 nm laser with cryogen cooling vs cryogen cooling alone. Subjects had similar inflammatory lesions in their bilateral upper back and selection of treatment and control

Table 19.1 Major randomized controlled trials of narrowband light therapy for acne vulgaris.

	Papageorgiou et al. [16]	Elman et al. [41]	Tzung et al. [17]	Gold et al. [18]	Na and Suh [39]
Treatment	Daily treatments for 12 weeks in 4 parallel groups: 1) blue light 2) blue/red light 3) cool white light 4) 5% BPO	Twice weekly treatments for 4 weeks with blue light in a split-face double-blind trial	Twice weekly treatments for 4 weeks with blue light in a split-face trial	Twice weekly treatments for 4 weeks with blue light	Twice daily treatments for 8 weeks with a portable red-light-emitting device
Control(s)	Multiple parallel groups	Untreated side in split-face study	Untreated side in split-face study	Topical clindamycin 1% twice daily	Untreated side in split-face study
# of patients (age)	107 (14–50)	23 (mean 18.8)	31 (15–32)	34 (13–55)	30 (19–33)
Treated site	NA	Face	Face	Face	Face
Skin type	NA	NA	III–IV	NA	NA
Acne severity	Mild to moderate	Mild to moderate	Mild to moderate	Mild to moderate	Mild to moderate
Follow-up	Every 4 weeks for 12 weeks during treatment	2, 4, and 8 weeks after final treatment	4 weeks after final treatment	4 weeks after final treatment	At weeks 1, 2, 4, and 8 during treatment
Results	76% mean improvement in inflammatory lesions and 58% in comedones at 12 weeks in mixed light group, significantly better compared to BPO and white light groups ($P < 0.05$)	53% reduction in inflammatory lesions 8 weeks after final treatment ($P = 0.01$)	52% mean improvement on treated side vs 12% on control side, 4 weeks after final treatment ($P < 0.05$)	36% improvement in blue light group vs 14% in Clindamycin control group. Results were not statistically significant.	66% reduction vs 74% increase in inflammatory lesions and 59% reduction vs 3% increase in non-inflammatory lesions on treated vs control side, respectively, at 8 weeks ($P < 0.005$)
Side effects reported	Significantly more pruritus and dryness in BPO group (32%)	No side effects reported	Exacerbation of nodulocysts	NA	No significant side effects reported

NA: Information not available in the study.

Table 19.2 Major trials of the 1450 nm infrared diode laser for acne vulgaris.

	Paithankar et al. [9]	Friedman et al. [22][a]	Wang et al. [20]	Jih et al. [19][a]	Darne et al. [21]
Treatment	4 laser treatments with cryogen cooling vs cryogen cooling alone at 3-week intervals	3 laser treatments at 4–6-week intervals	4 laser treatments + microdermabrasion vs 4 laser treatments alone at 3-week intervals, in split-face study	3 laser treatments at fluences of 14 J/cm^2 vs 16 J/cm^2 at 3–4-week intervals, in split-face dose response study	3 laser treatments at 4-week intervals, in split-face study
Control(s)	Untreated side of upper back	None	Laser-treated only side of face	None	Untreated side of the face
# of patients (age)	27 (18–39)	19 (15–44)	20 (19–59)	20 (18–39)	38 (18–47)
Treated site	Upper back	Face	Face	Face	Face
Skin type	II–VI	II–IV	II–IV	II–VI	I–V
Acne severity	>20 inflammatory lesions	>5 inflammatory lesions	Moderate to severe	>20 inflammatory lesions	Moderate to severe
Randomization	Yes	No	Yes	Yes	Yes
Follow-up	6 months after final treatment	No follow-up after final treatment	3 months after final treatment	12 months after final treatment	12 months after final treatment
Results	98% reduction in lesion counts on laser-treated side compared to baseline ($P < 0.001$) vs 6% reduction on control side six months after final treatment	37% reduction in lesion counts after 1 treatment ($p < 0.01$), 58% after 2 treatments ($p < 0.01$), and 83% after 3 treatments ($p < 0.01$)	54.4% reduction in lesion counts in laser + microdermabrasion group vs 61.1% reduction in laser alone group, 3 months after final treatment ($P = 0.28$)	76.1% (in 14 J/cm^2 group) and 70.5% (in 16 J/cm^2 group), 12 months after final treatment ($P < 0.01$)	Change in lesion count and grade similar between the treated and control sides of the face, 12 months after final treatment
Side effects reported	Transient erythema, edema, and hyperpigmentation in laser + cryogen group	Transient edema and erythema.	Similar rates of erythema, edema, papules, and pain in both groups	Pain slightly higher with 16 J only after 1st treatment. Transient erythema and edema.	Transient post-op erythema which lasted for up to 36 hours

[a] Subjects were allowed to continue their topical or oral medications.
NA: Information not available in the study.

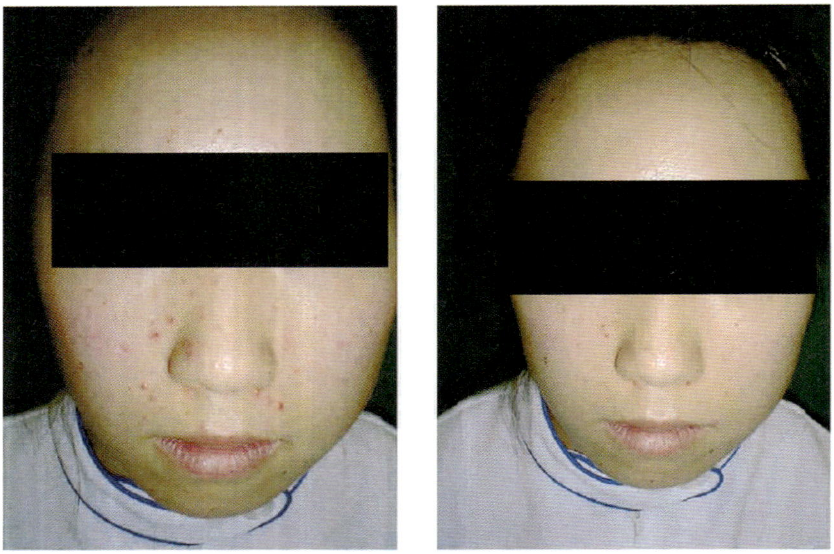

Figure 19.2 A patient with mild to moderate acne treated with narrowband blue light (peak 407–420 nm) twice weekly for five weeks, with marked improvement. *Source:* Kawada et al. [40]. Reprinted with permission of Elsevier Limited.

sides was randomized. At a six-month follow-up, the trial showed a statistically significant reduction in lesion counts on the treated side (98%) vs the control side (6%). Several other trials have since demonstrated the safety and efficacy of the 1450 nm diode laser in the treatment of mild to severe inflammatory acne (Table 19.2, Figures 19.3–19.6) [19–23].

19.3.3 Photodynamic Therapy

PDT relies on a photosensitizer and a light source to produce reactive oxygen species and damage sebaceous glands [12]. The most studied photosensitizers in PDT are topical 5-aminolevulinic acid (ALA) and methyl 5-aminolevulinate (MAL) (Figure 19.7). The efficacy of ALA and MAL has been compared for acne treatment in studies using long incubation periods and high fluence red light, with similar results [24–26]. Pain during treatment sessions was reported to be equal but worse with ALA after 24 hours.

The light source most studied and with the best results in long-term follow-up studies of PDT for acne is red light [27]. Sebaceous glands are located between 0.5 and 1 mm deep into the skin [28]. Therefore, although porphyrins have a maximal absorption peak in the blue light range, red light is used more often as it is able to penetrate deeper (up to 2 mm) and better reach the glands (Figure 19.8).

As most studies of PDT for acne to date have utilized different treatment parameters or have been poorly controlled, there is no consensus yet on appropriate treatment methods, and this modality has not yet received FDA approval for acne treatment.

19.3.4 Other Laser and Light Therapies

Pulsed Dye Laser: The first two randomized controlled trials (RCTs) to look at PDL in treating acne reported mixed results. In 2003 Seaton et al. reported 49% improvement in inflammatory acne lesions 12 weeks after one treatment with the 585 nm PDL compared to a sham-laser-treated control group [29]. However, shortly after, using similar laser settings in a split-face randomized trial,

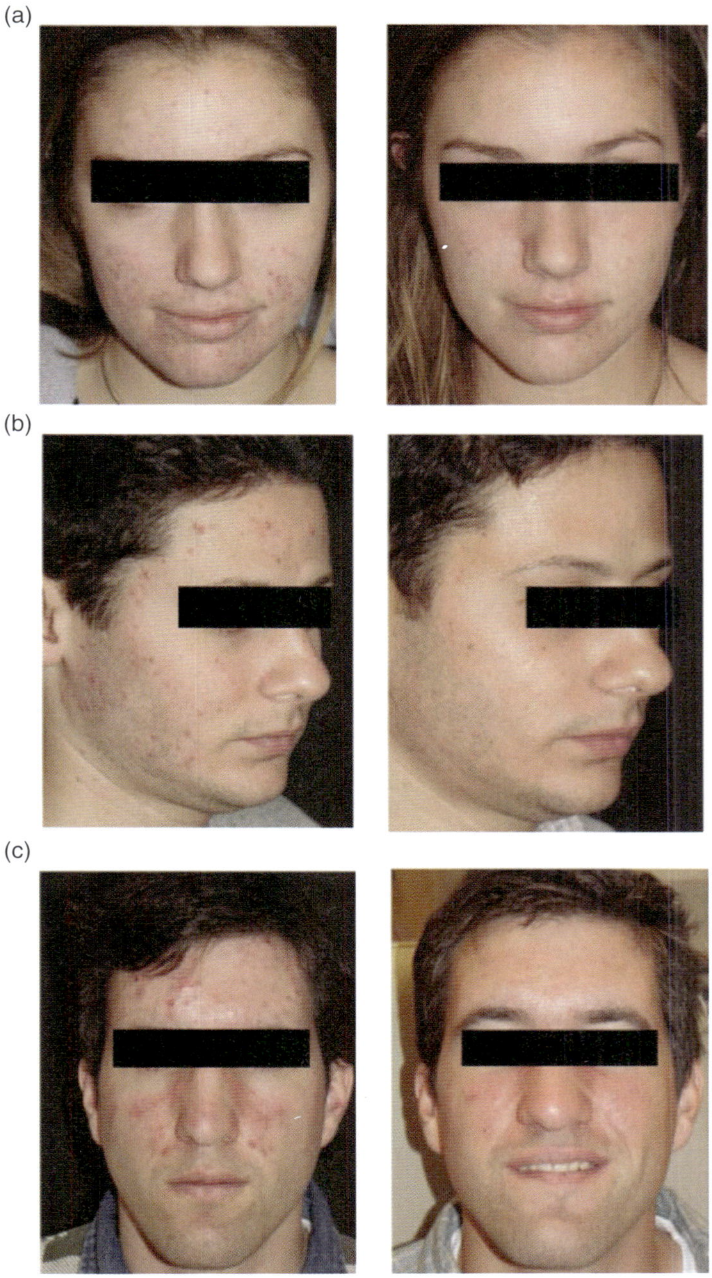

Figure 19.3 Patients treated with the 1450 nm diode laser for facial acne. Lesion counts were noted to decline with more treatment sessions. The follow-up pictures on the right are from one month after (a) two treatments, (b) three treatments, and (c) four treatments. *Source:* Mariwalla and Rohrer [7]. Reprinted with permission of John Wiley & Sons, Inc.

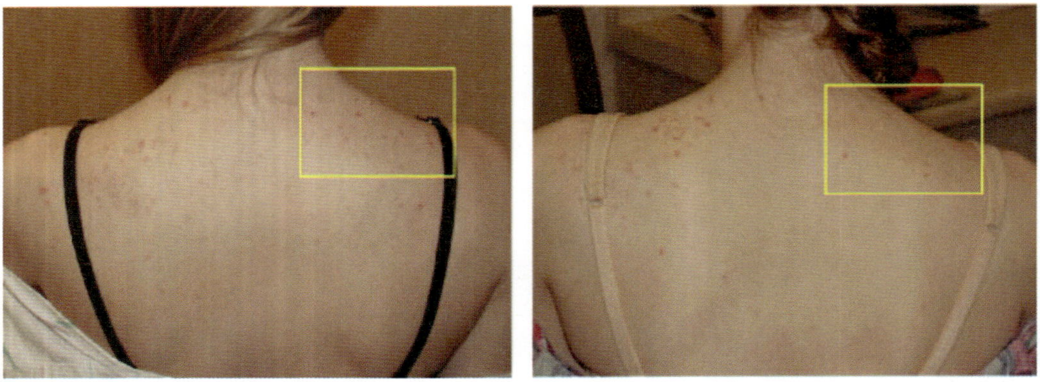

Figure 19.4 Patient response to one session of localized treatment with the 1450 nm diode laser over the marked area for back acne. *Source:* Mariwalla and Rohrer [7]. Reprinted with permission of John Wiley & Sons, Inc.

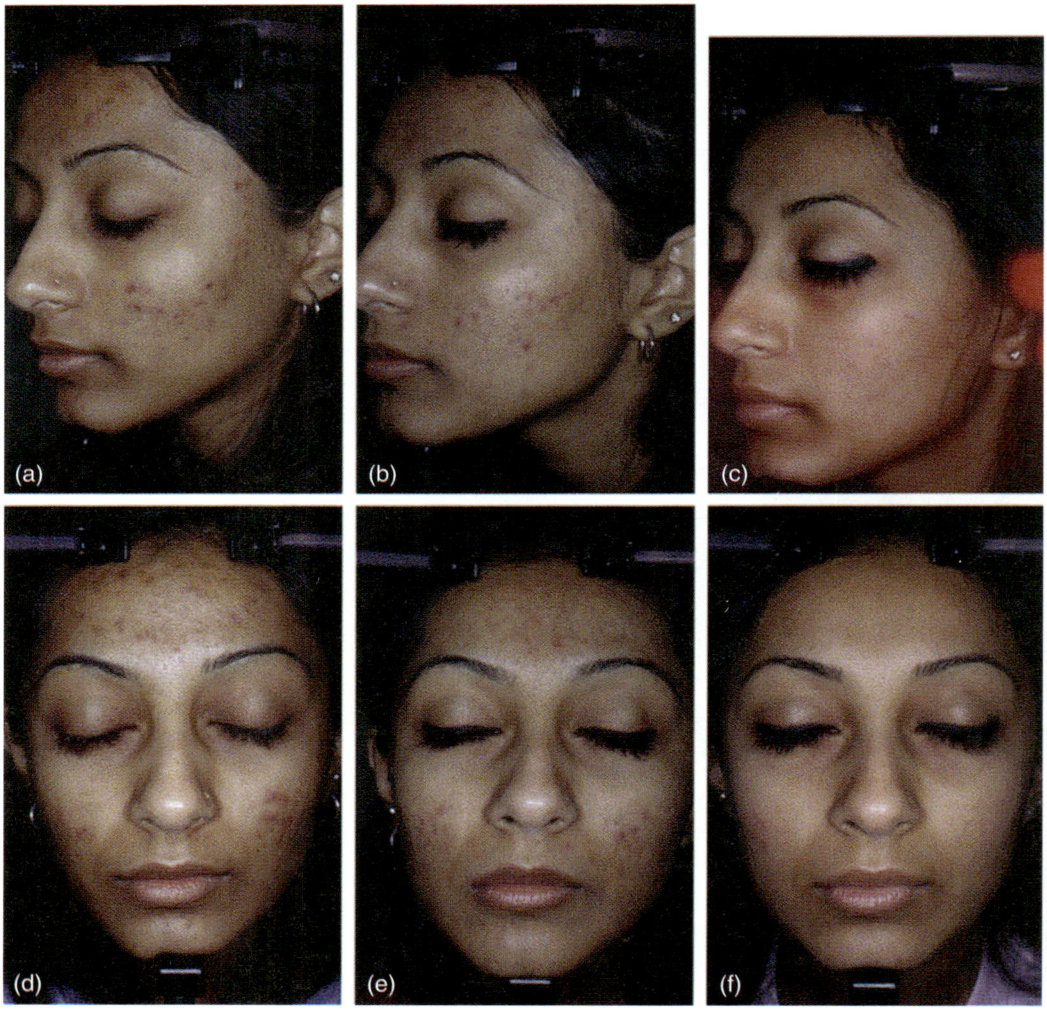

Figure 19.5 Left cheek in a patient treated with the 1450 nm diode laser three times at three- to four-week intervals, (a) before treatment, (b) after three treatments, and (c) at 12-month follow-up. Frontal view of the same patient, (d) before treatment, (e) at one-month follow-up, and (f) at 12-month follow-up. *Source:* Jih et al. [19]. Copyright 2006 American Academy of Dermatology, Inc. Reprinted with permission of Elsevier Limited.

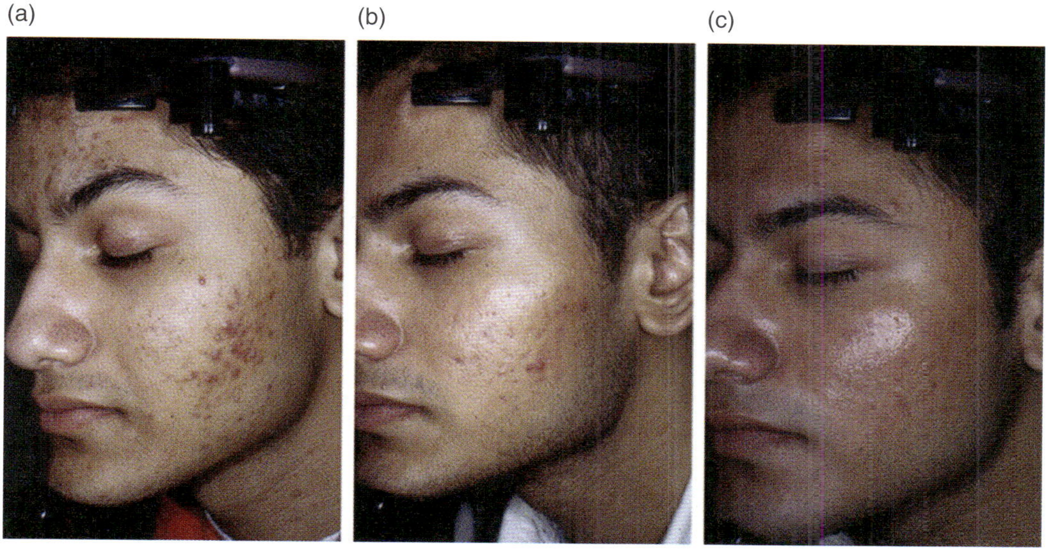

Figure 19.6 Another patient (a) before treatment, (b) after three treatments with the 1450 nm diode laser at three- to four-week intervals, and (c) at 12-month follow-up. *Source:* Jih et al. [19]. Copyright 2006 American Academy of Dermatology, Inc. Reprinted with permission of Elsevier Limited.

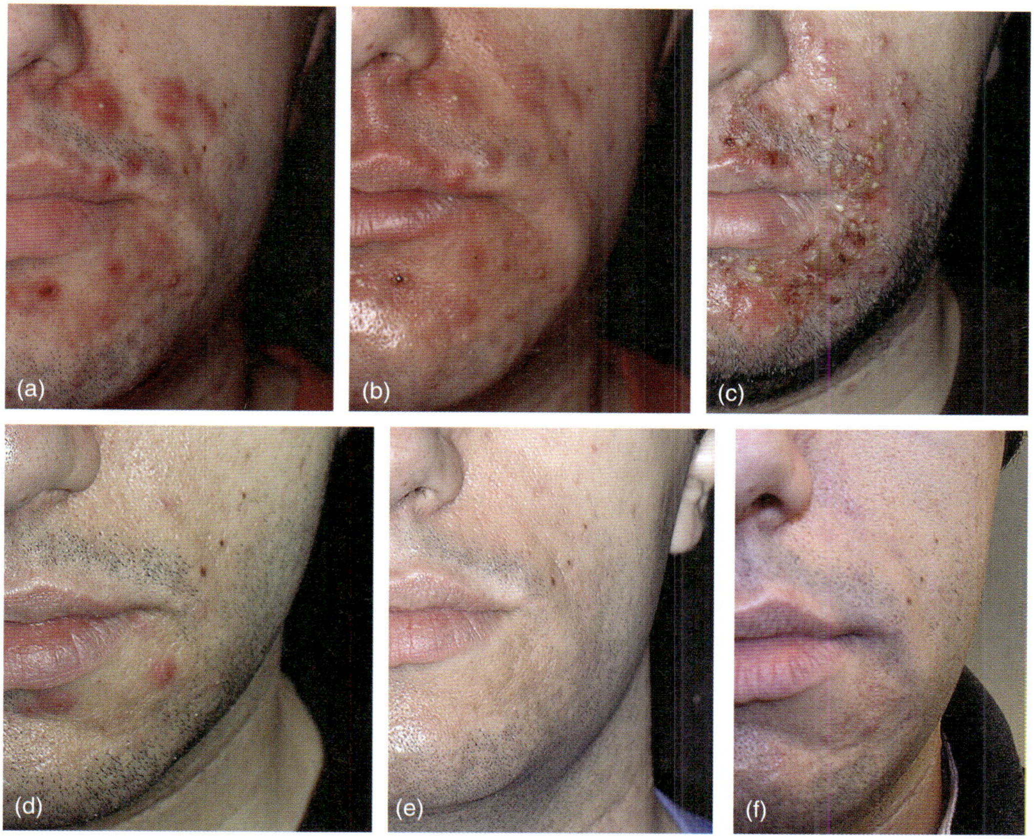

Figure 19.7 Patient with inflammatory acne treated with 20% 5-aminolevulinic acid and red light (633 nm) photodynamic therapy. Patient is seen (a) before treatment, (b) immediately after treatment, (c) two days after treatment, (d) seven months after treatment, (e) 10 months after initial and three months after second treatment, and (f) 12 months after initial treatment with four total treatments. (Courtesy R. Rox Anderson, MD). *Source:* Sakamoto et al. [27]. Copyright 2010 American Academy of Dermatology, Inc. Reprinted with permission of Elsevier Limited.

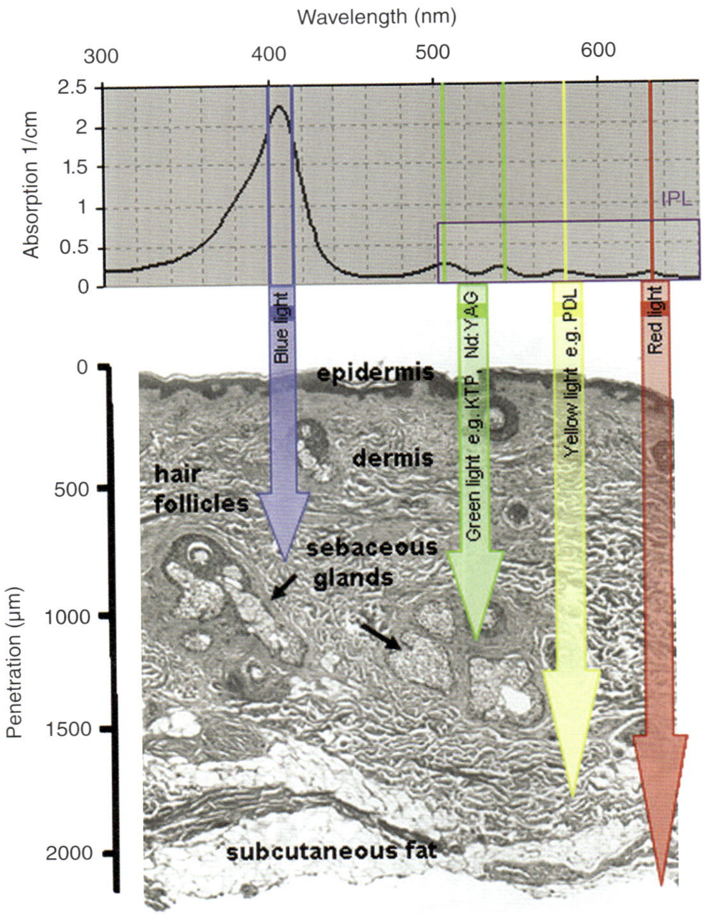

Figure 19.8 Red light is able to penetrate deeper into the dermis (compared to other common light sources used in photodynamic therapy) and activate porphyrins within more sebaceous glands, which offers a potential explanation for its superior efficacy in photodynamic therapy. IPL: Intense pulsed light, KTP: potassium titanyl phosphate, Nd:YAG: neodymium: yttrium aluminum garnet, PDL: pulsed dye laser. *Source:* Sakamoto et al. [27]. Copyright 2010 American Academy of Dermatology, Inc. Reprinted with permission of Elsevier Limited.

Orrigner et al. found no difference between treated vs untreated sides [30]. Karsai et al. compared treating patients with combination clindamycin 1% and benzoyl peroxide 5% gel alone vs in combination with the 585 nm PDL in a single-blinded RCT [31]. Both groups showed significant improvement but without any significant difference between them.

Intense Pulsed Light: Several studies have demonstrated that IPL is not any more effective than adapalene gel [32] or benzoyl peroxide [33] in the treatment of acne. IPL may be more effective in combination with topical photosensitizers in PDT [34, 35].

Potassium Titanyl Phosphate Laser: The 532 nm KTP laser has also been studied to a limited extent with variable results. Bowes et al. demonstrated mild efficacy in improving mild to moderate acne one month after treatment in a small controlled trial using the KTP laser [36]. Baugh et al. compared the KTP laser in a randomized split-face trial with sham treatment in 26 patients and observed significantly better results on the treated side at one week, but not at four weeks [37].

19.3.5 Lasers for Acne Scars

Lasers have also been successfully used for revision of atrophic acne scars. The most commonly studied lasers include the ablative CO_2 and Er:YAG lasers, the non-ablative 1450 nm diode and 1320 nm Nd:YAG lasers, as well as fractional photothermolysis with a 1550 nm erbium-doped fiber laser [4]. Chapter 18 covers the use of lasers in the treatment of scars in more depth.

19.4 Techniques

This section reviews the techniques for treating acne with narrowband light, infrared diode laser, and PDT, as established in some of the major studies utilizing these treatment options. It should be noted that certain challenges are unique to laser surgery in the pediatric population, which most of these studies did not have to contend with due to the higher age range of participants. It is important to remember the following general principles when dealing with pediatric patients: laser settings may need to be adjusted to account for pediatric skin and the unpredictable nature of its scarring [38]. Moreover, the choice of suitable anesthesia, size-appropriate safety equipment, and proper management of patient and parent anxiety should be considered.

19.4.1 Narrowband Light

A detailed medical history and skin examination should be performed as the initial step in all patients scheduled to undergo treatment with laser or light therapy [39]. Before treatment with any narrowband light sources, proper eye protection with goggles and a gentle facial wash is recommended [17].

Studies of narrowband light have used several different devices with different settings. Blue light (400–420 nm) has been studied the most among narrowband light sources; techniques in selected studies are as follows [16, 17, 40–44]:

- Treatments are usually delivered twice weekly for four to eight weeks.
- Treatment times range from 8 to 20 minutes.
- Light is delivered at a distance of 5–30 cm.
- Fluences range from 24 to 81 J/cm^2.
- Irradiances range from 40 to 90 mW/cm^2.
- Cumulative dose is usually 320 J/cm^2 but can range from 192 to 768 J/cm^2.
- One study applied skin cooling during light exposure with a built-in cooling system [41].

Red light (635–670 nm) has also been studied in treatment of mild to moderate acne [16, 39]:

- Red light can be administered alone or in combination with blue light.
- Treatments can be delivered daily for 8–12 weeks using portable LEDs.
- Treatment times are 15 minutes once or twice daily.
- Fluences range from 2.4 to 5.4 J/cm^2.
- Irradiances range from 2.67 to 6 mW/cm^2.
- Cumulative treatment dose ranges from 202 to 604.8 J/cm^2.

19.4.2 Infrared 1450 nm Diode Laser

The infrared 1450 nm diode laser Smoothbeam (Candela Corporation, Wayland, MA) has an integrated dynamic cooling device that provides cryogen spray cooling to preserve the epidermis while the infrared wavelength penetrates deeper to induce thermal damage of sebaceous glands. A summary of techniques used in different studies of this laser follows [9, 19–22]:

- The treatment regimen entails three to four treatments separated by three- to six-week intervals.
- Prior to treatment, topical anesthesia may be provided using topical lidocaine 5%, applied 30 minutes to an hour before laser treatment.

- Treatment is then performed on the entire face (or the entire selected area for back acne) from forehead to the jawline with non-overlapping pulses.
- A spot size of 6 mm is most often used.
- Four equal laser pulses are delivered which are preceded, separated by, and followed by cryogen spray for cooling.
- Pulse durations range from 160 to 210 ms, with cryogen spray durations ranging from 15 to 45 ms.
- Fluences range from 8 to 22 J/cm^2.
- Immediately following treatment, application of a moisturizing cream and sunscreen to the treated skin surface is carried out. Moreover, patients should be counseled on avoiding sun exposure and using a sunscreen with a sun protection factor of at least 30 on a daily basis post treatment [9, 19–22].
- Results are usually appreciated within two to four treatments [38].

19.4.3 Photodynamic Therapy

To administer PDT, the physician must first decide on the type of topical photosensitizer, light source, and treatment parameters.

- Prior to the application of the photosensitizer cream, the skin should be cleansed. This can be accomplished with alcohol, salicylic acid, soap, or an acetone scrub [11, 45–49].
- Some studies recommended curettage of inflammatory lesions [24] and perforation of nodulocysts with a cannula [26] prior to treatment.
- Topical anesthesia should not be applied because it may precipitate into a salt when combined with ALA and weaken treatment effectiveness [27]. Injectable anesthesia can be used without epinephrine.
- The topical photosensitizer (ALA or MAL) should be equally distributed on the area to be treated with incubation for three hours under occlusion.
- During the procedure, the patient may feel stinging pain. This pain can be reduced by decreasing the irradiance and adding a cooling device, such as a fan blowing cool air or spritzing cool water on the skin.
- After treatment is performed the patient should be instructed that complete healing is usually seen after a week of treatment but that the erythema and hyperpigmentation may persist for up to four weeks.
- Since porphyrins can be present in the skin for another 24–48 hours, intense visible light avoidance is recommended.
- Several treatment sessions may be required for some patients.

19.5 Complications

- Narrowband light sources can result in mild pain, erythema, dry skin, and pruritus.
- The infrared diode laser can result in mild pain, transient erythema, and edema. There are few reports of self-limited hyperpigmentation, especially in darker skin types.
- PDT can result in mild pain, transient erythema, and edema. Hyperpigmentation is uncommon and occurs more often in darker skin types. Localized photosensitivity can last for up to 48 hours.

Overall, laser and light therapies used in the treatment of acne have been well-tolerated, with few, short-lived adverse effects reported. Narrowband light sources such as blue and red light have had very minimal reports of adverse effects or patient discomfort. These include mild and self-limited burning after treatment [39], slight redness after treatment [42, 43], dryness of skin, and mild pruritus [43]. One study found that nodulocystic acne worsened during a trial of blue light therapy, which they suggested may have resulted from the natural course of the disease, and progression of comedones and papulopustules to nodulocysts [17]. The study concluded that "acne patients without nodulocysts are better candidates for blue light treatment."

The infrared diode laser has likewise been associated with minimal adverse effects, chief among them mild pain, transient postoperative erythema and edema [9, 19–22] which resolved in a day or two. A few reports of hyperpigmentation exist, especially in darker skin types [9]. These episodes all resolved spontaneously during follow-ups.

PDT is also fairly well-tolerated, with a low rate of serious adverse events. The most common adverse events include pain and stinging during light treatment, which can be ameliorated by spritzing cool water or providing ventilation with a fan [27]. Cessation of light exposure relieves this acute pain. Postoperative erythema and edema usually last for several days. An acute inflammatory reaction and transient tanning following therapy are also common. The risk of permanent scarring or ulceration is extremely low. Patients have localized photosensitivity for up to 48 hours after treatment and should be counseled to avoid bright visible light for that time. Most patients show complete healing one week after photodynamic therapy, but erythema and hyperpigmentation can last for a few weeks longer, especially in darker skin types.

19.6 Conclusion

Lasers and lights have shown promise in treating inflammatory acne. They are safe and offer the benefit of few adverse events. However, further studies are needed to establish their efficacy in comparison to standard therapy with a combination of topical and oral medications. Larger-sized RCTs with long-term follow-ups are necessary. Specifically, there is a need for more study in the pediatric population and to identifying patients who stand to benefit the most from laser therapy, which is important considering the significant cost burden of laser surgery.

References

1 Dreno, B. and Poli, F. (2003). Epidemiology of acne. *Dermatology* 206: 7–10.

2 Rademaker, M., Garioch, J., and Simpson, N. (1989). Acne in school children: no longer a concern for dermatologists. *BMJ* 298: 1217–1219.

3 Layton, A., Henderson, C., and Cunliffe, W. (1994). A clinical evaluation of acne scarring and its incidence. *Clin. Exp. Dermatol.* 19: 303–308.

4 Thiboutot, D., Gollnick, H., Bettoli, V. et al. (2009). New insights into the management of acne: an update from the Global Alliance to improve outcomes in acne group. *J. Am. Acad. Dermatol.* 60: S1–S50.

5 US Food and Drug Administration web site. ClearLight phototherapy device, model CL 420. http://www.accessdata.fda.gov/cdrh_docs/pdf/K013623.pdf (accessed 8 October 2013).

6 US Food and Drug Administration web site. Candela Smoothbeam Laser System. http://www.accessdata.fda.gov/cdrh_docs/pdf4/K041242.pdf (accessed 8 October 2013).

7 Mariwalla, K. and Rohrer, T. (2005). Use of lasers and light-based therapies for treatment of acne vulgaris. *Lasers Surg. Med.* 37: 333–342.

8 Elman, M. and Lebzelter, J. (2004). Light therapy in the treatment of acne vulgaris. *Dermatol. Surg.* 30: 139–146.

9 Paithankar, D., Ross, E., Saleh, B. et al. (2002). Acne treatment with a 1,450 nm wavelength laser and cryogen spray cooling. *Lasers Surg. Med.* 31: 106–114.

10 Perez-Maldonado, A., Runger, T., and Kreju-Papa, N. (2007) The 1,450-nm diode laser reduces sebum production in facial skin: a possible mode of action of its effectiveness for the treatment of acne vulgaris. *Lasers Surg. Med.* 39: 189–192.

11 Hongcharu, W., Taylor, C., Chang, Y. et al. (2000). Topical ALA-photodynamic therapy for the treatment of acne vulgaris. *J. Invest. Dermatol.* 115: 183–192.

12 Sakamoto, F., Lopes, J., and Anderson, R. (2010). Photodynamic therapy for acne

vulgaris: a critical review from basics to clinical practice: part I. Acne vulgaris: when and why consider photodynamic therapy? *J. Am. Acad. Dermatol.* 63: 183–193.
13 US Food and Drug Administration web site. NLite System. http://www.accessdata.fda.gov/cdrh_docs/pdf2/K024189.pdf (accessed 10 October 2013).
14 US Food and Drug Administration web site. ARAMIS II Dermatological Laser. http://www.accessdata.fda.gov/cdrh_docs/pdf3/K032260.pdf (accessed 8 October 2013).
15 Shalita, A., Harthy, Y., and Elman, M. (2001). Acne phototherapy using UV-free high-intensity narrow-band blue light: a three-center clinical study. *Proc. SPIE* 4244: 61–73.
16 Papageorgiou, P., Katsambas, A., and Chu, A. (2000). Phototherapy with blue (415 nm) and red (660 nm) light in the treatment of acne vulgaris. *Br. J. Dermatol.* 142: 973–978.
17 Tzung, T., Wu, K., and Huang, M. (2004). Blue light phototherapy in the treatment of acne. *Photodermatol. Photoimmunol. Photomed* 20: 266–269.
18 Gold, M., Rao, J., Goldman, M. et al. (2005). A multicenter clinical evaluation of the treatment of mild to moderate inflammatory acne vulgaris of the face with visible blue light in comparison to topical 1% clindamycin antibiotic solution. *J. Drugs Dermatol.* 4: 64–70.
19 Jih, M., Friedman, P., Goldberg, L. et al. (2006). The 1450-nm diode laser for facial inflammatory acne vulgaris: dose-response and 12-month follow-up study. *J. Am. Acad. Dermatol.* 55: 80–87.
20 Wang, S., Counters, J., Flor, M. et al. (2006). Treatment of inflammatory facial acne with the 1,450 nm diode laser alone versus microdermabrasion plus the 1,450 nm laser: a randomized, split-face trial. *Dermatol. Surg.* 32: 249–255.
21 Darne, S., Hiscutt, E., and Seukeran, D. (2011). Evaluation of the clinical efficacy of the 1,450 nm laser in acne vulgaris: a randomized split-face, investigator-blinded clinical trial. *Br. J. Dermatol.* 165: 1256–1262.
22 Friedman, P., Jih, M., Kimyai-Asadi, A. et al. (2004). Treatment of inflammatory facial acne vulgaris with the 1450-nm diode laser: a pilot study. *Dermatol. Surg.* 30: 147–151.
23 Mazer, J. (2004). Treatment of facial acne with a 1450 nm diode laser: a comparative study. *Lasers Surg. Med.* 34: S67.
24 Wiegell, S. and Wulf, H. (2006). Photodynamic therapy of acne vulgaris using methyl aminolaevulinate: a blinded, randomized, controlled trial. *Br. J. Dermatol.* 154: 969–976.
25 Wiegell, S. and Wulf, H. (2006). Photodynamic therapy of acne vulgaris using 5-aminolevulinic acid versus methyl aminolevulinate. *J. Am. Acad. Dermatol.* 54: 647–651.
26 Horfelt, C., Funk, J., Frohm-Nilsson, M. et al. (2006). Topical methyl aminolaevulinate photodynamic therapy for treatment of facial acne vulgaris: results of a randomized, controlled study. *Br. J. Dermatol.* 155: 608–613.
27 Sakamoto, F., Torezan, L., and Anderson, R. (2010). Photodynamic therapy for acne vulgaris: a critical review from basics to clinical practice: part II. *J. Am. Acad. Dermatol.* 63: 195–211.
28 Sakamoto, F., Tannous, Z., Doukas, A. et al. (2009). Porphyrin distribution after topical aminolevulinic acid in a novel porcine model of sebaceous skin. *Lasers Surg. Med.* 41: 154–160.
29 Seaton, E., Charakida, A., Mouser, P. et al. (2003). Pulsed-dye laser treatment for inflammatory acne vulgaris: randomised controlled trial. *Lancet* 362: 1347–1352.
30 Orringer, J., Kang, S., Hamilton, T. et al. (2004). Treatment of acne vulgaris with a pulsed dye laser: a randomized controlled trial. *JAMA* 291: 2834–2839.
31 Karsai, S., Schmitt, L., and Raulin, C. (2010). The pulsed-dye laser as an adjuvant treatment modality in acne vulgaris: a randomized controlled single-blinded trial. *Br. J. Dermatol.* 163: 395–401.

32 Yeung, C., Shek, S., Bjerring, P. et al. (2007). A comparative study of intense pulsed light alone and its combination with photodynamic therapy for the treatment of facial acne in Asian skin. *Lasers Surg. Med.* 39: 1–6.

33 Chang, S., Ahn, S., Rhee, D. et al. (2007). Treatment of facial acne papules and pustules in Korean patients using an intense pulsed light device equipped with a 530- to 750-nm filter. *Dermatol. Surg.* 33: 676–679.

34 Santos, M., Belo, V., and Santos, G. (2005). Effectiveness of photodynamic therapy with topical 5-aminolevulinic acid and intense pulsed light versus intense pulsed light alone in the treatment of acne vulgaris: comparative study. *Dermatol. Surg.* 31: 910–915.

35 Rojanamatin, J. and Choawawanich, P. (2006). Treatment of inflammatory facial acne vulgaris with intense pulsed light and short contact of topical 5-aminolevulinic acid: a pilot study. *Dermatol. Surg.* 32: 991–996.

36 Bowes, L., Manstein, D., and Rox Andersen, R. (2003). Effects of 532 nm KTP laser exposure on acne and sebaceous glands. *Lasers Med. Sci.* 18: S6–S7.

37 Baugh, W. and Kucaba, W. (2005). Nonablative phototherapy for acne vulgaris using the KTP 532 nm laser. *Dermatol. Surg.* 31: 1290–1296.

38 Chapas, A. and Geronemus, R. (2005). Our approach to pediatric dermatologic laser surgery. *Lasers Surg. Med.* 37: 255–263.

39 Na, J. and Suh, D. (2007). Red light phototherapy alone is effective for acne vulgaris: randomized, single-blinded clinical trial. *Dermatol. Surg.* 33: 1228–1233.

40 Kawada, A., Aragane, Y., Kameyama, H. et al. (2002). Acne phototherapy with a high-intensity, enhanced, narrowband, blue light source: an open study and in vitro investigation. *J. Dermatol. Sci.* 30: 129–135.

41 Elman, M., Slatkine, M., and Harth, Y. (2003). The effective treatment of acne vulgaris by a high-intensity, narrow band 405–420 nm light source. *J. Cosmet. Laser Ther.* 5: 111–117.

42 Omi, T., Bjerring, P., Sato, S. et al. (2004). 420 nm intense continuous light therapy for acne. *J. Cosmet. Laser Ther.* 6: 156–162.

43 Morton, C., Scholefield, R., Whitehurst, C. et al. (2005). An open study to determine the efficacy of blue light in the treatment of mild to moderate acne. *J. Dermatolog. Treat.* 16: 219–223.

44 Tremblay, J., Sire, D., Lowe, N. et al. (2006). Light-emitting diode 415 nm in the treatment of inflammatory acne: an open label, multicentric, pilot investigation. *J. Cosmet. Laser Ther.* 8: 31–33.

45 Yung, A., Stables, G., Fernandez, C. et al. (2007). Microbiological effect of photodynamic therapy (PDT) in healthy volunteers: a comparative study using methyl aminolaevulinate and hexyl aminolaevulinate cream. *Clin. Exp. Dermatol.* 32: 716–721.

46 Hong, S. and Lee, M. (2005). Topical aminolevulinic acid-photodynamic therapy for the treatment of acne vulgaris. *Photodermatol. Photoimmunol. Photomed.* 21: 322–325.

47 Goldman, M. and Boyce, S. (2003). A single-center study of aminolevulinic acid and 417 NM photodynamic therapy in the treatment of moderate to severe acne vulgaris. *J. Drugs Dermatol.* 2: 393–396.

48 Taub, A. (2004). Photodynamic therapy for the treatment of acne: a pilot study. *J. Drugs Dermatol.* 3: S10–S14.

49 Akaraphanth, R., Kanjanawanitchkul, W., and Gritiyarangsan, P. (2007). Efficacy of ALA-PDT vs blue light in the treatment of acne. *Photodermatol. Photoimmunol. Photomed.* 23: 186–190.

20

Laser for Verrucae

Ariel Eber[1], Marina Perper[1], Sebastian Verne[1], Robert Magno[1], Mana Alharbi[2], Ibrahim Alomair[2], Abdulkareem Alfuraih[2], Ali Rajabi-Estarabadi[1], and Keyvan Nouri[3]

[1] *Department of Dermatology & Cutaneous Surgery, University of Miami Miller School of Medicine, Miami, FL, USA*
[2] *Al-Imam Mohammad Ibn Saud Islamic University (IMSIU), Riyadh, Saudi Arabia*
[3] *Department of Dermatology, Ophthalmology, Otolaryngology & Surgery, University of Miami Leonard M. Miller School of Medicine, Miami, FL, USA*

20.1 Introduction

Viral warts are one of the most common skin disorders in the pediatric and adolescent population. In fact, up to one third of primary school children have warts, representing one of the most common reasons for referral to a dermatologist in this population [1]. Warts, or verrucae, are caused by infection with human papilloma virus (HPV). Warts can be embarrassing and result in physical discomfort, so it is important for the physician to discuss with both the parent and child about potential outcomes [2]. In immunocompetent children, they are usually benign and tend to resolve in a number of months. However, some verrucae are persistent and can be very difficult to treat and may require a combination of modalities to completely eradicate [3]. Additionally, treatment can be very practitioner-dependent, requiring what many refer to as the "art of medicine" in addition to the science of such [4].

Transmission of HPV usually occurs through skin-to-skin contact with infected individuals or through contact with fomites. Self-inoculation also commonly occurs. There are several types of verrucae, including common warts (verrucae vulgaris), flat warts (verrucae plana), plantar warts (verrucae plantaris), and, less commonly in the pediatric population, genital warts (condyloma acuminatum). While sexual abuse must always be considered in the pediatric patient with genital warts, especially in those under three years old, condyloma acuminatum may certainly be acquired in other ways including perinatally [5] or from the mother's hands.

20.2 Indications

Extra consideration must be taken in treating warts for the unique population that is pediatrics. The capacity for verrucae to spontaneously resolve in children means that the costs of treatment must be carefully weighed [6]. Watchful waiting is an option for new warts, because treatment does not decrease transmissibility of the virus [7]. Additionally, clearance rates after treatment can vary greatly between practitioners, as most modalities for verrucae are highly user-dependent [2]. Factors to consider include: patient discomfort, cost, psychological trauma, and potential scarring [6]. The necessary cooperation of young patients paired with the uncertainty that complete healing

Pediatric Dermatologic Surgery, First Edition. Edited by Keyvan Nouri, Latanya Benjamin, Jasem Alshaiji, and Jan Izakovic.

will take place are unique challenges that modify the treatment algorithm [4]. Laser therapy also usually requires local anesthesia and can even require general anesthesia in certain cases, which is yet another consideration for practitioners when selecting a treatment modality. Currently, there are innumerable options for verrucae with a combination of therapies usually the preferred approached [8]. The use of lasers, PDT and combination therapy for veruccae is discussed below.

20.3 Types of Laser

Verrucae, commonly referred to as warts, is a common problem in children that often requires multiple therapies to eliminate [2]. The difficulty involved with treating viral warts has resulted in a wealth of treatment options and a dearth of literature comparing modalities. Because therapies are user-dependent, variation in success among individual practitioners further obfuscates the ideal therapy [1]. In recent years, technological advancements have made laser therapy a more viable and common treatment modality [9]. The pulsed dye laser (PDL) and carbon dioxide laser are two of the most commonly used lasers in treatment of verrucae.

20.3.1 Carbon Dioxide Laser

CO_2 lasers have been used for several decades to treat warts in patients of all ages [10]. More recently this approach has fallen out of favor because of its association with infection, postoperative pain, and protracted healing [4, 11]. Compared to the pulsed dye laser, the CO_2 laser causes substantial nonselective damage to the surrounding tissue [1]. Despite this, studies have demonstrated the carbon dioxide laser as an efficient way to clear recalcitrant warts on the hands, arms, and legs [12]. Also, the CO_2 laser has been used to treat genital and anogenital warts in children and adolescents with good clearance rates [13, 14]. Many studies have been examined and reports from a recent systematic review describe spot sizes ranging from 0.2 to 1.0 mm and power ranging from 8 to 25 W for focused mode and a spot size of 2 mm with power ranging from 3 to 25 W for the defocused mode. Although the carbon dioxide laser has been shown to be very effective (above 50% clearance in two different studies), the complications linked to, as well as the sometimes severe pain caused by treatment, make the CO_2 laser poorly suited for treatment of pediatric verrucae [11]. For these reasons the CO_2 laser should primarily be reserved for use in recurrent or recalcitrant warts or genital warts. It is not a recommended first-line therapy.

Overall, CO_2 laser is less favorable compared to PDL, producing nonselective thermal tissue destruction with wounds left to heal by secondary intension [2]. Other adverse effects include scarring, hypo- or hyperpigmentation, and postoperative pain [15].

20.3.2 Pulsed Dye Laser

The pulsed dye laser functions by causing selective thermal damage to wart vasculature [16]. Additionally, it presents a lower risk of infection, post-operative pain, and scarring than the CO_2 laser [4, 11]. One of the few studies exclusively on children, in which common warts, periungual warts, plantar warts, and flat warts were treated with PDL, concluded that PDL is a safe and moderately effective treatment option [17]. The study only achieved a 48.1% clearance rate indicating that PDL therapy should be considered as an additional therapy combined with other treatments [17]. The high cost of PDL therapy in addition to the aforementioned drawbacks suggest that cheaper and less aggressive modalities should be considered and the costs and benefits weighed with the family. Another study focused on recalcitrant warts in children and achieved a 75% clearance rate [11]. Authors concluded that PDL is the best treatment available if conventional therapies fail [11]. Both studies used a 585 nm wavelength, 5–7 mm spot size, high fluence (6.5–10 J/cm^2), and required 3.1 treatments on average to achieve clearance [11, 17]. Interestingly, another study examining "conventional therapy" (cryotherapy with cantharidin) versus PDL for the treatment of warts demonstrated no statistically significant difference between the two experimental groups [18].

Complications associated with PDL included pigment changes, blistering, and mild scarring [2]. Additionally, local pain during and after the procedure, bullae, crusting, scarring, and temporary pigment changes may occur [15]. Although multiple treatment sessions are generally necessary for remission, PDL has significantly fewer adverse effects than the CO_2 laser. Furthermore, compared with cryotherapy, PDL has a lower incidence of pain and bulla formation [15].

20.3.3 Nd: YAG Laser

The neodymium-doped yttrium aluminum garnet or Nd:YAG laser is postulated to work similarly to PDL. The wavelength emitted by Nd:YAG, 1064 nm, targets hemoglobin's modest absorption peak between 800 and 1100 [15]. A recent review discusses its use for verrucae as the longer wavelength and lower hemoglobin and melanin absorption coefficients permit for deeper penetration into the hyperkeratotic epidermis within warts compared to PDL [15]. The largest study on the utility of Nd:YAG for warts included pediatric patients and demonstrated simple and recalcitrant common, palmoplantar, and periungual warts treated with Nd:YAG displayed a clearance rate of 96% after a mean of 1.49 treatments [19]. While there are no established optimal laser parameters, Han et al. demonstrated a high success rate, but many side effects, with a pulse duration of 20 ms, at a fluence of 20 J/cm^2 [19].

Complications associated with the Nd:YAG laser include serious pain, hemorrhagic bullae, transient numbness, pigment changes, and nail dystrophy if used periungually [15].

20.4 Photodynamic Therapy

Photodynamic therapy (PDT) is an effective treatment option for various types of warts occurring in pediatric populations including recalcitrant hand and foot warts, plantar warts, recalcitrant plantar warts, and facial flat warts [2]. Further, a case study has demonstrated that topical 5-aminolaevulinic acid mediated photodynamic therapy successfully treated a 9-year-old girl with vulvar condyloma acuminatum and is a promising treatment for genital warts in children [20]. Results of PDT are generally equivalent to or superior to other therapies [21]. The therapy uses light of a wavelength absorbed by photosensitizing molecules that are exogenously placed on target tissue [21]. The photosensitizing agent is usually 5-aminolaevulinic acid [22], and is applied topically. It is then absorbed by hyperkeratotic wart keratinocytes. Following light stimulation, accrued porphyrins from ALA produce a photooxidation cascade damaging cells treated with PDT [2]. To cover the porphyrin excitation peak, the PDT light can be produced from different light sources including lasers, photoemitting diodes, and white light [21].

PDT induces minimal adverse events; in one study no nail dystrophy, wounds, inflammation, or scarring occurred after PDT treatment of periungual warts with 20% δ-aminolevulinic acid [4]. Also minor pain, itching, and mild hypopigmentation can be seen with the use of PDT [2].

20.5 Combination Therapy with Lasers

Various combination therapies exist for the effective treatment of pediatric verrucae.

Mitsuishi et al. conducted a clinical trial using combination treatment involving the CO_2 laser (spot size, 0.2 mm; 8–10 W) followed by artificial dermis application for the treatment of verrucae. This study involved patients ranging from 7 to 65, including the pediatric population. Results indicated an 89% clearance rate for plantar warts after one treatment session and undetectable HPV DNA at the postoperative site three months following treatment. Recurrence was reported in 11% of patients, but minor recurrences cleared with salicylic acid [15]. An advantage of using the CO_2 laser is that it can excise lesional skin including adipose tissue and at least a 1 mm margin including nonlesional skin, allowing the efficient removal of HPV DNA and viral particles. Further, the application of the artificial dermis to the wound facilitates rapid wound healing and minimizes severe tenderness in scars [23]. A single case report also explored combination treatment for verruca with the CO_2 laser. Two CO_2 laser treatments (spot size, 0.2–0.4 mm; 1–3 W) with a one-month interval between treatments followed by imiquimod 5% application was effective in treating recalcitrant warts on the external ear [15].

Recalcitrant cutaneous warts in pediatric populations may also be treated with a combination of the PDL and intralesional bleomycin. In a clinical trial performed by Dobson et al., 60% of 27 patients receiving this combination therapy achieved a complete response. This study included patients aged 13–62, also including both adults and pediatric patients. The use of anesthetic and repeat treatment sessions resulted in better clearance rates. A complete response of 75% was achieved with anesthetic, and additional treatment sessions resulted in a 92% clearance rate. Reported adverse events with this treatment option include painful hemorrhagic blistering and superficial ulceration [24]. Additional clinical trials with a larger sample size should be conducted to further determine the effectiveness of the use of the pulsed dye laser in combination with intralesional bleomycin.

Other combination therapies include the pretreatment of verrucae with salicylic acid before initiating PDL. This may decrease the number of laser treatments required for treating verrucae, potentially decreasing costs. A trial involving 19 patients reported that a group pretreated with salicylic acid received an average of 2.2 treatments, while a group that only received PDL treatment needed an average of 3.1 treatments [2].

20.6 Other Combination Therapies

Another potential combination therapy involving the use of eutectic lidocaine/prilocaine cream 5% (EMLA), a topical anesthetic, prior to liquid nitrogen cryotherapy aims to decrease the pain of cryotherapy. There was no overall statistical difference in the pain of cryotherapy following the application of the cream versus placebo. However, in subset analyses, it was found that it may help reduce pain specifically in cases of verrucae on hardened skin surfaces like the palms and soles [25]. Cryotherapy is also frequently used in combination with salicylic and lactic acid. Nevertheless, it is more effective when used alone (33–93% clearance) as compared to its use with the acids (29–75% clearance) [26].

In another study, combination therapy using cantharidin 1%, salicylic acid 30%, and podophyllotoxin 5% followed by surgical debridement after treatment has shown a very high cure rate for plantar warts (95.8%) at six months. It should be noted that cantharidin is not FDA-approved in the United States, so must be compounded by a pharmacist. Further, cantharidin-containing products may cause significant blistering within 24 hours [2].

20.7 Conclusion/Future Direction

Ultimately, the literature suggests lasers constitute a useful and effective therapy for verrucae. As of now there are not sufficient studies comparing lasers to conventional therapy or lasers to one another, however, the current literature suggests that PDL is at least as effective as conventional therapy, cryotherapy and cantharidin. Furthermore, CO_2, PDL, and Nd:YAG are the lasers most represented in the literature, and of these PDL remains the one with the least adverse effect. Treatment guidelines are still needed in the arena of lasers for wart treatment.

References

1 Kuwabara, A.M., Rainer, B.M., Basdag, H. et al. (2015). Children with warts: a retrospective study in an outpatient setting. *Pediatric Dermatology* 32: 679–683.

2 Boull, C. and Groth, D. (2011). Update: treatment of cutaneous viral warts in children. *Pediatric Dermatology* 28: 217–229.

3 Gladsjo, J.A., Alio Saenz, A.B., Bergman, J. et al. (2009). 5% 5-fluorouracil cream for treatment of verruca vulgaris in children. *Pediatric Dermatology* 26: 279–285.

4 Torrelo, A. (2002). What's new in the treatment of viral warts in children. *Pediatric Dermatology* 19: 191–199.

5 Jayasinghe, Y. and Garland, S.M. (2006). Genital warts in children: what do they mean? *Archives of Disease in Childhood* 91: 696–700.

6 Esterly, N. (1987). Management of warts in children. *Pediatric Dermatology* 4: 36–54.

7 Rivera, A. and Tyring, S.K. (2004). Therapy of cutaneous human papillomavirus infections. *Dermatologic Therapy* 17: 441–448.

8 Douglass, M.C.K., Moroz, B., Heskel, N.S. et al. (1987). Management of warts in children. *Pediatric Dermatology* 4: 36–54.

9 Cordisco, M.R. (2009). An update on lasers in children. *Current Opinion in Pediatrics* 21: 499–504.

10 Logan, R.A. and Zachary, C.B. (1989). Outcome of carbon dioxide laser therapy for persistent cutaneous viral warts. *The British Journal of Dermatology* 121: 99–105.

11 Sethuraman, G., Richards, K.A., Hiremagalore, R.N. et al. (2010). Effectiveness of pulsed dye laser in the treatment of recalcitrant warts in children. *Dermatologic Surgery: Official Publication for American Society for Dermatologic Surgery [et al]* 36: 58–65.

12 Serour, F. and Somekh, E. (2003). Successful treatment of recalcitrant warts in pediatric patients with carbon dioxide laser. *European Journal of Pediatric Surgery: Official Journal of Austrian Association of Pediatric Surgery [et al] = Zeitschrift fur Kinderchirurgie* 13: 219–223.

13 Collet-Villette, A.M., Gaudy-Marqueste, C. et al. (2007). Carbon dioxide laser therapy for anogenital warts in children. *Annales de dermatologie et de venereologie* 134: 829–832.

14 Krakowski, A.C., Feldstein, S., and Shumaker, P.R. (2015). Successful treatment of pearly penile papules with carbon dioxide laser resurfacing after local anesthesia in an adolescent patient. *Pediatric dermatology* 32: 433–435.

15 Nguyen, J., Korta, D.Z., Chapman, L.W. et al. (2016). Laser treatment of nongenital verrucae: a systematic review. *JAMA Dermatology* 152: 1025–1034.

16 Tosti, A. and Piraccini, B.M. (2001). Warts of the nail unit: surgical and nonsurgical approaches. *Dermatologic Surgery: Official Publication for American Society for Dermatologic Surgery [et al]* 27: 235–239.

17 Park, H.S., Kim, J.W., Jang, S.J. et al. (2007). Pulsed dye laser therapy for pediatric warts. *Pediatric Dermatology* 24: 177–181.

18 Robson, K.J., Cunningham, N.M., Kruzan, K.L. et al. Pulsed-dye laser versus conventional therapy in the treatment of warts: a prospective randomized trial. *Journal of the American Academy of Dermatology* 43: 275–280.

19 Han, T.Y., Lee, J.H., Lee, C.K. et al. (2009). Long-pulsed Nd:YAG laser treatment of

warts: report on a series of 369 cases. *Journal of Korean Medical Science* 24: 889–893.
20 Chen, M., Xie, J., and Han, J. (2010). Photodynamic therapy of condyloma acuminatum in a child. *Pediatric Dermatology* 27: 542–544.
21 Lipke, M.M. (2006). An armamentarium of wart treatments. *Clinical Medicine & Research* 4: 273–293.
22 Malavige, G.N., Fernando, S., Fernando, D.J. et al. (2004). Dengue viral infections. *Postgraduate Medical Journal* 80: 588–601.
23 Mitsuishi, T., Sasagawa, T., Kato, T. et al. (2010). Combination of carbon dioxide laser therapy and artificial dermis application in plantar warts: human papillomavirus DNA analysis after treatment. *Dermatologic Surgery: Official Publication for American Society for Dermatologic Surgery [et al]* 36: 1401–1405.
24 Dobson, J.S. and Harland, C.C. (2014). Pulsed dye laser and intralesional bleomycin for the treatment of recalcitrant cutaneous warts. *Lasers in surgery and medicine* 46: 112–116.
25 Gupta, A.K., Koren, G., and Shear, N.H. (1998). A double-blind, randomized, placebo-controlled trial of eutectic lidocaine/prilocaine cream 5% (EMLA) for analgesia prior to cryotherapy of warts in children and adults. *Pediatric Dermatology* 15: 129–133.
26 Munoz Garza, F.Z., Roe Crespo, E., Torres Pradilla, M. et al. (2015). Intralesional Candida antigen immunotherapy for the treatment of recalcitrant and multiple warts in children. *Pediatric Dermatology* 32: 797–801.

21

Lasers and Lights for Onychomycosis

Elizabeth Yim[1], Leyre A. Falto-Aizpurua[1], Jennifer Ledon[1], and Keyvan Nouri[2]

[1] *Department of Dermatology & Cutaneous Surgery, University of Miami Miller School of Medicine, Miami, FL, USA*
[2] *Department of Dermatology, Ophthalmology, Otolaryngology & Surgery, University of Miami Leonard M. Miller School of Medicine, Miami, FL, USA*

21.1 Introduction

Onychomycosis is a fungal infection of the nail that causes the nail to thicken, discolor, disfigure, or split. There are different types of onychomycosis, with distal subungual onychomycosis being the most common. Typically, the infective organism originates in the nail bed, leading to an infection of the hyponychium, and slowly spreads proximally to the nail plate, resulting in opaque, yellowish discoloration, and distortion of the nail. These changes can also be accompanied by accumulation of hyperkeratotic debris subungually (subungual hyperkeratosis) as well as separation of the nail plate from the nail bed (onycholysis). The causative organism is *Trichophytum phyton* in approximately 90% of cases [1] and the global prevalence of onychomycosis is estimated to be 2–8% [2]. It is most commonly seen in the elderly, diabetics, and individuals with trauma to the nail [2]. In recent years, however, there has been an increase in frequency of onychomycosis among children [3, 4].

Onychomycosis is not only a cosmetic concern, but occasionally also a significant medical one as it may lead to painful cutaneous bacterial infections such as paronychia or erysipelas, greatly affecting one's quality of life [5, 6]. Traditional treatment options include topical or systemic antifungal medications as well as surgical or chemical nail avulsions. Topical antifungals, such as ciclopirox olamine and amorolfine, however, have low to moderate efficacy in the vast majority of patients because these are unable to fully penetrate the nail plate into the nail bed where the fungal growth originates [7, 8]. Systemic antifungal agents, such as terbinafine, itraconazole and griseofulvin, have increased efficacy but can cause intolerable side effects, such as kidney or liver damage. Laser and light therapies are becoming increasingly popular options as these can be utilized in the clinic and require little patient compliance. Furthermore, lasers and light therapy are minimally invasive and require relatively few sessions. This chapter will discuss in depth the principles behind laser and light therapy, as well as their indications, techniques, and complications.

21.1.1 Summary

- Fungal infection begins in the hyponychium and spreads onto the nail plate, resulting (most commonly) in subungual hyperkeratosis and onycholysis.
- The incidence of onychomycosis in the pediatric population is increasing

Pediatric Dermatologic Surgery, First Edition. Edited by Keyvan Nouri, Latanya Benjamin, Jasem Alshaiji, and Jan Izakovic.

- Systemic antifungal therapies have high efficacy rates but carry significant side effects and should be used with caution.

21.2 Indications and Contraindications

The following are indications for laser therapy:

- recalcitrant onychomycosis
- patients unresponsive to topical and systemic antifungals, or cannot tolerate them due to side effects
- poor patient compliance to topical treatment options, as these often require multiple daily applications. Laser therapy requires only a certain number of appointments and may be a better alternative for these patients.

The following are contraindications for laser therapy:

- pregnancy (never been studied; effects to the fetus are unknown)
- neuropathies causing loss of sensation in the extremities
- current or past use (6 months) of isotretinoin
  patients unable to tolerate light or laser therapy, such as patients:
  - who have seizure disorders triggered by light
  - with lupus erythematosus
  - who have received or are receiving gold therapy
  - on medications that increase their sensitivity to light.

21.3 Mechanism of Action

The exact mechanism of laser treatment for onychomycosis is still under investigation, but it is based on the principle of selective photothermolysis [9]. The absorption of light energy by the fungi is converted into heat or mechanical energy [9]. Fungi are heat-sensitive above 55 °C and therefore sustained absorption of laser energy by the mycelium is likely to result in fungicidal effects [9]. However, heating dermal tissue above 40 °C can cause pain and necrosis. In order to prevent tissue damage, the laser energy format must be either pulsed to allow dissipation of heat or delivered at a moderate energetic level [10]. Laser therapy may also play a role in modulating the immune system or changing the local microenvironment [10]. In addition, lasers may cause destruction of pathogenic micro-organisms and stimulate reparative processes [11].

Many variables contribute to the mechanism and effectiveness of laser function, each differing on the type of laser used. It is important to discuss these variables before presenting the different types of lasers that are currently commercially available to treat onychomycosis.

21.4 Devices

Laser parameters have to be appropriately understood in order to establish the settings for each patient.

- *Wavelength:* The maximum tissue penetrance in the nail is found in the near-infrared spectrum [12]. There are a number of options for both solid state and diode lasers. For instance, Neodymium-doped yttrium aluminum garnet (Nd:YAG) laser crystals can be designed to produce wavelengths at 1064, 1320, and 1540 nm [12], in addition to being frequency-doubled to produce wavelengths at 532 nm.
- *Pulse duration:* Normal tissue damage occurs at temperatures greater than 40 °C, therefore laser energy must be confined to short pulse durations as increased pulse duration leads to increased thermal energy. There are three primary classes of pulse durations available commercially: long-pulse systems with millisecond pulse durations; short-pulse systems with microsecond pulse durations; and Q-switched lasers

with nanosecond pulse durations. The Q-switched laser has the highest peak energy per pulse, as the pulse energy is inversely related to pulse duration [13].

- *Frequency or repetition rate:* The principle of selective photothermolysis requires temporal spacing between energetic pulses to allow for dispersal of any heat energy to prevent damage to the dermal tissue. A higher frequency decreases the time frame, and allows more laser pulses per second [12].
- *Spot size:* The spot size represents the diameter of the laser beam. A small spot results in greater scattering of laser energy than a larger spot size [14].
- *Energy:* The required energy needed to produce a photothermal effect varies based on the pulse duration of the laser. This measurement is usually an average based on the maximum pulse energy and the spot size [12].

21.4.1 Carbon Dioxide Laser

One of the earliest lasers to be used in dermatology was the carbon dioxide (CO_2) laser. Functioning more as an ablation device, the CO_2 laser targets water within the skin, ultimately leading to tissue vaporization. CO_2 lasers are therefore able to penetrate through the nail plate to the nail bed where the fungi grow. Spot diameter may vary from 0.5 to 1.55 mm, with total power up to 25 W [15]. Clearance rates vary from 66% to 75% [15–17]. Nails can be debulked prior to laser treatment to expose the underlying hyperkeratotic nail bed. The advantages of using CO_2 lasers are selective tissue ablation, intra-treatment hemostasis, sterilization of the surgical site by intense heat production, and marked diminution of postoperative pain and edema [15, 17]. While CO_2 lasers can be used as primary treatment or as an adjunct to topical antifungals, the results are largely unpredictable [17]. For these reasons these have largely been replaced by other less-invasive laser treatment options.

When using CO_2 lasers, protective eyeglasses should be worn. Instruments must also have a dull or matte finish to prevent reflection and adjacent tissues should be protected with a moist gauze [15]. The laser beam is passed side to side on the involved portion of the nail, ablating evenly and precisely. After the nail bed has been entirely ablated, remove the charred tissue with a curette [17]. A repeat pass can be done if there is still hyperkeratotic material that has not been ablated, which can be done under local anesthesia. A postoperative dressing of antibacterial or antibiotic cream with mild compression is recommended for the first 24 hours after the procedure [17]. Once the nail bed has healed, patients should be instructed to clean the nail bed with soap and water [17]. Afterwards, regular follow-up visits should be performed to monitor the nail as it grows.

21.4.2 Solid State Lasers

Solid-state lasers use solid crystal rods to produce certain wavelengths. These include the Nd:YAG and titanium sapphire (Ti:Sapphire) lasers [10] and can be used as continuous lasers or as pulsed lasers with pulse durations in the millisecond, microsecond, nanosecond or femtosecond ranges [10]. Different pulse formats may result in greater nonspecific healing to the nail plate, or require longer treatment lengths to produce a fungicidal effect.

21.4.2.1 Long-Pulse Nd:YAG Lasers [5]

These lasers have a pulse duration in the millisecond range and can cause a high degree of non-specific heating, thus a cooling system to prevent thermal spread is required [10]. These lasers typically emit a 1064 nm wavelength, which allows deep penetration to the nail bed where the fungus grows. They can also operate at frequency-doubled wavelengths like 532 nm, which can target the endogenous red pigment in Trichophyton rubrum [12]. The 1064 nm wavelength emitted by the Nd:YAG laser is primarily absorbed

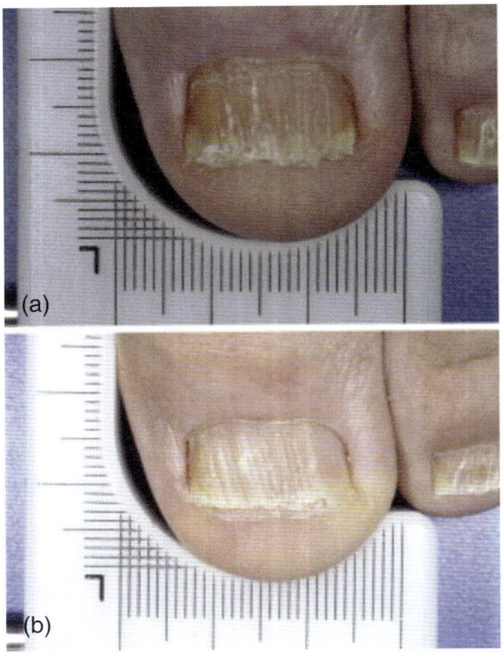

Figure 21.1 Onychomycosis. Photography of 1064 nm Nd:YAG laser-treated nail 1 at baseline (a) and 24 weeks (b). *Source:* From Carney et al. [19]. Copyright 2013 American Academy of Dermatology, Inc. Reprinted with permission of Elsevier Limited.

by dark pigments, such as melanin, which is found in the cell walls of *Trichophyton* species. There are several clinical trials using Nd:YAG 1064 nm for treatment of onychomycosis (Figure 21.1) [5, 18, 19]. Some studies have shown clearance can be achieved in 95.8% of patients after four treatments at one-week intervals [5]. These lasers have shown to be safe and effective with minimal adverse events [18].

21.4.2.2 Short Pulse Nd:YAG Lasers

These lasers have a pulse duration in the microsecond range [12]. The shorter pulse duration allows rapid cooling and therefore do not require cooling systems. These lasers have the ability to cause quick, safe, and precise targeting of chromophores. According to some studies, negative fungal cultures have been obtained in 87.5% of cultures after the second or third session [20]. This laser is also typically well tolerated by patients.

21.4.2.3 Q-Switched Nd: YAG Laser

These lasers have pulse duration in the nanosecond range. They emit the highest peak power per pulse of all the Nd:YAG lasers [10]. The short pulse induces microcavitation, acoustic shock waves that could result in significant inhibition of the fungal colonies [21]. Short pulses will also induce thermal shocks in the target chromophore via rapid healing and cooling. It is speculated that these very short pulses generate mechanical damage to the fungal colony [22]. Unlike photodynamic therapy with UV radiation, there are no teratogenic risks, and no toxic photoablation effects deriving from Nd:YAG lasers [23]. In 2011 the Q-Clear™ Compact Laser System (Light Age, Inc.) laser received FDA approval for the clearance of nails infected by onychomycosis. In their clinical trial an increase in clear nail growth was observed in 95% of patients.

Vural et al. demonstrated *in vitro* that Q-switched Nd:YAG (532 nm) had significant inhibitory effect on *T. rubrum* colony growth [22]. They hypothesized that growth inhibition of *T. rubrum* was due to specific sensitivity to 532 nm energy rather than nonspecific thermal damage. This is because it is known that the 532 nm wavelength is well absorbed by red pigment, which can be found in abundant quantities in *T. rubrum* due its xanthomegnin content [22].

Q-switched Nd:YAG laser with 1064 nm is also capable of inhibiting *T. rubrum* growth. Although this setting is beyond the absorption spectrum of xanthomegnin, its effectiveness is postulated to be due to another absorbing chromophore, such as melanin, present in the cell walls of *T. rubrum* [22].

21.4.2.4 Titanium Sapphire Laser

With a pulse duration in the femtosecond range, the titanium sapphire laser selectively delivers energy into the deep layers of the nail bed, without damaging the surrounding tissue [23]. Thought to break down transparent or semitransparent biological tissues due to nonlinear absorption of laser energy, the titanium sapphire laser functions with minimal thermal and mechanical effects [6]. The laser is usually operated at a wavelength of 800 nm, which could effectively traverse the nail, thus eliminating dermatophytes at any level [6].

Studies have shown that the use of a femtosecond laser with laser fluences of 7×10^{31} photons/m^{2}s can selectively eliminate *T. rubrum* from infected toenails, as evidenced by clear nail clippings [6]. However, laser intensities above 1.7×10^{32} photons/m^{2}s are capable of damaging the structure of the nail plate.

21.4.3 Near-Infrared Diode Lasers

Near-infrared diode lasers use semiconductors for the optical gain medium as an alternative to solid crystals. They utilize dual wavelengths of 870 and 930 nm, which are near – infrared light that have unique photolethal effects on fungal pathogens, as *T. rubrum*, *Candida albicans*, *Phaeoannellomyces*, and *Rhodotorula* [24, 25]. Neuman et al. observed these effects under confocal microscopy, noting that these specific wavelengths destroyed both eukaryotic and prokaryotic cells [26]. One advantage of using this type of laser is that it operates at physiologic temperatures that are thermally safe for human tissue [25]. In a randomized controlled study, 85% of infected toenails treated showed clinical improvement after four months of treatment [25]. Bornstein et al. achieved 100% inactivation of *T. rubrun in vitro* 91 hours after treatment [24]. The wavelengths are delivered simultaneously for four minutes, followed by a second exposure of 930 nm alone for two minutes [25]. This device is a safe and reliable alternative for treatment of onychomycosis.

The 980 nm laser has also been demonstrated to disrupt fungal growth *in vitro*, and results were comparable to 1064 nm system [27]. A clinical study performed in Italy showed that a Blueshine Gold series 980 nm diode laser® cleared 37 out of 48 toenails [28]. Three to four treatments were done with 30-day intervals, with two alternating passes, first one vertical and second was horizontal (Figure 21.2).

There have been reports in the literature that excessive exposure to near-infrared light can cause an oxidative stress response that can lead to premature photo-aging and decrease in type I collagen [29].

21.4.4 Summary

- The CO_2 laser is one of the earlier lasers. The nails are usually debulked prior to treatment to expose the hyperkeratotic nail bed. Clearance rates for onychomycosis vary from 66 to 75%.
- Solid state lasers include the Nd:YAG and Ti:Sapphire lasers. Different pulse formats of these lasers may result in greater nonspecific healing to the nail plate, or require longer treatment lengths to produce a fungicidal effect.
- Near-infrared diode lasers use semiconductors for the optical gain medium as an alternative to solid crystals. It utilizes dual wavelengths of 870 and 930 nm that have unique photolethal effects on fungal pathogens.

21.5 Technique

The nail area should be cleaned thoroughly with alcohol to remove contaminants prior to laser treatment [30]. For distal subungual onychomycosis, the infected nail can be clipped proximally, and the nail bed and underside of the nail plate scraped with a serrated curette (1–2 mm) [30]. For proximal subungual onychomyosis, the normal surface of the nail plate should be pared down with number 15 scalpel at the lunula. If the nails are thicker than 2 mm, patients have pretreatment with urea to debride nails prior to laser therapy [12, 30, 31]. This helps the laser to penetrate through the hyperkeratotic region.

The patient should be seated in a position so that nails are easily accessible to the physician. Protective eyewear should be worn by both the patient and physician to prevent ocular damage from accidental laser exposure [12].

Laser energy should be applied in a spiral or grid pattern to ensure complete coverage of the nail plate [12]. After the entire nail

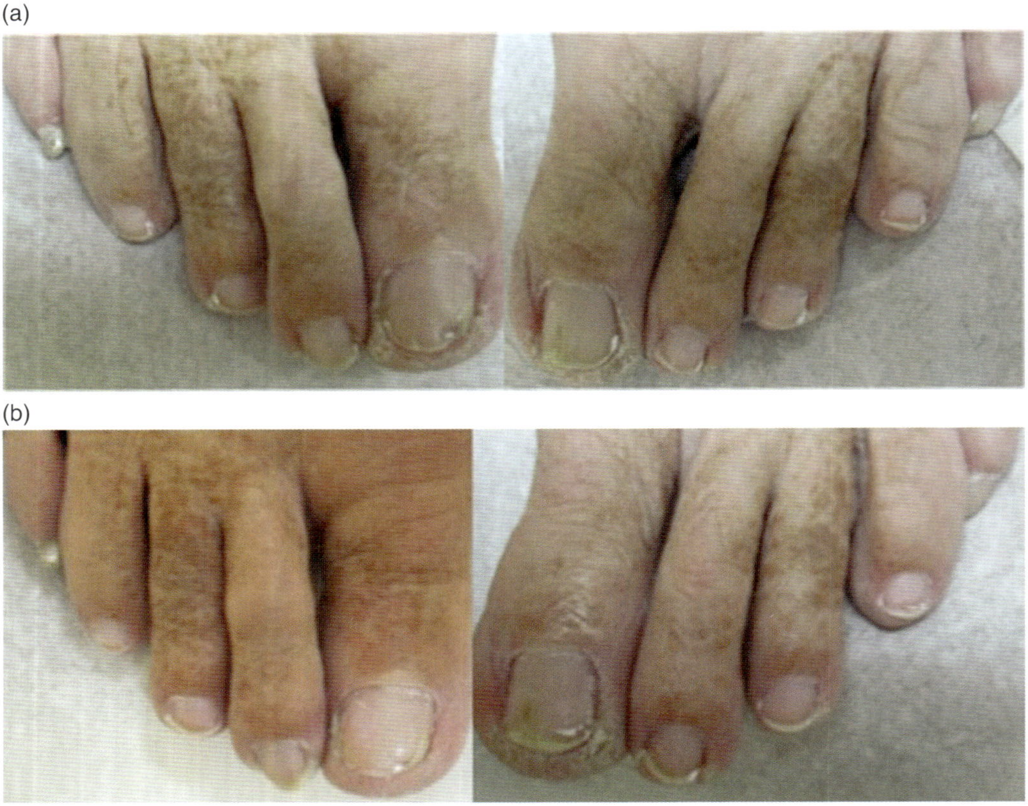

Figure 21.2 A total of seven patients with onychomycosis were treated with a 980 nm diode laser for two to six sessions. The pictures above are representative for one of the study patients before (a) and after treatment (b).

plate is irradiated, pause for two minutes, then repeat one to three more times depending on which toe is being treated [12, 30]. For long-pulse lasers, a cooling system is needed while in short-pulse laser treatment cooling is not necessary. The available types of lasers and their parameters are listed in Table 21.1.

Afterwards, a topical antifungal cream may be applied. The number of laser treatment varies, but usually ranges from one to four sessions, with one- to three-week intervals [23, 30, 31]. Most treatments last 15–30 minutes each. Patients should be followed up at one, three and six months to look for relapse [12].

The success of laser therapy largely depends upon the wavelength, output power, pulse duration, exposure time, spot size, and thickness of hyperkeratotic tissue.

21.5.1 Summary

- *Improving nail penetration:* For distal subungual onychomycosis, the infected nail can be clipped proximally, and the nail bed and underside of the nail plate scraped with a serrated curette. For proximal subungual onychomyocis, the normal surface of the nail plate pared down with number 15 scalpel at the lunula. If the nails are thicker than 2 mm, pretreatment with urea to debride nails prior to laser therapy is recommended.
- Laser energy should be applied in a spiral or grid pattern to ensure complete coverage of the nail plate. This can be repeated 1–3 times with a 2-minute pause between them.
- Treatment sessions will vary (1–4) with 1–3 weeks intervals.

Table 21.1 Commercially available lasers for onychomycosis treatment and their parameters [10].

Type of Laser	System Name	Wavelength (nm)	Energy (J/cm^2)	Spot Size (mm)	Pulse Length	Pulse Frequency (Hz)	International Approvals for Onychomycosis
Long-pulse Nd:YAG	Dualis SP™, Fotona [30]	1064	35–40	4	35 ms	1	EU, US
Short-pulse Nd:YAG	PinPointe™ FootLaser™, Nuvolase	1064	25.5	2.5	100–3000 μs	1	US, Canada, EU, Australia
	GenesisPlus™, Cutera	1064	16	5	300 μs	2	US, Canada, EU
	VARIA™, CoolTouch	1064	—	—	600 μs	—	US, EU
	JOULE ClearSense™, Sciton	1064	13	—	0.3–200 ms	6	US
Ti:Sapphire	Mira® 900, Coherent Laser Group	800	10^{31} to $10^{33}\ m^{-2}\ s^{-1}$	0.12–0.45	200 fs	76 MHz	—
Diode	Noveon®, Nomir Medical Technologies	870, 930	212/424	15	—	—	EU
Q-switched. Nd:YAG [12]	Q-Clear, Light Age	1064	4–12	2.5–6	3–10 ns		US, EU

21.6 Photodynamic Therapy (PDT)

The use of PDT for the treatment of onychomycosis is currently off-label. PDT uses visible spectrum light to activate a topically applied photosensitizing agent, which generates reactive oxygen species (ROS) that causes selective destruction of dermatophytes and yeast [12, 32, 33].

There are two types of photosensitizing agents, 5-aminolevulinic acid (5-ALA) and methyl ester methylaminolevulate (MAL). ALA and MAL are precursors in the heme biosynthesis pathway, which cause an accumulation of protoporphyrin IX (PpIX), an optically active molecule that possess peak wavelength absorption between 630 and 700 nm [12]. PpIX is an effective inhibitor of *T. rubrum* when used in conjunction with red-spectrum light [34]. Blue light may also be used, but red light is often used as it penetrates deeper than blue light. A Wood's lamp can be used to confirm absorption of the photosensitizer with the presence of strong red fluorescence. When the photosensitizing agent is absorbed by red light makes the fungi more susceptible to destruction than the surrounding healthy tissue. This has led to significant reduction in its growth [34, 35]. Sylsens B, an investigational photosensitizer, is a non-heme porphyrin that is photodynamically active but is not commercially available [36].

In addition, ALA may have a direct toxic effect to fungi. Infected nails exposed to 100 mmol of 5-ALA for six hours, showed reduced viability of *Candida* in culture [37]. However, a maximum incubation period of six hours with 100 mM ALA plus red light resulted in only 79% reduction in *T. interdigitale* viability, indicating that onychomycosis resulting from dermatophyte infection may be more difficult to treat with PDT than from *Candida* infection.

The nail is pretreated for 10–12 hours (or 7–10 evenings) with a keratinolytic urea solution (20–40%), followed by occlusion for 5 hours with a photosensitizer agent [6]. The nail is then irradiated with a red light source. Some disadvantages of using PDT include discomfort during irradiation, and local phototoxic reactions. In addition, PDT requires a minimum of three and up to seven sessions, in addition to long pretreatment periods, making PDT a more impractical method. Some contraindications include allergy to peanuts or MAL (MAL contains peanut oil) and the presence of invasive squamous cell carcinoma or morpheaform basal cell carcinoma at the treatment field) [38].

Several case reports described successful resolution of onychomycosis with PDT [39–41]. However, larger studies have not been able to replicate their success. In Sotiriou et al. there was only 43% cure rate at 12-month follow-up after three treatments of 20% 5-ALA followed by delivery of red light (570–670 nm) at 40 J/cm^2 [1]. This rate dropped to 37% at 18 months. Better fungicidal effect may be achieved by application of a second treatment within 24–48 hours, a time interval in which hyphal tip morphology could not change into more resistant globular structures [34].

21.6.1 Summary

- PDT uses visible spectrum light to activate a topically applied photosensitizing agent (ALA or MAL), which generates ROS, causing selective destruction of dermatophytes and yeast.
- Currently PDT is an off-label use for the treatment of onychomycosis.
- The nail is pretreated for 10 to 12 hours (or 7–10 evenings) with a keratinolytic urea solution (20–40%), followed by occlusion for 5 hours with a photosensitizer agent [6]. The nail is then irradiated with a red light source.

21.7 Light Therapy

Ultraviolet (UV) irradiation, in particular 200–280 nm wavelengths, has germicidal effects and these have led scientists to investigate its potential use in the treatment of onychomycosis [42]. The xenon flash lamp is a gas-discharge lamp designed to produce extremely intense, full-spectrum white light, including UV. However, it is well known that UV radiation is damaging to human tissue, particularly to skin [43]. UVB irradiation has been well studied and accepted as a main cause of skin cancer such as squamous and basal cell carcinomas. UVC irradiation causes DNA damage by inducing formation of pyrimidine dimers. Despite this, several studies have shown promising results with the use of UVA and UVC light for treating onychomycosis [43]. UVA light (340–355 nm) in conjunction with a synthetic photosensitizer, was demonstrated to be fungicidal to *T. rubrum* independent of fungal growth stage [34]. However, care must be taken to protect the surrounding skin, such as perinychium, hyponychium, and cuticle. A UV blocking agent with dimethyl sulfoxide or glycerol should be used to scatter UV light. In addition, careful calculation of dosimetry must be made with reference to patient's nail thickness. However, the mutagenic potential of UV light has limited its use in treating onychomycosis and other potentially safer alternatives are often chosen.

21.7.1 Summary

- The mutagenic potential of UV light has limited its use in treating onychomycosis and other potentially safer alternatives are often chosen.

21.8 Complications

21.8.1 Lasers

Complications of laser therapy include adverse events related to treatment, such as mild discomfort and burning sensation. Some level of pain is expected, but can also result from inadequate anesthesia, insufficient cooling, or inappropriate laser settings (excess fluence) [44]. A slight yellowish discoloration of the nail plate has been reported. However, no serious adverse events have been reported [29]. Frequent exposure to near-infrared wavelengths can accelerate photoaging and decrease type I collagen. Nd:YAG lasers have been shown to damage healthy tissue by excessive heating when pulses are delivered in high doses.

21.8.2 PDT

In PDT, redness, swelling, blistering, and bruising may result [12]. MAL and ALA should be removed after PDT to reduce continuous synthesis of porphyrin, which increases sensitivity to visible light [38]. Patients should avoid sun exposure, bright light exposure 48 hours after the procedure to avoid hyperpigmentation. One concern with PDT is that treatment may not be fungicidal and only delays the progression of infection [45].

21.8.3 UV

As mentioned above, the use of UV radiation increases the risk of cancers, particularly that of the skin. This may pose an unnecessary risk, and other alternatives are recommended.

21.9 Conclusion/Future Directions

There are many factors that contribute to fungal nail infection, such as diabetes, trauma, increase risk of recurrence, and other underlying dermatologic conditions that may lead to nail pathology such as psoriasis or atopic dermatitis, which the physician should consider when treating the patient. The success of lasers largely depends on the chosen parameters and the thickness of hyperkeratotic tissue. It is important that patients are informed about the procedure itself, expected side effects as well as any potential risks and complications of the procedure. In addition, it is important that patients are aware that nail plates take about 7 to 10 months to fully grow as toenails grow at 1 mm/month [12].

Most lasers have been approved for "temporary increase in clear nail" [46]. Further studies, particularly randomized controlled trials, are needed in investigating the efficacy of lasers for eradicating onychomycosis.

References

1 Sotiriou, E., Koussidou-Eremonti, T., Chaidemenos, G. et al. (2010). Photodynamic therapy for distal and lateral subungual toenail onychomycosis caused by Trichophyton rubrum: preliminary results of a single-centre open trial. *Acta Dermato-Venereologica* 90 (2): 216–217.

2 Gupta, A.K., Jain, H.C., Lynde, C.W. et al. (2000). Prevalence and epidemiology of onychomycosis in patients visiting physicians' offices: a multicenter Canadian survey of 15,000 patients. *Journal of the American Academy of Dermatology* 43 (2 Pt 1): 244–248.

3 Lange, M., Roszkiewicz, J., Szczerkowska-Dobosz, A. et al. (2006). Onychomycosis is no longer a rare finding in children. *Mycoses* 49 (1): 55–59.

4 Sigurgeirsson, B., Kristinsson, K.G., and Jonasson, P.S. (2006). Onychomycosis in Icelandic children. *Journal of the European Academy of Dermatology and Venereology: JEADV* 20 (7): 796–799.

5 Kozarev, J. and Vizintin, Z. (2010). Novel laser therapy in treatment of onychomycosis. *Journal of the Laser and Health Academy* 2010 (1): 1–8.

6 Manevitch, Z., Lev, D., Hochberg, M. et al. (2010). Direct antifungal effect of femtosecond laser on Trichophyton rubrum onychomycosis. *Photochemistry and Photobiology* 86 (2): 476–479.

7 Baran, R., Gupta, A.K., and Pierard, G.E. (2005). Pharmacotherapy of onychomycosis. *Expert Opinion on Pharmacotherapy* 6 (4): 609–624.

8 Kumar, S. and Kimball, A.B. (2009). New antifungal therapies for the treatment of onychomycosis. *Expert Opinion on Investigational Drugs* 18 (6): 727–734.

9 Altshuler, G.B., Anderson, R.R., Manstein, D. et al. (2001). Extended theory of selective photothermolysis. *Lasers in Surgery and Medicine* 29 (5): 416–432.

10 Gupta, A. and Simpson, F. (2012). Device-based therapies for onychomycosis treatment. *Skin Therapy Letter* 17 (9): 4–9.

11 Dayan, S., Damrose, J.F., Bhattacharyya, T.K. et al. (2003). Histological evaluations following 1064-nm Nd:YAG laser resurfacing. *Lasers in Surgery and Medicine* 33 (2): 126–131.

12 Gupta, A.K. and Simpson, F.C. (2012). Medical devices for the treatment of onychomycosis. *Dermatologic Therapy* 25 (6): 574–581.

13 Welch, A.J., Torres, J.H., and Cheong, W.F. (1989). Laser physics and laser-tissue interaction. *Texas Heart Institute Journal/from the Texas Heart Institute of St. Luke's Episcopal Hospital, Texas Children's Hospital* 16 (3): 141–149.

14 Patil, U.A. and Dhami, L.D. (2008). Overview of lasers. *Indian Journal of Plastic Surgery: Official Publication of the Association of Plastic Surgeons of India* 41 (Suppl): S101–S113.

15 Apfelberg, D.B., Rothermel, E., Widtfeldt, A. et al. (1984). Preliminary report on use of carbon dioxide laser in podiatry. *Journal of the American Podiatry Association* 74 (10): 509–513.

16 Borovoy, M. and Tracy, M. (1992). Noninvasive CO_2 laser fenestration improves treatment of onychomycosis. *Clinical Laser Monthly* 10 (8): 123–124.

17 Rothermel, E. and Apfelberg, D.B. (1987). Carbon dioxide laser use for certain diseases of the toenails. *Clinics in Podiatric Medicine and Surgery* 4 (4): 809–821.

18 Kimura, U., Takeuchi, K., Kinoshita, A. et al. (2012). Treating onychomycoses of the toenail: clinical efficacy of the submillisecond 1064 nm Nd: YAG laser using a 5 mm spot diameter. *Journal of Drugs in Dermatology: JDD* 11 (4): 496–504.

19 Carney, C., Cantrell, W., Warner, J. et al. (2013). Treatment of onychomycosis using a submillisecond 1064-nm neodymium:yttrium-aluminum-garnet laser. *Journal of the American Academy of Dermatology* 69 (4): 578–582.

20 Hochman, L.G. (2011). Laser treatment of onychomycosis using a novel 0.65-millisecond pulsed Nd:YAG 1064-nm laser. *Journal of Cosmetic and Laser Therapy: Official Publication of the European Society for Laser Dermatology* 13 (1): 2–5.

21 Suthamjariya, K., Farinelli, W.A., Koh, W. et al. (2004). Mechanisms of microvascular response to laser pulses. *The Journal of Investigative Dermatology* 122 (2): 518–525.

22 Vural, E., Winfield, H.L., Shingleton, A.W. et al. (2008). The effects of laser irradiation on Trichophyton rubrum growth. *Lasers in Medical Science* 23 (4): 349–353.

23 Tchernev, G., Penev, P.K., Nenoff, P. et al. (2013). Onychomycosis: modern diagnostic and treatment approaches. *Wiener Medizinische Wochenschrift* 163 (1–2): 1–12.

24 Bornstein, E., Hermans, W., Gridley, S. et al. (2009). Near-infrared photoinactivation of bacteria and fungi at physiologic temperatures. *Photochemistry and Photobiology* 85 (6): 1364–1374.

25 Landsman, A.S., Robbins, A.H., Angelini, P.F. et al. (2010). Treatment of mild, moderate, and severe onychomycosis using 870- and 930-nm light exposure. *Journal of the American Podiatric Medical Association* 100 (3): 166–177.

26 Neuman, K.C., Chadd, E.H., Liou, G.F. et al. (1999). Characterization of photodamage to Escherichia coli in optical traps. *Biophysical Journal* 77 (5): 2856–2863.

27 Paasch, U., Mock, A., Grunewald, S. et al. (2013). Antifungal efficacy of lasers against dermatophytes and yeasts in vitro. *International Journal of Hyperthermia: The Official Journal of European Society for Hyperthermic Oncology, North American Hyperthermia Group* 29 (6): 544–550.

28 510 k Summary Blushine's Gold Series. online: FDA; 2011 : 11

29 Schroeder, P., Haendeler, J., and Krutmann, J. (2008). The role of near-infrared radiation in photoaging of the skin. *Experimental Gerontology* 43 (7): 629–632.

30 Kozarev, J. (2010). Novel laser therapy in treatment of onychomycosis. *Journal of the Laser and Health Academy* 1: 1–8.

31 The Medical Letter (2013). Laser treatment of onychomycosis. *The Medical Letter on Drugs and Therapeutics* 55 (1410): 15.

32 Calzavara-Pinton, P.G., Venturini, M., and Sala, R. (2005). A comprehensive overview of photodynamic therapy in the treatment of superficial fungal infections of the skin. *Journal of Photochemistry and Photobiology. B, Biology* 78 (1): 1–6.

33 Donnelly, R.F., McCarron, P.A., and Tunney, M.M. (2008). Antifungal photodynamic therapy. *Microbiological Research* 163 (1): 1–12.

34 Smijs, T.G., Pavel, S., Talebi, M. et al. (2009). Preclinical studies with 5,10,15-Tris(4-methylpyridinium)-20-phenyl-[21H,23H]-porphine trichloride for the photodynamic treatment of superficial mycoses caused by Trichophyton rubrum. *Photochemistry and Photobiology* 85 (3): 733–739.

35 Kamp, H., Tietz, H.J., Lutz, M. et al. (2005). Antifungal effect of 5-aminolevulinic acid PDT in Trichophyton rubrum. *Mycoses* 48 (2): 101–107.

36 Gupta, A.K. and Simpson, F.C. (2014). Investigational drugs for onychomycosis. *Expert Opinion on Investigational Drugs* 23 (1): 97–106.

37 Donnelly, R.F., McCarron, P.A., Lightowler, J.M. et al. (2005). Bioadhesive patch-based delivery of 5-aminolevulinic acid to the nail for photodynamic therapy of onychomycosis. *Journal of Controlled Release: Official Journal of the Controlled Release Society* 103 (2): 381–392.

38 Bissonnette, R. (2011). Photodynamic therapy. In: *Lasers in Dermatology and Medicine* (ed. K. Nouri), 221–229. London: Springer-Verlag.

39 Piraccini, B.M., Rech, G., and Tosti, A. (2008). Photodynamic therapy of onychomycosis caused by Trichophyton rubrum. *Journal of the American Academy of Dermatology* 59 (5 Suppl): S75–S76.

40 Watanabe, D., Kawamura, C., Masuda, Y. et al. (2008). Successful treatment of toenail onychomycosis with photodynamic therapy. *Archives of Dermatology* 144 (1): 19–21.

41 Gilaberte, Y., Aspiroz, C., Martes, M.P. et al. (2011). Treatment of refractory fingernail onychomycosis caused by nondermatophyte molds with methylaminolevulinate photodynamic therapy. *Journal of the American Academy of Dermatology* 65 (3): 669–671.

42 Cutler, T.D. and Zimmerman, J.J. (2011). Ultraviolet irradiation and the mechanisms underlying its inactivation of infectious agents. *Animal Health Research Reviews/ Conference of Research Workers in Animal Diseases* 12 (1): 15–23.

43 Dai, T., Tegos, G.P., Rolz-Cruz, G. et al. (2008). Ultraviolet C inactivation of dermatophytes: implications for treatment of onychomycosis. *The British Journal of Dermatology* 158 (6): 1239–1246.

44 Moore, R.L., Martinez, J., and Lee, K.K. (2011). Prevention and treatment of laser comoplications. In: *Lasers in Dermatology and Medicine* (ed. K. Nouri), 365–377. London: Springer-Verlag.

45 Becker, C. and Bershow, A. (2013). Lasers and photodynamic therapy in the treatment of onychomycosis: a review of the literature. *Dermatology Online Journal* 19 (9): 19611.

46 Clearances UFMDk. 510(k) number: K113810. Decision date: Mar 8, 2012. Modified Alma Lasers Harmony 1064 (Nd:YAG), Alma Lasers, Inc. www.accessdata.fda.gov/cdrh_docs/pdf11/K113810.pdf (accessed 21 October 2013).

22

Lasers for Pigmented Lesions

Harleen Arora[1], Leyre Falto-Aizpurua[2], Ali Rajabi-Estarabadi[2], and Keyvan Nouri[3]

[1] University of Miami, Coral Gables, FL, USA
[2] Department of Dermatology & Cutaneous Surgery, University of Miami Miller School of Medicine, Miami, FL, USA
[3] Department of Dermatology, Ophthalmology, Otolaryngology & Surgery, University of Miami Leonard M. Miller School of Medicine, Miami, FL, USA

22.1 Introduction

Pigmented lesions present in the pediatric population are usually benign. Common benign pigmented lesions found among children include congenital nevi, café au lait macules, Becker's nevi, and nevus of Ota/Ito. Lesions such as lentigines are often a result of years of sun exposure and therefore are more commonly found in adults.

Despite the benign nature of these lesions, it may be wished to remove them for cosmetic reasons. For this reason, several removal methods have been employed throughout history, including laser therapy. In 1963, Leon Goldman and his colleagues discovered that pigmented skin selectively absorbed 0.5 ms pulses of ruby laser radiation [1, 2]. Despite these findings, ablative, continuous wave (nonselective) lasers continued to be used. It was not till after the1980s that the quality-switched (QS) lasers began to be used to selectively target pigment. Research performed during these years, along with the development of new technologies, improved significantly the efficacy and side effect profile of laser treatment for pigmented lesions [3]. Currently, both pulsed lasers and intense pulsed light (IPL) have become the treatment of choice for epidermal lesions, while pulsed lasers are the choice for dermal pigmented lesions.

The characteristics and composition of many pigmented lesions change as a child grows older, often resulting in the lesion being more resistant to treatment. Thus, in many cases it is appropriate to start treatment of these lesions at a younger age, likely resulting in fewer treatment sessions needed for improvement, with fewer complications [4]. In this chapter, we will focus on laser treatment for congenital melanocytic nevi, café au lait macules (CALMs), Becker's nevus, and nevus of Ota/Ito.

22.1.1 Congenital Nevi

Congenital melanocytic nevi (CMN) are generally benign, pigmented skin growths, which are a result of tissue malformation in the neuroectoderm [5]. These lesions may be present at birth or within the first few months of life. CMN are generally categorized based on size (maximal diameter) and classified as either small, medium, large, or giant [6] (Table 22.1).

Pediatric Dermatologic Surgery, First Edition. Edited by Keyvan Nouri, Latanya Benjamin, Jasem Alshaiji, and Jan Izakovic.

Table 22.1 Congenital melanocytic nevi classification by size.

Classification	Size	
Small	<1.5 cm	
Medium	1.5–10 cm	M1
	10–20 cm	M2
Large	20–30 cm	L1
	30–40 cm	L2
Giant	40–60 cm	G1
	>60 cm	G2

22.1.2 Café Au Lait Macules

CALMs are light brown homogeneously pigmented macules with well-circumscribed borders, commonly presenting in children. These macules often occur as isolated lesions and their sizes can range from 1 to 2 mm to more than 20 cm in diameter [7]. CALMs can occur as multiple lesions as well, but in this case are often associated with neurofibromatosis syndrome. Histologically, CALMs show hypermelanosis in keratinocytes and melanocytes, giant melanin granules, and a higher number of melanocytes in the basal layer.

22.1.3 Becker's Nevus

Becker's nevi are benign hyperpigmented epidermal lesions commonly located on the upper trunk or shoulder of males. The nevi may be acquired or congenital and could have macular or popular presentations [8], although they are often hypertrichotic with dark, coarse hair [9]. They may also present as smooth muscle hamartomas of the dermis. In adult males, a pathogenic role is known to be played by androgenic stimulation while sun exposure does not seem to have much of a role. The incidence of Becker's nevus in children is frequent and the sites of occurrence are similar to those seen in adults. However, hypertrichosis is rare in children since androgenic stimulation is minimal [10].

22.1.4 Nevus of Ota/Ito

Nevi of Ota are dermal pigmented lesions presenting with blue-gray mottled macules occurring in females versus males in a 5:1 ratio. Also known as oculodermal melanoma or nevus fuscoceruleus opthalmomaxillaris, a nevus of Ota tends to be located within the distribution of the trigeminal nerve's first and second branches. This implies that a nevus of Ota may affect mucosal surfaces of the eye, nose, ear, and mouth. Occurrences are frequently reported among Asians, with 1 out of every 500 being reported in Japan [11]. Histological analysis shows elongated melanocytes within the upper dermis extending dendritically. Congenital nevi of Ota appear in 50% of the cases, with acquired nevi appearing by the second decade of life. Occurrences of melanoma in nevi of Ota are rare but have been reported [12].

Nevus of Ito, also called nevus fuscocaeruleus acromiodeltoideus, is a dermal melanocytic condition similar to nevus of Ota, affecting the shoulder area innervated by the posterior supraclavicular and lateral brachiocutaneous nerves [13]. Although also common in the Asian population, it is less frequent than nevus of Ota. It usually presents unilaterally, although bilateral presentations and in association with nevus of Ota have been reported [14].

22.1.5 Summary

- Pigmented lesions present in the pediatric population are usually benign, although it might be wished to remove them for cosmetic concerns.
  We will discuss in this chapter the laser treatment for:
  - congenital melanocytic nevi
  - café au lait macules
  - Becker's nevus
  - nevus of Ota and Ito.

22.2 Types of Lasers

Theoretically, pigmented lesions can be removed with several laser systems because of melanin's wide absorption range

(500–1100 nm). The more accepted lasers for pigment removal are the QS ruby laser or QSRL (694 nm), the QS alexandrite laser or QSAL (755 nm) and the QS Neodymium Yttrium Aluminum Garnet or QS Nd:YAG laser (1064 nm), which can be frequency-doubled (532 nm) [15]. These lasers work by specifically targeting the melanosome as a chromophore, based on the theory of selective photothermolysis [16]. With QS technology, energy is delivered in rapid pulsed bursts (nanosecond domain), matching melanin's thermal relaxation time. [8] The absorption capacity of melanin decreases as wavelength increases but a longer wavelength is desirable for deeper skin penetration [16]. With increasing wavelengths, increased dosage is required for the laser treatment to be effective [17,18].

Advances in laser technology have allowed for other laser and light sources, such as the long-pulsed ruby, diode and IPL sources, to be efficient in removing certain pigmented lesions. These can only remove superficial pigment due to their limited skin penetration [1]. IPL sources have a non-coherent filtered flash lamp that emits a broad band of visible light (400–1200 nm) inducing a photothermal effect on pigment [19]. It has demonstrated efficacy when treating superficial pigmented lesions with no significant post-inflammatory hyperpigmentation [20]. This device, as well as the long-pulsed lasers, have millisecond domains producing thermal effects.

Pigment non-selective lasers can also be used to remove certain lesions. For example, the carbon dioxide – CO_2 – (10 600 nm) and erbium-doped yttrium aluminum garnet – Er:YAG – (2940 nm) lasers ablate the epidermis by targeting water, removing some epidermal pigment. Although some pigment will be removed, the side effects are increased when compared to pigment-specific lasers. Fractionated forms of these lasers that are available work in a similar way. However, interspersed areas of skin remain unaffected, resulting in faster healing [1].

22.2.1 Summary

- Several lasers can be effective for the removal of pigmented lesions given melanin's wide absorption range.
- Pigment selectivity is based on the principle of selective photothermolysis.
  The more accepted lasers for pigment removal are:

- QS ruby laser (694 nm)
- QS alexandrite laser (755 nm)
- QS Nd:YAG laser (532 nm or 1064 nm).

22.3 Indications and Contraindications

Epidermal pigmented lesions usually respond to laser and light treatments; CALMs and Becker's nevus are included in this category. Short laser wavelengths are sufficient for epidermal lesions as deep tissue penetration is not necessary [1, 21]. On the other hand, dermal lesions can be treated with longer laser wavelengths to ensure deep tissue penetration with minimal epidermal damage, but any signs of atypia in such lesions should be ruled out prior to treatment of any pigmented lesion. Laser therapy for atypical dermal lesions can be dangerous due to the potential for malignant change, which may be less detectable if the pigmentation is diminished through treatment [22–24]. CMN and nevus of Ota/Ito fall into the category of dermal lesions [1].

Patients who have suntanned should not be treated because lasting postoperative spotty hypopigmentation may occur. Those with significant post-inflammatory hyperpigmentation should not be treated either as this may result in scarring [25]. Laser treatment for patients who are currently on or have undergone isotretinoin therapy within the past six months may result in keloid formation [26]. Although parenteral gold therapy for other medical conditions such as juvenile rheumatoid arthritis is not commonly used in children, caution should be advised to patients with any past gold

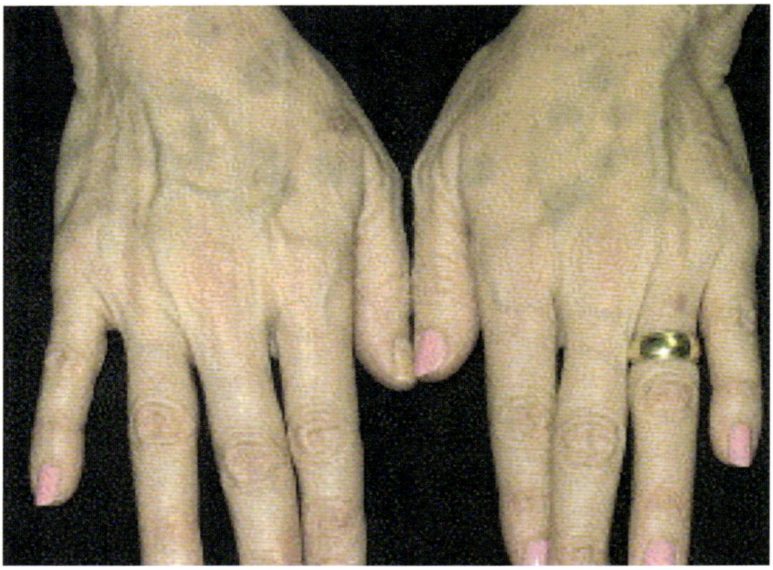

Figure 22.1 Dorsal hands chrysiasis. *Source:* From Geist et al. [28]. Copyright 2006 American Academy of Dermatology, Inc. Reprinted with permission of Elsevier Limited.

therapy because localized chrysiasis can be induced by QS lasers (Figure 22.1) [27–31].

22.3.1 Summary

- Epidermal pigmented lesions, such as CALMs and Becker's nevus, can be treated with shorter wavelengths.
- Dermal pigmented lesions, such as CMN and nevus of Ota/Ito, need longer wavelengths laser treatment to ensure tissue penetration.
- Malignancy should always be ruled out prior to laser treatment.
- Suntanned patients, those with significant post-inflammatory hyperpigmentation, those that are on or have undergone isotretinoin therapy in the past six months and those on gold therapy should not have laser therapy performed.

22.4 Techniques

Prior to treatment several things should be discussed with the patient and their parents or guardians. Treatment expectations should be established to assure if laser treatment is a realistic option. The procedure should be explained in detail as well as common side effects and possible adverse reactions. In addition, both patient and parents may experience anxiety which should be appeased by proper physician care and treatment description. The type and size of the lesion to be treated will be evaluated by the physician to determine the best laser source to be used, considering the nature of the child's skin. The need for anesthesia and delivery method will also be determined at this point depending on the age of the patient, pain tolerance and anxiety level. The physician also should provide safety equipment of the appropriate size during the procedure [4].

When using QS lasers, the spot size and fluence will be determined based on the type of lesion and the Fitzpatrick skin type of the patient. Afterwards, spot testing might be performed to ensure no acute adverse reactions occur. To determine the appropriate fluence, the physician will observe for an adequate threshold response when firing the first one to two pulses at the lesion. An appropriate threshold response will be marked by an immediate thin and uniform whitening of the lesion with no signs of epidermal damage. When the fluence level is too low, the threshold whitening will be barely visible and when it is too high, the whitening will be confluent and bright. The minimal fluence that produces an adequate threshold response should be used; any higher or lower than this may produce negative side effects. Since there is a higher density of melanin in darker skin types, threshold responses will occur at lower fluence levels [32]. When determining the appropriate spot size, it is important to remember that larger spot sizes allow the use of less energy and is less damaging for the epidermis and dermo-epidermal junction. To ensure deeper skin penetration, a dermal lesion will require a larger spot size along with a higher fluence.

When optimal settings are determined, rapid pulses can be delivered with a frequency of up to 10 Hz (laser-dependent), with a 10% overlap to ensure confluent whitening. Lesions usually require multiple treatments for maximal clearance and the frequency will be determined on an individual basis, although treatment sessions are typically performed at least every six weeks. When treating children, laser settings may need to be modified to account for children's skin, which is more sensitive and unpredictable with respect to scarring [4]. To avoid postoperative dyspigmentation and ensure appropriate dermal penetration, longer wavelength lasers such as the QS Nd:YAG (1064 nm) laser should be used to treat darker skin types.

Following treatment, patients will observe darkening of lesions for a few days and it will later develop crusting. The amount of crusting depends on treatment intensity and will usually flake off within a week to 10 days after treatment. The patient should be instructed to gently wash the treated area with mild soap and water and to apply an occlusive ointment twice daily. Sun exposure should be minimized and sunscreen with a minimal SPF of 30 used in the post-procedural months. Post-procedural discomfort may be alleviated by ice packs, gauzes soaked in cold water, or hydro-occlusive dressings. If needed, antihistamines and or analgesics may be given following laser treatment.

IPL and other millisecond domain lasers can be used to treat epidermal pigmented lesions, but have a different clinical endpoint from that of QS lasers. For such lasers, the pigmented lesion may darken immediately after treatment and have surrounding erythema. It will develop a dark scale that usually flakes off in a few days. IPL treatment is usually performed with active skin cooling to protect the epidermis from excessive thermal damage. As with QS laser, several IPL treatments may be necessary for optimal clearance.

22.4.1 Summary

- Before treatment, discuss with the patient and/or parents a detailed procedure, possible side effects, adverse reactions, number and frequency of treatments, post-procedural care and establish realistic expectations.
- Determine the most useful laser device and set the appropriate parameters.

22.5 Congenital Nevi

Treatment of congenital pigmented nevi is a controversial topic in the United States and most European countries. Physicians are wary in treating CMN with lasers due to their ability to mask potential malignancies. However, in several Asian countries such as Japan, laser treatments for CMN are performed. Pigment-specific lasers, resurfacing lasers, and a combination of both are used for CMN.

QSRL [24] and QS Nd:YAG lasers have been used most for treatment [33], although one study found QSRL to be more effective than QS Nd:YAG [34] (Figure 22.2). Several studies confirm that the combined use of QSRL and normal mode ruby laser (NMRL) [35–37] is also effective, perhaps more than either alone, although in children this combination has shown negative results [38]. Another study, however, showed that QSRL was effective in decreasing upper dermal pigmentation

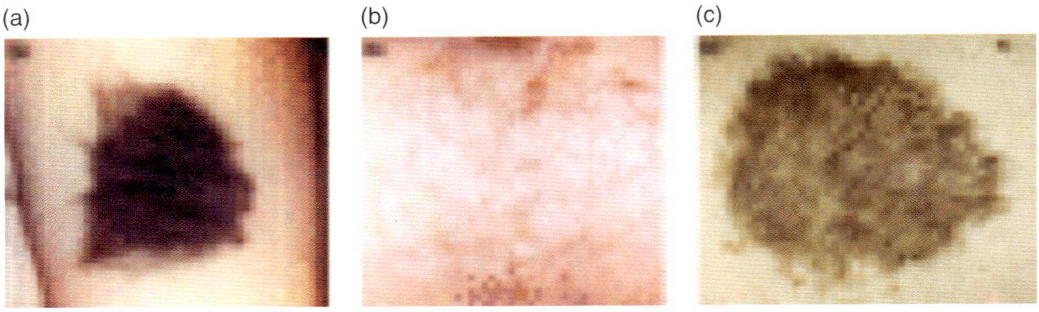

Figure 22.2 (a) A six-year-old boy with a medium-sized congenital melanocytic naevus on his left upper arm; (b) the lesion significantly improved in color and cosmetic appearance after five sessions of normal-mode ruby laser and 10 of Q-switched ruby laser therapy; (c) recurrence of the lesion at the age of 21 years. *Source:* From Minakawa et al. [5] Copyright 2011. Reprinted with permission of John Wiley and Sons.

without significant scarring in prepubertal children [39]. Side effects included temporary erythema, hypopigmentation, and eventual repigmentation. QS alexandrite has also been found to be partially effective [40, 41], as has its combination with QSRL [33, 42] or CO_2 lasers [40]. QSRL [43] and Er:YAG [44] lasers have shown to be relatively safe and effective in treating neonates and infants. Minimal repigmentation, scarring, dyspigmentation, or operative bleeding was encountered. Treatment of pigmented nevi such as CMN beginning in infancy may be beneficial because the pigmented nevi nests can be better identified through the more transparent skin of an infant [43]. Partial repigmentation many times results from the use of QS lasers, leading to about 50% total clearance [24]. Laser treatment may also aid with the hypertrichosis present in CMN.

22.5.1 Summary

- Pigment-specific lasers, resurfacing lasers, and a combination of both are used for CMN, QSRL and QS Nd:YAG lasers having been used most.
- Combination therapies include QSAL with QSRL or CO_2 laser, as well as QSRL with Er: YAG laser.
- Treatment of pigmented nevi in infancy, although controversial, may be beneficial.

22.6 Café Au Lait Macules

Traditional treatments for CALMs include dermabrasion, cryotherapy, or excision, all bearing the risk of scarring and dyspigmentation as side effects [9]. Laser treatment has been looked into as an alternative but, unfortunately, has not been found to be very successful for CALMs and often shows unpredictable results. Multiple treatments are needed for temporary lightening or clearing to be achieved. However, there is a refractory rate of about 50% [9]. The 510 nm pulsed dye laser (PDL) has shown some effectiveness in the treatment of CALMs while Er:YAG resurfacing has shown elimination of CALMs [9, 45]. Lasers such as the QS Nd:YAG (Figures 22.3 and 22.4), QSAL, and QSRL have also been reported to be used to treat CALMs but have shown less clearing [9, 20, 46–48], varied response, and a higher rate of repigmentation [49]. Wang et al., however, reported that the use of the QSAL showed a relatively high efficacy, especially among male patients [50]. Somvos et al. found that copper vapor laser treatment was also effective in treatment of CALMs [51]. Unfortunately, laser treatment of CALMs is often associated with negative side effects such as post-inflammatory hyperpigmentation, especially in darker skin types.

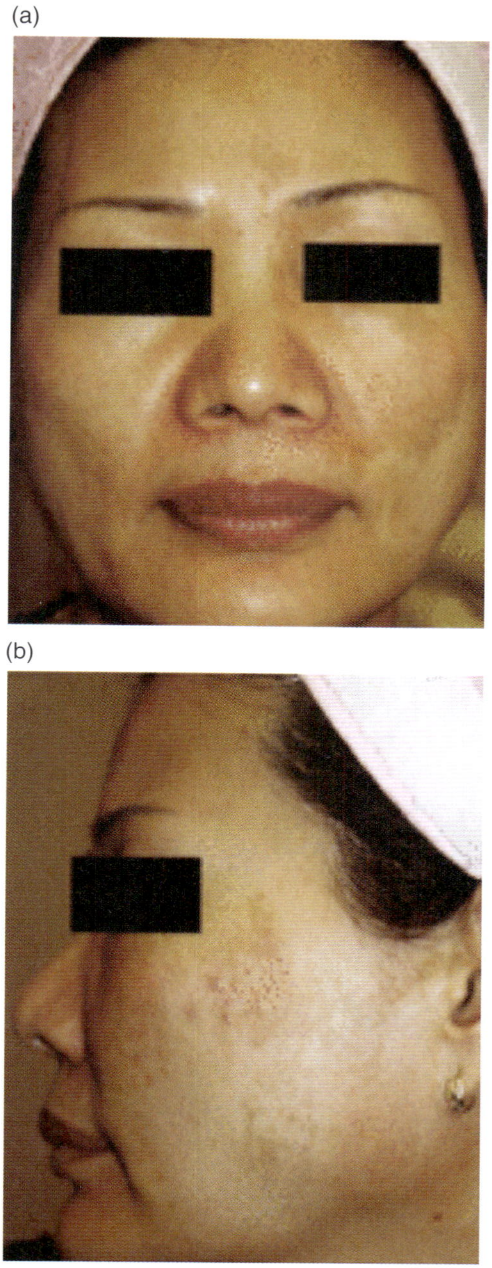

Figure 22.3 (a) Café au lait macule spreading from the left side of the forehead to the nose and cheek on the left side of the face, and several discrete brownish macules; (b) side profile. *Source:* From Kim et al. Treatment of segmental Café au lait macules using 1064 nm Q-switched Nd:YAG laser with low pulse energy. Copyright 2009 Reprinted with permission of John Wiley and Sons.

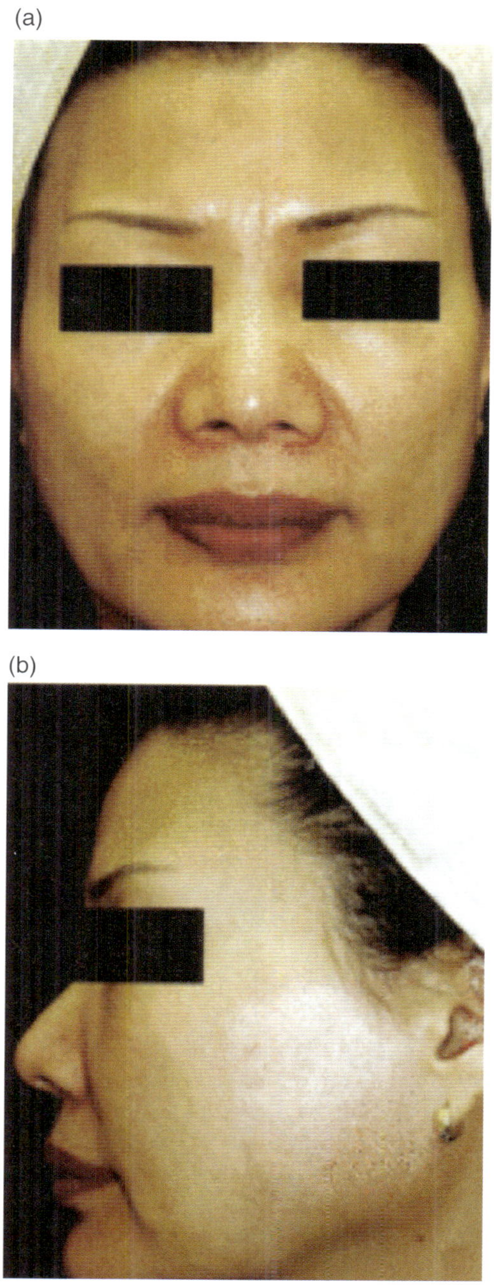

Figure 22.4 (a) Clinical improvement after 10 sessions of laser treatment with QS Nd:YAG; (b) side profile of the same patient. *Source:* From Kim et al. Treatment of segmental Café au lait macules using 1064 nm Q-switched Nd:YAG laser with low pulse energy. Copyright 2009 Reprinted with permission of John Wiley and Sons.

22.6.1 Summary

- Overall, laser therapy for CALMs has not been as effective.
- Er YAG and PDL have shown some improvement. Lasers like QS Nd: YAG, QSAL, and QSRL have varied responses but generally are less effective.

22.7 Becker's Nevus

QS lasers, Er:YAG lasers, and 1550 nm fractional erbium-doped fiber lasers have been found to improve the pigmented portions of Becker's nevus. Although complete clearance with lasers is rare, partial pigment clearance has been observed. A comparative study of QSRL laser and QS Nd:YAG found the QSRL laser to be slightly more effective, although both laser treatments led to improvement [9, 52]. Long-pulsed ruby and alexandrite lasers have also been used to treat Becker's nevi. Both of these lasers can decrease hair density, although the long-pulsed alexandrite laser has been used in patients with Fitzpatrick skin types III to IV and demonstrated positive results with no repigmentation at follow-up [53]. In 2005, a comparative study of the Er:YAG versus the QS Nd:YAG laser concluded that a single treatment with the Er:YAG laser was more effective than three treatments with the Nd:YAG laser (Figures 22.5–22.7) [54]. The 1550 nm nonablative fractional erbium-doped fiber laser has also shown to lead to significant clearance with several treatments [55], and may present as a new mode of treatment for Becker's nevus [56]. The hyperpigmented portions of Becker's nevi, however, often respond to laser treatment similarly to CALMs, with a high refractory rate and postoperative hyperpigmentation [57].

22.7.1 Summary

- Although complete clearance is rare, QS lasers, Er: YAG, and 1550 nm fractional erbium-doped fiber lasers have shown improvement for Becker's nevi to different degrees.

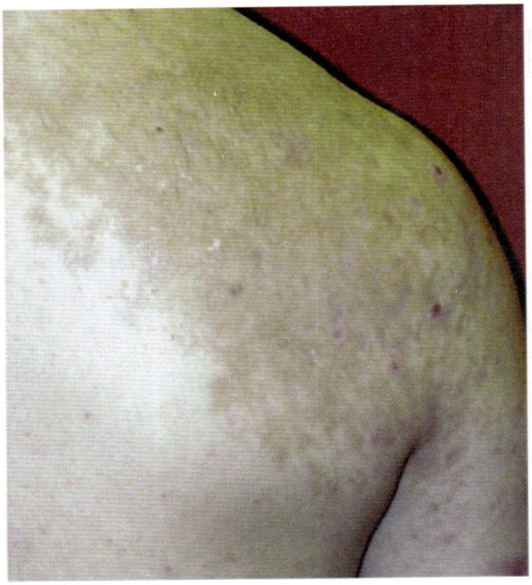

Figure 22.5 Becker's nevus on the right shoulder of a Caucasian 23-year-old male shows characteristic dark brown pigmentation and localized hypertrichosis. *Source:* From Trelles et al. [53]. Copyright 2004 Reprinted with permission of John Wiley and Sons.

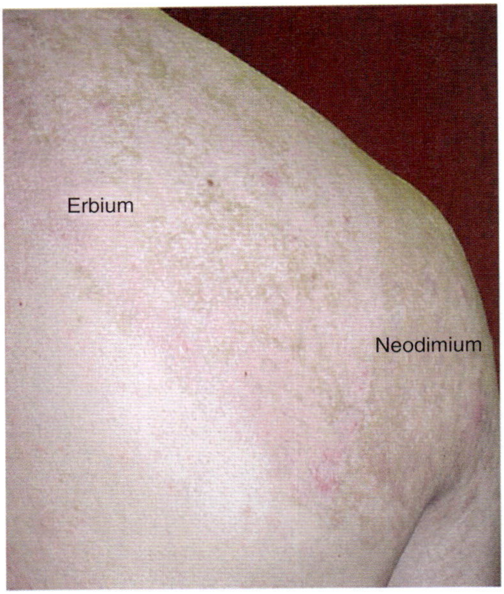

Figure 22.6 Six months post-treatment clinical evaluation showed substantial pigment clearance (>75%) in the area treated with the Er:YAG while pigment clearance of less than 25% was observed in the right half of the lesion treated with the Nd:YAG. *Source:* From Trelles et al. [53]. Copyright 2004 Reprinted with permission of John Wiley and Sons.

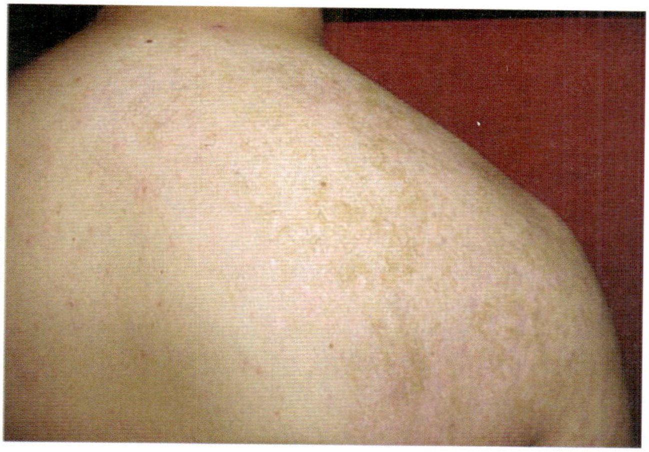

Figure 22.7 Complete clearance (100%) was observed two years after Er:YAG treatment. *Source:* From Trelles et al. [53], Copyright 2004 Reprinted with permission of John Wiley and Sons.

(a) (b)

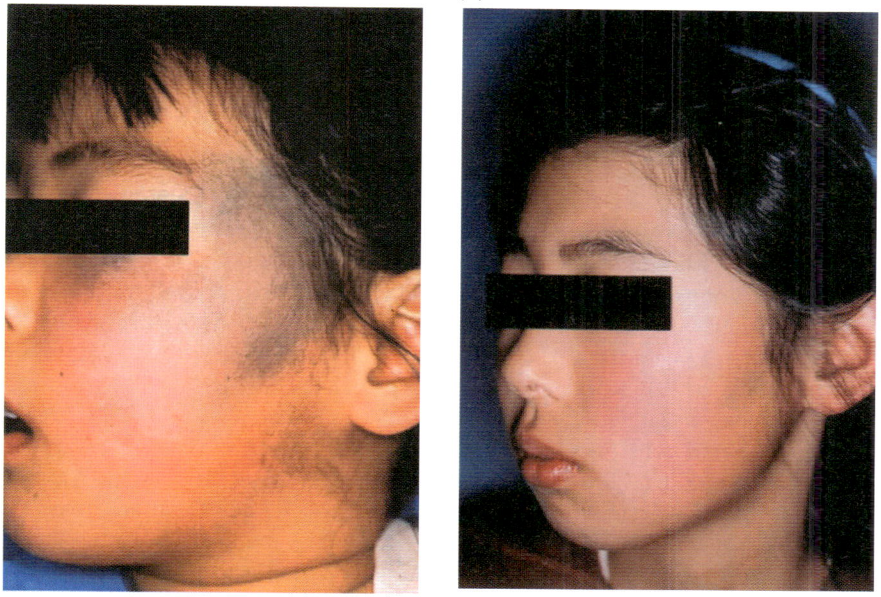

Figure 22.8 (a) A three-year-old patient with nevus of Ota before treatment with QSRL (b) Excellent response after three treatments and permanent result at the postoperative seventh year. *Source:* From Kono et al. [63]. Copyright 2003. Reprinted with permission of John Wiley and Sons.

22.8 Nevus of Ota/Ito

A retrospective study on laser treatments for nevus of Ota in 104 children determined that early laser treatment provides better clearance with a reduced amount of treatment sessions, however, the younger the age of onset, the higher the recurrence rate [58]. Several studies have confirmed the effectiveness of QSRL laser in the treatment of nevus of Ota/Ito (Figure 22.8). Improvement can be seen in one treatment, but several treatments might be needed [59, 60] and hypopigmentation is the most common complication [61]. Ueda et al. found that QSRL laser treatment for nevi of Ota can be based on the predominant color of the lesion; a favorable outcome (greater than 75% improvement) was obtained within a year, but they found that the number of treatments depended on the predominant color of the lesion [62, 63]. According to this study, blue-green lesions are less responsive to treatment than brown-violet or violet-blue lesions, and thus take longer to treat. A study by Kono and colleagues assessed QSRL laser treatment of nevus of Ota in different age groups, showing that children need fewer treatment sessions to achieve clearance and have fewer complications when compared to adults [64]. Pretreatment with CO_2 laser in conjunction with QSRL has been shown to provide more clearance [65] and a combination of QSRL with IPL has also been shown to be effective [66].

QS Nd:YAG lasers are also used to treat these lesions, although comparative studies with the QSRL reveal that QSRL provides better clearance [52, 67]. The use of QS Nd:YAG can be useful when treating patients with darker skin types without serious side effects [68, 69] and an improvement of at least 50% in a majority of the patients [69, 70]. A retrospective study of 31 Korean patients with skin type 4 showed that patients younger than 10 years, treated with lower mean fluences with the 1064 Nd:YAG, had better overall results [71]. Fractionated Nd:YAG has also demonstrated clearance of nevus of Ota [9].

QSAL requires multiple sessions to treat nevus of Ota and Ito with the frequency of treatments being the primary factor affecting effectiveness [46, 72–74]. Five or more treatments tend to provide adequate positive results [46, 73–75], although nevi involving the eyelid seem to be relatively resistant to laser therapy [46]. A comparative study reported that QS Nd:YAG laser was slightly more effective than QS alexandrite, but the treatment combination was significantly more effective [70].

22.8.1 Summary

- Early treatment in nevus of Ota might lead to better results and fewer treatments.
- QSRL have been effective for nevus of Ota. Several treatments are often needed, with the number of treatments dependent on the color of the nevus. Combinations with CO_2 laser and IPL are also effective.
- QS Nd: YAG is also used to treat nevus of Ota but is less effective than QSRL. It is useful in treating patients with darker skin types.
- Five or more treatments with QSAL have also shown to be effective. QSAL is slightly less effective than QS Nd:YAG whereas a combination of both is more effective.

22.9 Complications

Side effects and complications after laser treatment for nevi include erythema [39, 76], repigmentation [24, 40, 41, 43, 77], dyspigmentation, rarely post-procedural pain or bleeding [44, 78], and the risk of a hidden malignancy. Swelling and erythema may occur, especially if high fluences were used to treat dermal lesions. Swelling is highly probable if the treated area was near the periorbital region. After laser therapy, repigmentation can occur due to several reasons: (i) subepidermal vacuolization or vesiculation can occur, depositing pigment in the cell periphery; (ii) residual melanocytes can migrate from adnexal structures or surrounding untreated skin; and (iii) the use of sub-threshold fluences can stimulate melanogenesis [79].

Hyper- or hypopigmentation can occur, as well as transient post-inflammatory hyperpigmentation [40, 80, 81] and, rarely, reactive hyperpigmentation [82]. The use of sub-threshold fluences may result in hyperpigmentation lasting several months, for which topical hydroquinone can be prescribed. Partial reactive hypopigmentation [5, 40, 42] or transient post-operative hypopigmentation [39, 76] can occur, often in tanned patients [1]. Textural changes may accompany dyspigmentation disorders [40, 42, 80]. Hypertrophic or depressed scarring may rarely occur after laser therapy [40, 80, 83]. Too-aggressive treatments can result in epidermal damage, sloughing of tissue, bleeding, prolonged healing and blistering, especially if a short wavelength device was used to treat a patient with a darker skin type.

Purpura is a common side effect when using the 532 nm QS Nd:YAG, because of its absorption by hemoglobin, causing blood vessels to rupture. This can last 5–10 days and should be avoided by firmly placing a microscope slide against the skin during laser treatment, compressing vessels and making hemoglobin less of a target. Urticarial reactions have been reported to occur and can last for several hours after treatment. These cannot be prevented but can be alleviated by administrating an antihistamine prior to procedure.

An important complication that the physician should always be aware of is the inadvertent disguise of potential malignancies. It is not common for nevi to be malignant, especially in the pediatric population [22, 23, 84–87]. However, lightening them using laser therapy might make difficult to detect malignancies within them [24]. Hence, long-term follow-ups are recommended to ensure the detection of a possible malignant change [33, 42].

22.9.1 Summary

- Side effects and complications of laser treatment depend on the device and intensity of the treatment.
- They might include erythema, pain, bleeding, dyspigmentation, scarring, purpura and urticarial reactions. There is always the possibility of repigmentation after laser treatment.
- The risk of a hidden malignancy can be minimized by doing a careful examination of the lesion prior to treatment.

22.10 Conclusion

Among the newer laser technologies are the shorter pulse duration (pico and femtosecond domain) lasers, which are being used to selectively and more effectively remove melanin from pigmented lesions. Lasers that penetrate deeper are also sought after in this field, to be able to treat dermal lesions effectively with minimal side effects. Laser technology currently available is also being modified to increase efficacy and diminish the side effect profile. For example, various epidermal cooling systems are being developed to protect the epidermis from further thermal damage and different studies are being performed to optimize laser treatment [1]. Other technologies of importance in this field are imaging devices that can accurately assess the depth of the lesion prior to treatment and residual pigmentation following treatment. Confocal microscopy and optical coherence tomography are promising technologies in this field.

References

1 Graber, E. and Dover, J.S. (2011). Lasers and lights for treating pigmented lesions. In: *Lasers in Dermatology and Medicine* (ed. K. Nouri), 63–82. London: Springer.

2 Goldman, L., Blaney, D.J., Kindel, D.J. Jr. et al. (1963). Effect of the laser beam on the skin preliminary report. *The Journal of Investigative Dermatology* 40: 121–122.

3 Arora, H., Falto-Aizpurua, L., Chacon, A. et al. (2015). Lasers for nevi: a review. *Lasers in Medical Science* 30 (7): 1991–2001.
4 Cantatore, J.L. and Kriegel, D.A. (2004). Laser surgery: an approach to the pediatric patient. *Journal of the American Academy of Dermatology* 50 (2): 165–184; quiz 185–168.
5 Minakawa, S., Takeda, H., Korekawa, A. et al. (2012). Q-switched ruby laser therapy and long-term follow-up evaluation of small to medium-sized congenital melanocytic naevi. *Clinical and Experimental Dermatology* 37 (4): 438–440.
6 Krengel, S., Scope, A., Dusza, S.W. et al. (2013). New recommendations for the categorization of cutaneous features of congenital melanocytic nevi. *Journal of the American Academy of Dermatology* 68 (3): 441–451.
7 Shah, K.N. (2010). The diagnostic and clinical significance of cafe-au-lait macules. *Pediatric Clinics of North America* 57 (5): 1131–1153.
8 Cohen, P.R. (1988). Becker's nevus. *American Family Physician* 37 (5): 221–226.
9 Polder, K.D., Landau, J.M., Vergilis-Kalner, I.J. et al. (2011). Laser eradication of pigmented lesions: a review. *Dermatologic Surgery: Official Publication for American Society for Dermatologic Surgery [et al]* 37 (5): 572–595.
10 Patrizi, A., Medri, M., Raone, B. et al. (2012). Clinical characteristics of Becker's nevus in children: report of 118 cases from Italy. *Pediatric Dermatology* 29 (5): 571–574.
11 Hidano, A., Kajima, H., Ikeda, S. et al. (1967). Natural history of nevus of Ota. *Archives of Dermatology* 95 (2): 187–195.
12 Jay, B. (1965). Malignant melanoma of the orbit in a case of oculodermal melanosis. (Naevus of Ota). *The British Journal of Ophthalmology* 49 (7): 359–363.
13 Ito, M. (1954). Studies on Melanin XXII. Nevus fuscocaeruleus acromio-deltoideus. *The Tohoku Journal of Experimental Medicine* 60: 10.
14 Mukhopadhyay, A.K. (2013). Unilateral nevus of Ota with bilateral nevus of Ito and palatal lesion: a case report with a proposed clinical modification of Tanino's classification. *Indian Journal of Dermatology* 58 (4): 286–289.
15 Bukvic Mokos, Z., Lipozencic, J., Ceovic, R. et al. (2010). Laser therapy of pigmented lesions: pro and contra. *Acta Dermatovenerologica Croatica: ADC* 18 (3): 185–189.
16 Anderson, R.R. and Parrish, J.A. (1983). Selective photothermolysis: precise microsurgery by selective absorption of pulsed radiation. *Science* 220 (4596): 524–527.
17 Margolis, R.J., Dover, J.S., Polla, L.L. et al. (1989). Visible action spectrum for melanin-specific selective photothermolysis. *Lasers in Surgery and Medicine* 9 (4): 389–397.
18 Anderson, R.R., Margolis, R.J., Watenabe, S. et al. (1989). Selective photothermolysis of cutaneous pigmentation by Q-switched Nd: YAG laser pulses at 1064, 532, and 355 nm. *The Journal of Investigative Dermatology* 93 (1): 28–32.
19 Lin, J.Y. and Chan, H.H. (2006). Pigmentary disorders in Asian skin: treatment with laser and intense pulsed light sources. *Skin Therapy Letter* 11 (8): 8–11.
20 Moreno-Arias, G.A., Bulla, F., Vilata-Corell, J.J. et al. (2001). Treatment of widespread segmental nevus spilus by Q-switched alexandrite laser (755 nm, 100 nsec). *Dermatologic Surgery: Official Publication for American Society for Dermatologic Surgery [et al]* 27 (9): 841–843.
21 Tanghetti, E.A., Hoffmann, K.A., and Hoffmann, K. (2017). Short-pulsed laser for the treatment of tattoos, pigmented lesions, scars and rejuvenation. *Seminars in Cutaneous Medicine and Surgery* 36 (4): 148–154.
22 Konz, B. (2007). Therapy of congenital melanocytic nevi. Excision, dermabrasion, laser. *Der Hautarzt; Zeitschrift fur Dermatologie, Venerologie, und verwandte*

Gebiete 58 (8): 659–660, 662–656, 668–670.

23 Ferguson, R.E. Jr. and Vasconez, H.C. (2005). Laser treatment of congenital nevi. *The Journal of Craniofacial Surgery* 16 (5): 908–914.

24 Marghoob, A.A., Borrego, J.P., and Halpern, A.C. (2007). Congenital melanocytic nevi: treatment modalities and management options. *Seminars in Cutaneous Medicine and Surgery* 26 (4): 231–240.

25 Bernstein, E.F. (2006). Laser treatment of tattoos. *Clinics in Dermatology* 24 (1): 43–55.

26 Kent, K.M. and Graber, E.M. (2012). Laser tattoo removal: a review. *Dermatologic Surgery: Official Publication for American Society for Dermatologic Surgery [et al]* 38 (1): 1–13.

27 Giannini, E.H. and Cawkwell, G.D. (1995). Drug treatment in children with juvenile rheumatoid arthritis. Past, present, and future. *Pediatric Clinics of North America* 42 (5): 1099–1125.

28 Almoallim, H., Klinkhoff, A.V., Arthur, A.B. et al. (2006). Laser induced chrysiasis: disfiguring hyperpigmentation following Q-switched laser therapy in a woman previously treated with gold. *The Journal of Rheumatology.* 33 (3): 620–621.

29 Geist, D.E. and Phillips, T.J. (2006). Development of chrysiasis after Q-switched ruby laser treatment of solar lentigines. *Journal of the American Academy of Dermatology* 55 (2 Suppl): S59–S60.

30 Trotter, M.J., Tron, V.A., Hollingdale, J. et al. (1995). Localized chrysiasis induced by laser therapy. *Archives of Dermatology* 131 (12): 1411–1414.

31 Yun, P.L., Arndt, K.A., and Anderson, R.R. (2002). Q-switched laser-induced chrysiasis treated with long-pulsed laser. *Archives of Dermatology* 138 (8): 1012–1014.

32 Kossida, T., Farinelli, W., Flotte, T. et al. (2006). Mechanism of immediate whitening during tattoo removal. *Lasers in Surgery and Medicine* 18: 70.

33 Reda, A.M., Taha, I.R., and Riad, H.A. (1999). Clinical and histological effect of a single treatment of normal mode alexandrite (755 nm) laser on small melanocytic nevi. *Journal of Cutaneous Laser Therapy* 1 (4): 209–215.

34 Grevelink, J.M., van Leeuwen, R.L., Anderson, R.R. et al. (1997). Clinical and histological responses of congenital melanocytic nevi after single treatment with Q-switched lasers. *Archives of Dermatology* 133 (3): 349–353.

35 Kono, T., Ercocen, A.R., and Nozaki, M. (2005). Treatment of congenital melanocytic nevi using the combined (normal-mode plus Q-switched) ruby laser in Asians: clinical response in relation to histological type. *Annals of Plastic Surgery* 54 (5): 494–501.

36 Kono, T., Nozaki, M., Chan, H.H. et al. (2001). Combined use of normal mode and Q-switched ruby lasers in the treatment of congenital melanocytic naevi. *British Journal of Plastic Surgery* 54 (7): 640–643.

37 Kono, T., Ercocen, A.R., Chan, H.H. et al. (2002). Effectiveness of the normal-mode ruby laser and the combined (normal-mode plus q-switched) ruby laser in the treatment of congenital melanocytic nevi: a comparative study. *Annals of Plastic Surgery* 49 (5): 476–485.

38 Helsing, P., Mork, G., and Sveen, B. (2006). Ruby laser treatment of congenital melanocytic naevi – a pessimistic view. *Acta Dermato-Venereologica* 86 (3): 235–237.

39 Waldorf, H.A., Kauvar, A.N., and Geronemus, R.G. (1996). Treatment of small and medium congenital nevi with the Q-switched ruby laser. *Archives of Dermatology* 132 (3): 301–304.

40 Kim, S. and Kang, W.H. (2005). Treatment of congenital nevi with the Q-switched alexandrite laser. *European Journal of Dermatology: EJD* 15 (2): 92–96.

41 Sohn, S., Kim, S., and Kang, W.H. (2004). Recurrent pigmented macules after q-switched alexandrite laser treatment of congenital melanocytic nevus. *Dermatologic Surgery: Official Publication for American*

Society for Dermatologic Surgery [et al] 30 (6): 898–907; discussion 907.

42 Kono, T., Ercocen, A.R., Kikuchi, Y. et al. (2003). A giant melanocytic nevus treated with combined use of normal mode ruby laser and Q-switched alexandrite laser. *The Journal of dermatology* 30 (7): 538–542.

43 Kishi, K., Okabe, K., Ninomiya, R. et al. (2009). Early serial Q-switched ruby laser therapy for medium-sized to giant congenital melanocytic naevi. *The British Journal of Dermatology* 161 (2): 345–352.

44 Ostertag, J.U., Quaedvlieg, P.J., Kerckhoffs, F.E. et al. (2006). Congenital naevi treated with erbium:YAG laser (Derma K) resurfacing in neonates: clinical results and review of the literature. *The British Journal of Dermatology* 154 (5): 889–895.

45 Alora, M.B. and Arndt, K.A. (2001). Treatment of a cafe-au-lait macule with the erbium:YAG laser. *Journal of the American Academy of Dermatology* 45 (4): 566–568.

46 Kagami, S., Asahina, A., Watanabe, R. et al. (2007). Treatment of 153 Japanese patients with Q-switched alexandrite laser. *Lasers in Medical Science* 22 (3): 159–163.

47 Kilmer, S.L., Wheeland, R.G., Goldberg, D.J. et al. (1994). Treatment of epidermal pigmented lesions with the frequency-doubled Q-switched Nd:YAG laser. A controlled, single-impact, dose-response, multicenter trial. *Archives of Dermatology* 130 (12): 1515–1519.

48 Suh, D.H., Han, K.H., and Chung, J.H. (2001). The use of Q-switched Nd:YAG laser in the treatment of superficial pigmented lesions in Koreans. *The Journal of Dermatological Treatment* 12 (2): 91–96.

49 Shimbashi, T., Kamide, R., and Hashimoto, T. (1997). Long-term follow-up in treatment of solar lentigo and cafe-au-lait macules with Q-switched ruby laser. *Aesthetic Plastic Surgery* 21 (6): 445–448.

50 Wang, Y., Qian, H., and Lu, Z. (2012). Treatment of cafe au lait macules in Chinese patients with a Q-switched 755-nm alexandrite laser. *The Journal of Dermatological Treatment* 23 (6): 431–436.

51 Somyos, K., Boonchu, K., Somsak, K. et al. (1996). Copper vapour laser treatment of cafe-au-lait macules. *The British Journal of Dermatology* 135 (6): 964–968.

52 Tse, Y., Levine, V.J., McClain, S.A. et al. (1994). The removal of cutaneous pigmented lesions with the Q-switched ruby laser and the Q-switched neodymium: yttrium-aluminum-garnet laser. A comparative study. *The Journal of Dermatologic Surgery and Oncology* 20 (12): 795–800.

53 Choi, J.E., Kim, J.W., Seo, S.H. et al. (2009). Treatment of Becker's nevi with a long-pulse alexandrite laser. *Dermatologic Surgery: Official Publication for American Society for Dermatologic Surgery [et al]* 35 (7): 1105–1108.

54 Trelles, M.A., Allones, I., Moreno-Arias, G.A. et al. (2005). Becker's naevus: a comparative study between erbium: YAG and Q-switched neodymium:YAG; clinical and histopathological findings. *The British Journal of Dermatology* 152 (2): 308–313.

55 Glaich, A.S., Goldberg, L.H., Dai, T. et al. (2007). Fractional resurfacing: a new therapeutic modality for Becker's nevus. *Archives of Dermatology* 143 (12): 1488–1490.

56 Cordisco, M.R. (2009). An update on lasers in children. *Current Opinion in Pediatrics* 21 (4): 499–504.

57 Goldberg, D.J. (1993). Benign pigmented lesions of the skin. Treatment with the Q-switched ruby laser. *The Journal of Dermatologic Surgery and Oncology* 19 (4): 376–379.

58 Zong, W. and Lin, T. (2014). A retrospective study on laser treatment of nevus of Ota in Chinese children – a seven-year follow-up. *Journal of Cosmetic and Laser Therapy: Official Publication of the European Society for Laser Dermatology* 16 (4): 156–160.

59 Goldberg, D.J. and Nychay, S.G. (1992). Q-switched ruby laser treatment of nevus of Ota. *The Journal of Dermatologic Surgery and Oncology* 18 (9): 817–821.

60 Lowe, N.J., Wieder, J.M., Sawcer, D. et al. (1993). Nevus of Ota: treatment with high

energy fluences of the Q-switched ruby laser. *Journal of the American Academy of Dermatology* 29 (6): 997–1001.

61 Kono, T., Nozaki, M., Chan, H.H. et al. (2001). A retrospective study looking at the long-term complications of Q-switched ruby laser in the treatment of nevus of Ota. *Lasers in Surgery and Medicine* 29 (2): 156–159.

62 Ueda, S., Isoda, M., and Imayama, S. (2000). Response of naevus of Ota to Q-switched ruby laser treatment according to lesion colour. *The British Journal of Dermatology* 142 (1): 77–83.

63 Sardana, K., Chugh, S., and Garg, V. (2012). Are Q-switched lasers for nevus of Ota really effective in pigmented skin? *Indian Journal of Dermatology, Venereology and Leprology* 78 (2): 187–189; author reply 189–190.

64 Kono, T., Chan, H.H., Ercocen, A.R. et al. (2003). Use of Q-switched ruby laser in the treatment of nevus of Ota in different age groups. *Lasers in Surgery and Medicine* 32 (5): 391–395.

65 Manuskiatti, W., Sivayathorn, A., Leelaudomlipi, P. et al. (2003). Treatment of acquired bilateral nevus of Ota-like macules (Hori's nevus) using a combination of scanned carbon dioxide laser followed by Q-switched ruby laser. *Journal of the American Academy of Dermatology* 48 (4): 584–591.

66 Park, J.M., Tsao, H., and Tsao, S. (2008). Combined use of intense pulsed light and Q-switched ruby laser for complex dyspigmentation among Asian patients. *Lasers in Surgery and Medicine* 40 (2): 128–133.

67 Chang, C.J. and Kou, C.S. (2011). Comparing the effectiveness of Q-switched ruby laser treatment with that of Q-switched Nd:YAG laser for oculodermal melanosis (nevus of Ota). *Journal of Plastic, Reconstructive & Aesthetic Surgery: JPRAS* 64 (3): 339–345.

68 Fusade, T., Lafaye, S., and Laubach, H.J. (2011). Nevus of Ota in dark skin – an uncommon but treatable entity. *Lasers in Surgery and Medicine* 43 (10): 960–964.

69 Sharma, S., Jha, A.K., and Mallik, S.K. (2011). Role of q-switched Nd:YAG laser in nevus of Ota: a study of 25 cases. *Indian Journal of Dermatology* 56 (6): 663–665.

70 Chan, H.H., Leung, R.S., Ying, S.Y. et al. (2000). A retrospective analysis of complications in the treatment of nevus of Ota with the Q-switched alexandrite and Q-switched Nd:YAG lasers. *Dermatologic Surgery: Official Publication for American Society for Dermatologic Surgery [et al]* 26 (11): 1000–1006.

71 Seo, H.M., Choi, C.W., and Kim, W.S. (2014). Beneficial effects of early treatment of nevus of Ota with low-fluence 1,064-nm Q-switched Nd: YAG laser. *Dermatologic Surgery: Official Publication for American Society for Dermatologic Surgery [et al].*

72 Wang, H.W., Liu, Y.H., Zhang, G.K. et al. (2007). Analysis of 602 Chinese cases of nevus of Ota and the treatment results treated by Q-switched alexandrite laser. *Dermatologic Surgery: Official Publication for American Society for Dermatologic Surgery [et al]* 33 (4): 455–460.

73 Wang, H.W., Wang, J.B., Liu, Y.H. et al. (2006). Clinical efficacy of Q-switched alexandrite laser for pigmentary skin diseases in 4656 patients. *Zhongguo yi xue ke xue yuan xue bao Acta Academiae Medicinae Sinicae* 28 (2): 202–205.

74 Alster, T.S. and Williams, C.M. (1995). Treatment of nevus of Ota by the Q-switched alexandrite laser. *Dermatologic Surgery: Official Publication for American Society for Dermatologic Surgery [et al]* 21 (7): 592–596.

75 Mizuashi, M., Suetake, T., Aiba, S. et al. (2010). Dermal melanocytosis of the helix. *Pediatric Dermatology* 27 (3): 305–306.

76 Park, J.H., Hwang, E.S., Kim, S.N., and Kye, Y.C. (2004). Er:YAG laser treatment of verrucous epidermal nevi. *Dermatologic Surgery: Official Publication for American Society for Dermatologic Surgery [et al]* 30 (3): 378–381.

77 Martin, J.M., Monteagudo, C., Bella, R. et al. (2012). Complete regression of a melanocytic nevus under intense pulsed light therapy for

axillary hair removal in a cosmetic center. *Dermatology* 224 (3): 193–197.
78 Moser, C.M. and Hamsch, C. (2012). Successful treatment of cutaneous venous malformations in a patient with blue rubber bleb naevus syndrome by Nd:YAG laser. *The British Journal of Dermatology* 166 (5): 1143–1145.
79 Hruza, G.J., Dover, J.S., Flotte, T.J. et al. (1991). Q-switched ruby laser irradiation of normal human skin. Histologic and ultrastructural findings. *Archives of Dermatology* 127 (12): 1799–1805.
80 Thomas, J.L., Lister, T.S., Royston, S.L. et al. (2010). Adverse effects following Q-switched ruby laser treatment of pigmented lesions. *Journal of Cosmetic and Laser Therapy: Official Publication of the European Society for Laser Dermatology* 12 (2): 101–105.
81 Kar, H.K. and Gupta, L. (2011). 1064 nm Q-switched Nd: YAG laser treatment of nevus of Ota: an Indian open label prospective study of 50 patients. *Indian Journal of Dermatology, Venereology and Leprology* 77 (5): 565–570.
82 Kopera, D., Hohenleutner, U., and Landthaler, M. (1997). Quality-switched ruby laser treatment of solar lentigines and Becker's nevus: a histopathological and immunohistochemical study. *Dermatology* 194 (4): 338–343.
83 August, P.J., Ferguson, J.E., and Madan, V. (2011). A study of the efficacy of carbon dioxide and pigment-specific lasers in the treatment of medium-sized congenital melanocytic naevi. *The British Journal of Dermatology* 164 (5): 1037–1042.
84 Reynolds, N., Kenealy, J., and Mercer, N. (2003). Carbon dioxide laser dermabrasion for giant congenital melanocytic nevi. *Plastic and Reconstructive Surgery* 111 (7): 2209–2214.
85 Michel, J.L. (2003). Laser therapy of giant congenital melanocytic nevi. *European Journal of Dermatology: EJD* 13 (1): 57–64.
86 Helmbold, P., Rompel, R., Petres, J. et al. (1999). Congenital melanocytic nevi. *Der Hautarzt; Zeitschrift fur Dermatologie, Venerologie, und verwandte Gebiete.* 50 (11): 779–784.
87 Goldberg, D.J. and Stampien, T. (1995). Q-switched ruby laser treatment of congenital nevi. *Archives of Dermatology* 131 (5): 621–623.

23

Lasers for Tattoos

Stephanie Mlacker[1], Leyre Falto-Aizpurua[2], Colin McNamara[1], and Keyvan Nouri[3]

[1] Charles E. Schmidt College of Medicine, Florida Atlantic University, Boca Raton, FL, USA
[2] Department of Dermatology & Cutaneous Surgery, University of Miami Miller School of Medicine, Miami, FL, USA
[3] Department of Dermatology, Ophthalmology, Otolaryngology & Surgery, University of Miami Leonard M. Miller School of Medicine, Miami, FL, USA

23.1 Introduction

Tattooing developed independently for various religious, cultural, and decorative reasons throughout the world. As early as 2000 BCE, Egyptians were adorning their bodies with tattoos. However, in Western culture, tattoos were historically used to brand convicts and slaves, gaining associations with the lower socioeconomical classes [1, 2]. Consequently, various reasons for tattoo removal, and mechanisms of doing so, evolved. Some evidence of tattoo removal exists in Egyptian mummies, but it was the Greeks who provided the first written account of tattoo removal, using salt abrasives and specific pastes [3]. In 1928 an article listed surgical excision, electrolysis, and 50% tannic acid as methods for tattoo removal; however, these procedures caused adverse effects [4]. Other mechanisms used for tattoo removal were dermabrasion, thermal destruction and cryotherapy [5]. These modalities provided unpredictable results with significant side effects such as pain, skin discoloration, scarring, and prolonged healing. People in today's society get tattoos to decorate their bodies, to identify with particular groups or gangs, or to camouflage areas such as birthmarks or other tattoos [6–9].

Tattoos may be divided into five categories: professional, amateur, cosmetic, traumatic, and medical [10]. Professional tattoos have high artistic quality and are created by a professional using state-of-the-art technologies, materials, and standards of care [9]. Amateur tattoos are performed by nonprofessionals, often using decreased hygienic standards and using poor-quality inks that can often be removed in fewer treatment sessions than professional tattoos [9, 10]. Traumatic tattoos, probably the most common in the pediatric population, result from unintentional percutaneous implantation of particles via explosions or through scrapes in the skin [11]. Cosmetic tattoos can be used as permanent makeup or to conceal markings on the patient's skin. These are often difficult to remove due to the specific white and red pigments that they use [9, 12, 13]. Medical tattoos may function to mark areas treated with therapeutic radiation or to replace missing body parts such as an areola after radical mastectomy [12].

Today, in American culture, about 22–26% of adults have at least one tattoo, and it has been suggested that 10% of adolescents (aged 12–18) already have at least one. Of those with tattoos, about 17% have considered having one removed [11, 14]. Some people acquire tattoos impulsively while underage in

Pediatric Dermatologic Surgery, First Edition. Edited by Keyvan Nouri, Latanya Benjamin, Jasem Alshaiji, and Jan Izakovic.

an effort to express their unique identity and self-dominion, or while under the influence of drugs/alcohol – and regret their decision later [1, 2, 15]. People may seek tattoo removal for the purpose of improving self-esteem, becoming more socially accepted, assuaging family pressure, gaining higher levels of employment, moving on from a broken relationship, and for various other reasons [16, 17].

Tattoo removal in the past involved destroying both the tattoo and the surrounding skin. Laser affords the ability to practice selective photothermolysis, selectively destroying tattoo pigments while minimally affecting the surrounding skin [18]. The energy from laser light is converted to heat once absorbed by its target chromophore, resulting in its destruction [19]. Following the rules of selective photothermolysis, the target chromophore should be heated for as long as the duration of its thermal relaxation time (equivalent to the time necessary for a particle to lose half its heat), which is in the order of the nanosecond domain [4]. Lasers remove tattoos by altering the optic properties of their pigments. This is hypothesized to occur through a photoacoustic effect, which involves the transfer of heat energy thermally and mechanically destroying pigment particles and the cells that contain them, allowing macrophages to engulf and clear these particles [14, 18, 20]. Note thermal relaxation time increases with larger target sizes. For example, melanosomes and tattoo pigments are smaller structures and thus heat up more quickly than larger structures such as vessels [21, 22]. Smaller structures like tattoos must be removed by rapid heating; consequently, pulse durations must be short, ranging from nanoseconds to picoseconds [21]. Laser techniques have been around since the 1960s; however, early lasers were often no better than traditional tattoo removal methods, carrying many of the same risks and deficiencies. Only recently, with the invention of quality-switched (QS) lasers, has this field become a beneficial alternative to traditional tattoo removal methods [21, 23].

23.1.1 Summary

- Tattoos may be divided into five categories: professional, amateur, cosmetic, traumatic, and medical.
- 10% of adolescents (aged 12–18) already have at least one tattoo.
- Lasers that practice selective photothermolysis, selectively destroy tattoo pigments while minimally affecting the surrounding skin.

23.2 Indications and Contraindications

For laser tattoo removal to be effective several factors should be considered: the patient's Fitzpatrick skin type, the color of the tattoo to be removed, choosing the appropriate device, correctly performing the technique, and the number and frequency of treatments [5]. Certain wavelengths remove more effectively certain colors. The QS neodymium: yttrium-aluminum-garnet (Nd:YAG), 1064 nm laser is a better treatment option for darker skin types because it targets melanocytes deeper within tissue while sparing melanocytes and keratinocytes in the epidermal layer [4]. With the exception of the QS Nd:YAG (1064 nm) laser, treatment should be postponed for patients who present with suntanned skin [22].

Precautions should be taken when treating traumatic tattoos because these might contain flammable materials that were acquired into the skin via explosions or fireworks. These materials can combust during laser treatment; therefore, in order to avoid substantial scarring and any injury to the patient or practitioner, treatment of such tattoos must begin with a small, pretreatment spot test [11]. Laser treatment for patients who have undergone isotretinoin therapy within the last six months may result in keloid formation [22]. Although rarely see in the pediatric population, caution should be advised to patients taking parenteral gold therapy for other medical conditions because localized chrysiasis can be induced by QS lasers [24–27]. Chrysiasis is a rare, permanent, blue-gray skin discoloration in patients taking or that have ever taken gold salts that are exposed to UV light.

Before starting laser treatment, inspect the tattoo for hidden pigmented lesions. Several case reports have documented the development of malignant melanoma within tattoos [28]. It remains unclear if a correlation exists between tattoo placement, laser treatment, and malignant melanoma development. A study found that pigmented lesions treated with laser delays the diagnosis of melanoma and, consequently, appropriate therapy [29]. For this reason tattoos should not be placed over a pigmented lesion in the first place. If a pigmented lesion is present within a tattoo, the laser treatment will interfere with appropriate monitoring of the lesion, therefore excision of the lesion is recommended prior to laser treatment [28].

23.2.1 Summary

- QS 1064 nm Nd:YAG laser is recommended for tattoo removal in darker skin types.
- Precautions should be taken when treating certain traumatic tattoos.
- Laser treatment should be avoided in suntanned patients, those with significant post-inflammatory hyperpigmentation, and those with history of gold therapy or who have undergone isotretinoin therapy within the last six months.
- Caution is advised if a pigmented lesion is present within the tattoo that is desired to be removed.

23.3 Types of Lasers

Early laser tattoo removal methods included the argon laser and the carbon dioxide (CO_2) laser, both of which carried significant deficiencies and side effects [5, 30, 31]. The argon laser emits continuous energy at the 488 nm and the 514 nm wavelength. Although these wavelengths are preferentially absorbed by tattoo pigments rather than natural skin pigments, heat spreads from these tattoo pigments to the surrounding skin layers, resulting in scarring [8, 30]. The CO_2 laser emits either continuous or pulsed energy at the 10 600 nm, nonselectively ablating skin, removing tattoos while causing significant scarring with insufficient tattoo removal [30, 32].

More recent discoveries involving the use of QS lasers have allowed the production of nanosecond lasers, using high-powered pulses with very short duration, which decrease the incidence of thermal damage to surrounding skin layers [19, 33]. The production of nanosecond laser pulses is enabled because the Q-switching technique allows the sudden release of all exited-state energy sources from the laser in a single pulse during only the time in which it takes the light to travel across the laser [30]. The three main types of QS lasers include the ruby, alexandrite, and Nd:YAG lasers. Each QS laser has its own tattoo color range that it removes most efficiently [34] (See Table 23.1).

The QS ruby laser which emits laser energy at the range of 694 nm, best removes black and blue tattoo pigments while also effectively serving to remove green pigments, because it best absorbs light in the 600–800 nm range (Figure 23.1) [35]. This laser energy is pulsed to less than a 40 ns duration and uses energies from 8 to 10 J/cm^2 fluence range [36].

QS Nd:YAG lasers are capable of emitting laser energy with wavelengths of 1064 nm or, in the frequency-doubled version, 532 nm. These lasers can have a fluence of up to 12 J/cm^2 and have pulse durations of less than 10 ns. This allows it to remove black and blue pigments with the 1064 nm wavelength or red, orange and yellow pigments with the 532 nm wavelength (Figure 23.2) [4, 35, 36]. Longer wavelengths target superficial melanocytes less than shorter wavelengths of lights because they penetrate further into the dermis layer [35]. Since superficial melanocytes are less damaged using the QS Nd:YAG

Table 23.1 Lasers used for tattoo removal.

Laser	Wavelength (nm)	Pigment's Best Absorption Range: Red/Orange/Yellow 490–530	Blue/Green 600–800	Black/Dark Blue 700–1000	Comments
Flashlamp pulsed dye laser	510	X			
QS Ruby	694		X	X	All QS lasers can remove carbon and graphite present in traumatic tattoo
QS Alexandrite	755		X	X	
QS Nd:YAG	1064			X	
	532	X			

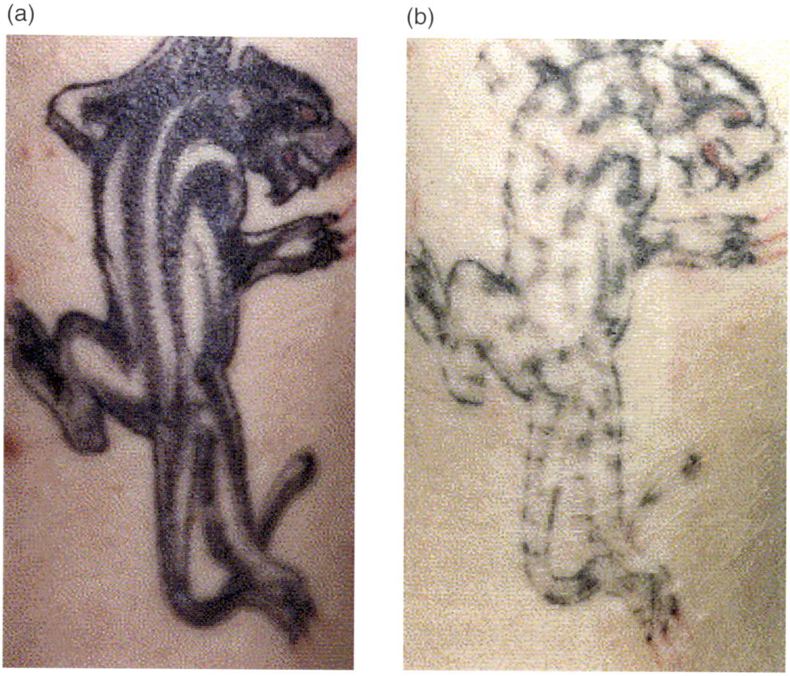

Figure 23.1 Before (a) and after (b) picture of black tattoo after one treatment session with the Q-switched ruby laser. *Source:* Bernstein et al. [8]. Reprinted with permission of Elsevier Limited.

(1064 nm) laser as opposed to the QS ruby, there is less hypopigmentation and blistering following treatment, making this laser the preferred treatment option for removing black and blue pigments in darker-skinned individuals [4, 22]. Melanin and, to a much lesser degree, hemoglobin compete with tattoo pigments to absorb energy from treatment lasers. Longer wavelengths generally penetrate deeper into the skin; therefore, lasers of higher wavelengths allow light to be preferentially absorbed by deeper tattoo inks rather than more superficial melanin layers. Furthermore, melanin is known to only weakly absorb at 1064 nm, making the QS Nd:YAG laser effective at minimizing side effects [35].

QS alexandrite lasers, which emit laser energy with a 755 nm wavelength, a pulse duration of 50–100 ns, and a fluence of 8 J/cm^2, best remove black and blue pigments and are more effective at removing green pigment than the QS ruby and QS Nd:YAG lasers [22,36].

All three QS lasers can effectively be used to remove traumatic tattoos, which usually contain carbon and graphite (Figure 23.3) [37]. The work of Zelickson et al. found that while all three QS lasers are equivalent in removing black pigments (because black pigment best absorbs red and infrared light, 700–1000 nm, red, brown, and orange pigments best respond to the Nd:YAG laser, while blue and green pigments best respond to the alexandrite laser, and purple and violet pigments best respond to the QS ruby laser) [12, 34, 38].

The flashlamp-pumped pulsed dye laser, which emits a 510 nm wavelength, has a longer pulse time of 300 ns and can only be used for red and certain orange and yellow pigments [32]. Three to seven treatment sessions may be needed for complete lightening of these pigment colors.

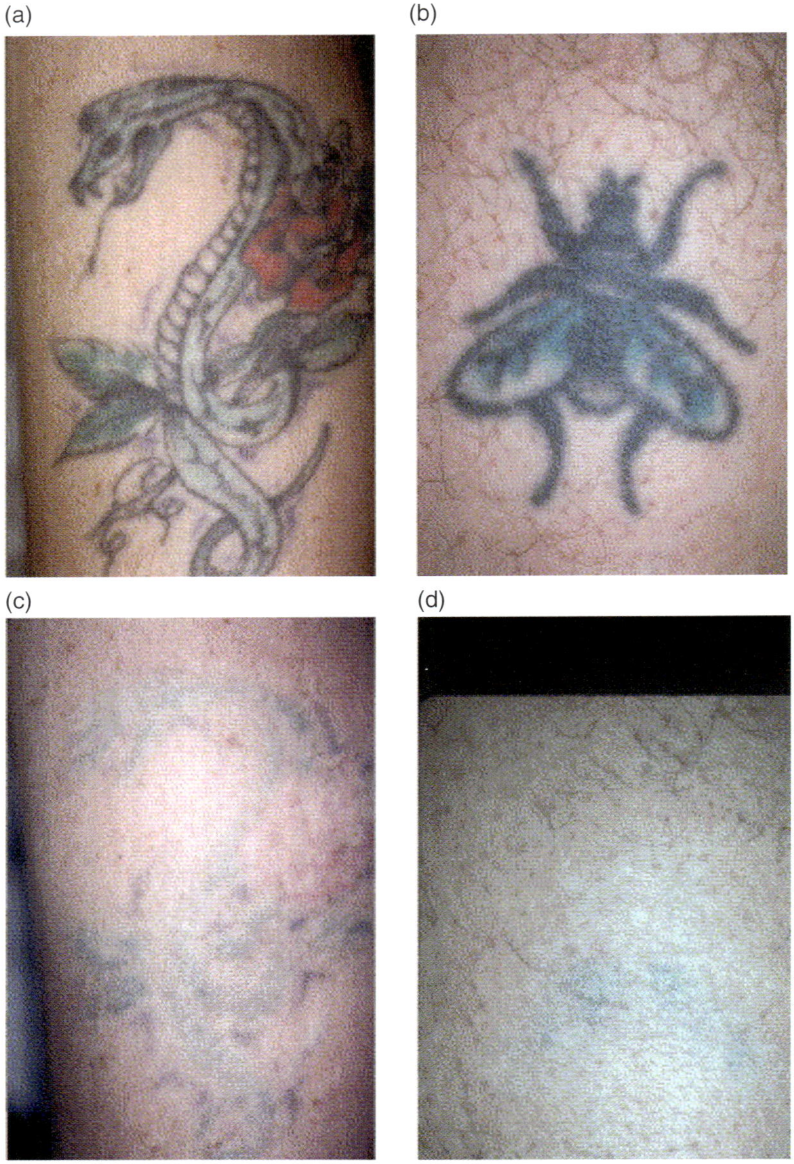

Figure 23.2 Tattoos containing green before (a, b) and after multiple treatments with a Q-switched Nd:YAG laser (c) or the Nd:YAG and alexandrite lasers (d). Residual green pigment can be seen in both cases. *Source:* Bernstein et al. [8] Reprinted with permission of Elsevier Limited.

On the other hand, light intensities emitted by an Intense Pulse Light (IPL) device are not specific to destroy tattoo ink and should not be used for this purpose [5]. These have long pulse duration (milliseconds) compared to the QS system, conducting the heat from the ink particles to the adjacent skin and skin appendages and resulting in thermal damage, reflected as scarring and discoloration [5, 26]. Second-degree burn in tattooed skin has been reported after photoepilation with an IPL device [39].

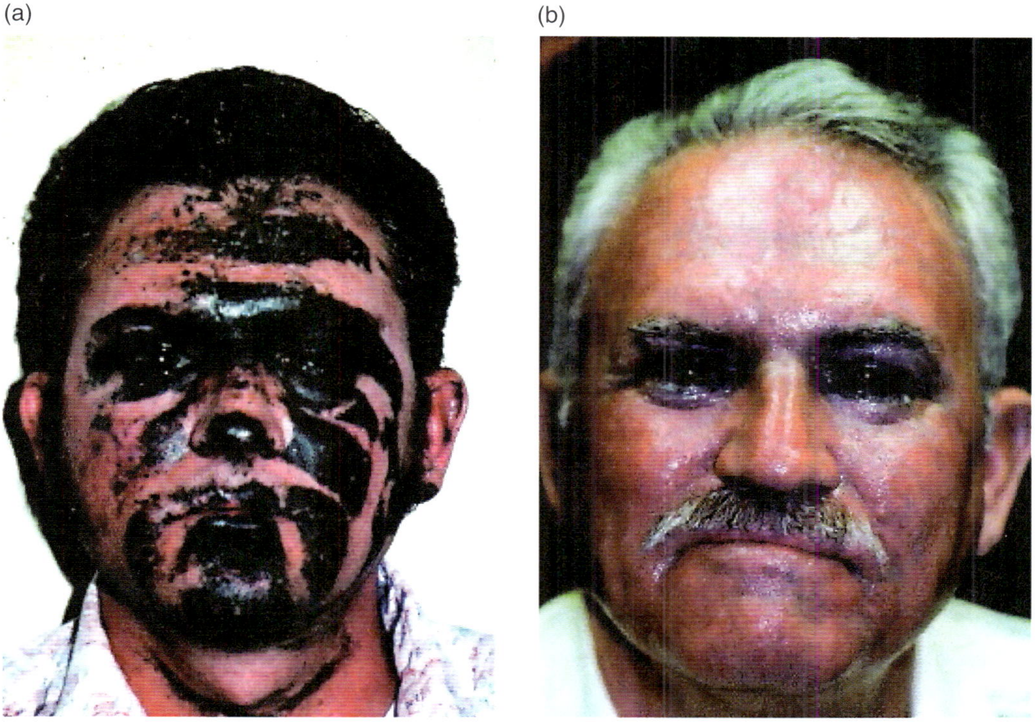

Figure 23.3 (a) Patient in 1974, five years after the explosion. (b) Patient in 2002, after 35 laser sessions. *Source:* Naversen et al. [37] Copyright 2004 American Academy of Dermatology, Inc. Reprinted with permission of Elsevier Limited.

23.3.1 Summary

- The 488 and 514 nm wavelengths emitted by the argon laser are preferentially absorbed by tattoo pigments, but the heat spread from these tattoo pigments to the surrounding skin layers may result in scarring.
- The CO_2 laser emits either continuous or pulsed energy at 10 600 nm wavelength, nonselectively removing tattoos while causing significant scarring with insufficient tattoo removal.
- QS lasers have allowed the production of nanosecond lasers, using high-powered pulses with very short duration, decreasing the incidence of thermal damage to surrounding skin.
- The three main types of QS lasers include the ruby, alexandrite, and Nd:YAG lasers. Each QS laser has its own tattoo color range that it removes most efficiently.
- The flashlamp-pumped pulsed dye laser emits a 510 nm wavelength, has a longer pulse time of 300 ns and can only be used for red and certain orange and yellow pigments.
- IPL is not recommended for tattoo removal.

23.4 Techniques

Treatment procedure should always be discussed in detail with the patient and their parents or guardian. Realistic expectations should also be established with them to improve patient compliance with treatment, maximizing results. Choosing the appropriate laser depends not only on the skin pigmentation and spot size but also the fluence, pulse duration, and wavelength necessary to remove the particular pigment color [22]. Larger laser beams should also be used in order to avoid scattering which occurs at the edge of the field and prevents a portion of the light from reaching significant depths [35].

Because many tattoos today use a myriad of colors, it is recommended that a practitioner use combinations of these three lasers in order to best remove colored tattoos [11]. Furthermore, to minimize the extent to which melanin absorbs energy from the treatment laser and the potential scarring associated with it, darker-skinned individuals should usually be first treated with a bleaching agent to skin overlaying the tattoo which will be removed [8, 32]. Local anesthesia, either via a topical cream 45 minutes prior to the procedure or via local infiltration 10 minutes prior to the procedure, should be administered to prevent significant levels of pain to the patient [8, 18]. Some children might require general anesthesia depending on the size and location of the tattoo [11]. Laser treatment should be performed through a clear hydrogel dressing in order to act as a heat sink in order to protect the epidermis, to prevent skin from becoming aerosolized during the procedure, and to prevent blood from spattering during the procedure. When applying a clear hydrogel dressing prior to the procedure, all plastic layers should be removed to avoid them heating up and damaging the patient's epidermis [8].

Laser treatment will produce an immediate white color response at the targeted site that resolves after 20 minutes (Figure 23.4). This reaction may not manifest if using an insufficient dose of laser exposure; however, it should be used as a means of determining endpoint of treatment [4]. Since too much energy absorbed by the epidermis can cause skin sloughing, blistering and greater risk of scarring, it is best to use the minimum fluence necessary to produce the whitening reaction [22]. In addition, the largest spot size which still delivers the necessary fluence in order to remove the tattoo should be used in order to minimize refractory effects [4]. Pinpoint bleeding observed intraoperatively is normal [22]. Furthermore, the targeted site may develop crusting and scabbing seven to 10 days following treatment. Thus, the patient should be advised to cover this area with an occlusive ointment and avoid sun exposure months post-treatment [22, 32].

On average, tattoo removal requires about four to 12 treatment sessions spaced six to eight weeks apart, which depends on the color, age, and type of tattoo used [11]. Regardless, treatment sessions and interval period should be determined for each patient. Too frequent an interval may increase side effects and decrease effectiveness of treatment; treatment intervals of a month can interfere with macrophages activity [5]. To maximize tattoo clearance, the Kirby-Desai Scale was proposed in 2009 to aid the clinician provide the patient with an estimate number of treatments needed [40]. This scale, developed for QS lasers, is based on a group of parameters, including patient's skin type, location, colors and density of the tattoo.

Frequently, tattoo inks are the result of a mixture of colors and ingredients, which formulations may not be uniform and are poorly regulated. For this reason, tattoos may not respond to laser treatment as it was originally anticipated [41]. For example, red and green ink may vary in their response to tattoo removal, while yellow and orange pigments are extremely resistant to treatment [2, 42]. Orange and yellow pigments are commonly difficult to remove because they minimally absorb current available wavelengths. Green pigment, although theoretically is absorbed well by QS ruby laser, it is speculated to be resistant to laser therapy because of the inherent quality of the ink mixture [43]. In general, professional tattoos are often more resistant when compared to amateur tattoos because they are usually deeper, densely packed and may contain multiple colors [44]. Pigments that are treatment-resistant or can darken may be removed with different wavelengths (attachable hand pieces with 585 and 650 nm wavelengths are available), ablative lasers or through surgical excision [5, 22]. Ink retention may also occur in patients in an immunosuppressed

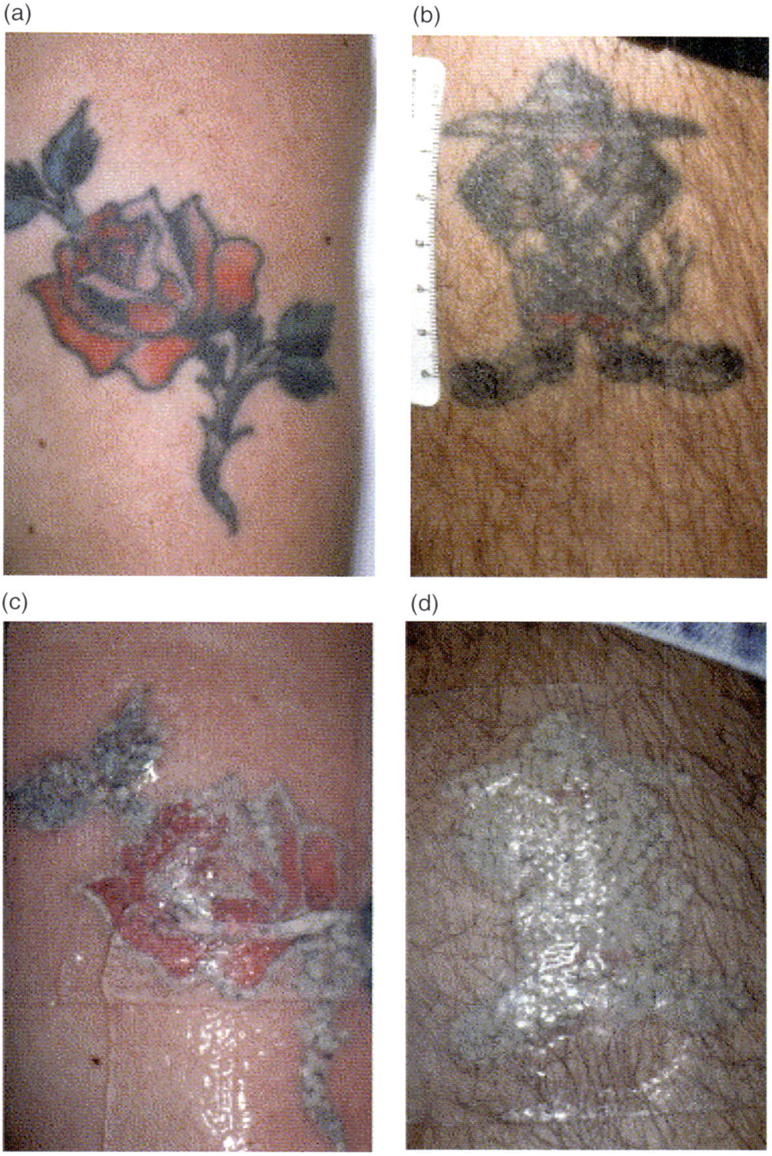

Figure 23.4 Normal immediate response of black tattoo pigment after treatment with QS ruby laser. Red pigment looks as if it had not been treated. *Source:* From Bernstein et al. [8] Copyright 2006 Reprinted with permission of Elsevier Limited.

state, because their lymphatic system will not clear the residual pigment particles appropriately [5].

For traumatic tattoos, it is important to remove the foreign particle whenever possible immediately after the incident. Several reports showed the QS ruby to effectively remove pencil and firework tattoos without significant scarring [11].

It is important to cease treatments once complete or significant clearance of tattoo ink is achieved. Transient hyperpigmentation may occur once complete resolution of tattoo ink is achieved following QS treatment, but is often misdiagnosed as ink retention [5, 45]. If this area continues to be treated, it will only prolong this phenomenon. If confusion exists between undesired hyperpigmentation and ink retention, treatment intervals should be prolonged, topical hydroquinone and sun avoidance considered [45].

23.5 Complications

The most common complications of laser tattoo removal include textural changes in the overlying epidermis, scarring (Figure 23.5), pruritus, hyperpigmentation, hypopigmentation, and allergic reactions [14]. Although the QS ruby laser has the highest clearance rate, it also has the highest incidence of hypopigmentation so should be avoided in darker-skinned individuals [35]. Like the QS ruby that emits shorter wavelengths, both the QS alexandrite and the QS Nd:YAG (532 nm) lasers may also result in post-treatment hypopigmentation [2, 35].

In some patients, partial tattoo removal may be the best option. If a tattoo cannot be fully removed, physicians should avoid increasing the fluence of the laser beyond standard levels because this would involve decreasing the laser's spot size, thereby increasing the amount of light scattered to the superficial layers of skin to dangerous levels [8, 35]. Some patients may experience blisters at the treatment site in the period immediately following treatment. Patients should be instructed to avoid rupturing these blisters in order to avoid infection [8].

Pigment-containing melanocytes in the epidermis absorb laser light and are therefore vulnerable to damage. For this reason, it is important that the patient avoid sun exposure before treatment, otherwise the procedure could result in short-term blistering, long-term scarring, hyperpigmentation, and hypopigmentation [22, 32].

Some patients may be allergic to particular tattoo pigments which could be exacerbated by the removal procedure. Furthermore, the laser may change certain tattoo pigments into materials to which a patient might experience an allergic reaction [19, 32]. Common pigments that patients may be allergic to include red pigments and cadmium derived yellow pigments [12]. Furthermore, Vasold et al. demonstrated that laser intensities cleave azo-containing tattoo inks, decomposing them into carcinogenic and cytotoxic byproducts [19]. Laser tattoo removal may also cause localized lymphadenopathy and elicit a cutaneous response in the patient following treatment [9, 22].

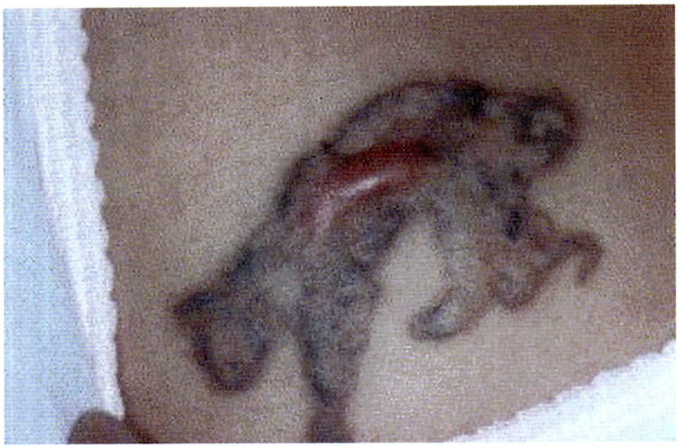

Figure 23.5 A tattoo treated with an intense pulsed light device having a millisecond domain pulse duration, with resultant keloidal scarring. *Source:* From Bernstein et al. [8] Copyright 2006 Reprinted with permission of Elsevier Limited.

Ortiz et al. have recently described a new complication termed "tattoo bleeding" whereby tattoo pigments travel into the surrounding skin during laser treatments. It is hypothesized that this effect may be due to channels created in the skin when injecting local anesthetics [22].

Laser treatment for patients who have undergone isotretinoin therapy within the last six months may result in keloid production post-treatment [22]. Chrysiasis can occur in patients treated with parenteral gold therapy in sun-exposed areas or secondary to QS laser treatment. A case report demonstrated effective clearance of this hyperpigmentation with normal mode ruby laser without inducing new hyperpigmentation in the surrounding area [25]. Another case report documented improvement of extensive intense chrysiasis after 595 nm pulsed dye laser treatment [46].

Paradoxical ink darkening can also occur after QS treatment [47–49]. Some colors (pink, yellow, white, peach) are more susceptible to this phenomenon due to the reduction of ferric to ferrous oxide, leading to darkening of the skin [5]. Another explanation for this phenomenon is the Tyndall effect, since the pigment is located in the dermis [47, 48]. If this occurs, additional treatments may be required, although the ink darkening may be a permanent consequence [50]. White tattoos often darken during treatment with QS lasers and will remain in this darkened state until fully removed after further treatments. This is due to Ti^{4+}, a common white pigment, changes states to Ti^{3+}, a blue-black pigment, when excited with laser energy [12, 13]. Red-brown ferric oxide pigments undergo a similar change to black ferrous oxide pigments [51]. In these circumstances, even though they pose a higher risk of scarring and generate more variable responses than the QS lasers, nonselective tissue ablation using the pulsed CO_2 (10 600 nm) or erbium-doped (Er):YAG (2940 nm) laser may be the preferred treatment option [22,31].

23.5.1 Summary

- Common complications of laser tattoo removal include textural changes in the overlying epidermis, scarring, pruritus, hyperpigmentation, hypopigmentation, among others.
- Other side effects include allergic reactions, "tattoo bleeding", and paradoxical ink darkening.

23.6 Conclusion and Future Directions

The development of picoseconds and even femtosecond lasers are being developed and tested to enable tattoo removal in fewer sessions and with fewer side effects [14, 52, 53]. Picosecond lasers emit shorter pulse durations than the QS lasers. This heats up the targeted area more quickly while using lower fluences, which results in not only less damage to surrounding tissue but also greater efficacy in targeting pigment material [21].

Beyond improving laser technology, efforts are also in place to improve the optical properties of skin, such as by using transdermal injections to avoid scattering and to increase penetration depth [42]. With more than 50 ink compounds used to create modern tattoos, common pigment colors may vary in composition and thus absorption spectra, causing variability in patient response to tattoo removal [54]. Consequently, paradoxical darkening and resistance to lightening may occur as significant side effects [5, 49, 51]. A proprietary tattoo pigment called the Freedom-2 solution has been developed based on the principle of bioresorbable pigments being encapsulated in microspheres, which completely rupture during only one laser treatment [12]. Certain creams, such as imiquimod, can enhance the results of laser tattoo removal treatments [55]. It is also hypothesized that fractional ablative resurfacing in conjunction with laser treatments may allow tattoo pigments to be removed transepidermally during treatments [18].

Research shows promise that treatments with an excimer laser may help reverse the effects of hypopigmentation after laser tattoo removal treatments [32].

If the tattoo industry were required to document injectable material, this would facilitate the efficacy of laser treatment, minimizing hazards and allowing for more predictable results [19, 54]. Infinitink tattoo ink, available in the US as of 2009, was produced for the purpose of easier removal. Thus, tattoos consisting of this pigment require fewer laser treatments than standard tattoo ink [22]. Knowledge is limited in the safety of tattoo colors and their decomposition products generated in response to laser treatment. Thus, further research in this area is warranted [19, 54].

Other studies performed in this area, intend to optimize laser treatment using current available technology. In a small prospective study, multiple passes within the first treatment session was studied with excellent results [56]. The authors compared a single-pass with four-pass treatment session separated by 20-minute intervals (R20 method) using QS Nd:YAG, during the first treatment session (Figure 23.6). Three months after treatment, results were compared and the R20 method demonstrated to be more effective than the traditional single-pass treatment session. Another study evaluated the safety and efficacy of topical perfluorodecalin (PFD) to facilitate the multi-pass treatment with QS Nd:YAG (R0 method) [57]. This randomized controlled study used PFD to clear the whitening reaction after laser treatment within a mean of 5 seconds, allowing for faster, multiple treatment passes in an average of a 5-minute session (compared to a 60-minute session with the R20 method). They demonstrated that the R0 method is equally effective than the R20 method with a significantly reduced treatment session time,

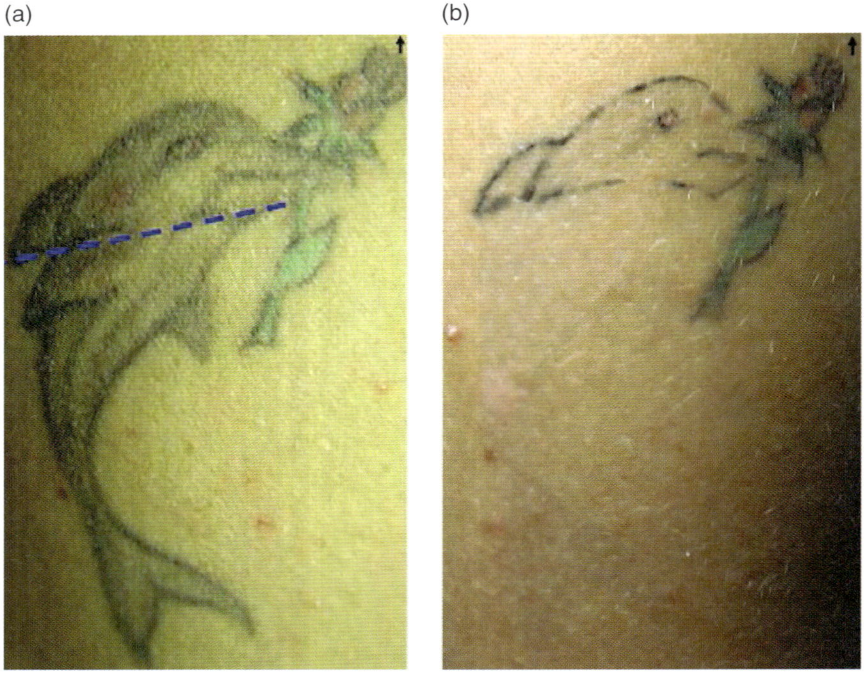

Figure 23.6 Five-year professional tattoo on deltoid of patient with skin type III. (a) Before treatment. (b) Three months after laser treatment session. *Upper part*: Conventional method. *Lower part*: R20 method, clearance. *Source:* Kossida et al. [56] Copyright 2012 American Academy of Dermatology, Inc. Reprinted with permission of Elsevier Limited.

and more effective than conventional single-pass session. This technique provides a safe, faster and effective method that should be further studied. Alternatively, a study analyzed the fragmentation response of black ink granules of a professional tattoo treated with QS Nd:YAG [20]. With this simulation they found that during initial treatment, larger granules reach higher temperatures allowing greater chance of fragmentation compared to smaller granules found in later treatments. For these smaller granules to reach an appropriate temperature for fragmentation to occur, larger spot sizes and higher fluencies are needed during following treatment sessions. The simulation predicted that these higher fluences could be used without increasing the risk of thermal damage to the neighboring tissue. Further studies are encouraged in this area.

References

1 Nicoletti, A. (2004). Perspectives on pediatric and adolescent gynecology from the allied health care professional. *J. Pediatr. Adolesc. Gynecol.* 17: 215–216.

2 Koch, J.R., Roberts, A.E., Armstrong, M.L. et al. (2010). Body art, deviance, and American college students. *Soc. Sci. J.* 47: 151–161.

3 Adatto, M.A., Halachmi, S., and Lapidoth, M. (2011). Tattoo removal. *Curr. Probl. Dermatol.* 42: 97–110.

4 Green, J.B. and Metelitsa, A.I. (2011). Optimizing outcomes of laser tattoo removal. *Skin Therapy Lett.* 16 (10): 1–3.

5 Kirby, W., Chen, C.L., Desai, A. et al. (2013). Causes and recommendations for unanticipated ink retention following tattoo removal treatment. *J. Clin. Aesthet. Dermatol.* 6 (7): 27–31.

6 Laumann, A.E. and Derick, A.J. (2006). Tattoos and body piercing in the united states: a national data set. *J. Am. Acad. Dermatol.* 55: 413–421.

7 Tiggemann, M. and Hopkins, L.A. (2011). Tattoos and piercings: bodily expressions of uniqueness? *Body Image* 8: 245–250.

8 Bernstein, E.F. (2006). Laser treatment of tattoos. *Clin. Dermatol.* 24: 43–55.

9 Mataix, J. and Silvestre, J.F. (2009). Cutaneous adverse reactions to tattoos and piercings. *Actas Dermosifiliogr.* 100: 643–656.

10 Kuperman-Beade, M., Levine, V.J., Ashinoff, R. et al. (2001). Laser removal of tattoos. *Am. J. Clin. Dermatol.* 2 (1): 21–25.

11 Sweeney, S.M. (2006). Tattoos: a review of tattoo practices and potential treatment options for removal. *Curr. Opin. Pediatr.* 18: 391–395.

12 Choudhary, S., Elsaie M.L., Leiva, A. et al. (2010). Lasers for tattoo removal: a review. *Lasers Med. Sci.* 25: 619–627.

13 Timko, A.L., Miller, C.H., Johnson, F.B. et al. (2001). In vitro quantitative chemical analysis of tattoo pigments. *Arch. Dermatol.* 137: 143–147.

14 Mariwalla, K. and Dover, J.S. (2006). The use of lasers for decorative tattoo removal. *Skin Therapy Lett.* 11 (5): 8–11.

15 Armstrong, M.L., Roberts, A.E., Owen, D.C. et al. (2004). Contemporary college students and body piercing. *J. Adolesc. Health* 35: 58–61.

16 Varma, S. and Lanigan, S.W. (1999). Reasons for requesting laser removal of unwanted tattoos. *Br. J. Dermatol.* 140: 483–485.

17 Cegolon, L., Baldo, V., Xodo, C. et al. (2011). VAHP Working Group. Tattoo removal in the typical adolescent. *BMC Res. Notes* 4: 209.

18 Ortiz, A.E. and Avram, M.M. (2012). Redistribution of ink after laser tattoo removal. *Dermatol. Surg.* 38: 1730–1731.

19 Vasold, R., Naarmann, N., Ulrich, H. et al. (2004). Tattoo pigments are cleaved by laser light – the chemical analysis in vitro provide evidence for hazardous

compounds. *Photochem. Photobiol.* 80: 185–190.
20 Humphries, A., Lister, T.S., Wright, P.A. et al. (2013). Finite element analysis of thermal and acoustic processes during laser tattoo removal. *Lasers Surg. Med.* 45: 108–115.
21 Saedi, N., Metelitsa, A., Petrell, K. et al. (2012). Treatment of tattoos with a picosecond alexandrite laser. *Arch. Dermatol.* 148 (12): 1360–1363.
22 Kent, K.M. and Graber, E.M. (2012). Laser tattoo removal: a review. *Dermatol. Surg.* 38: 1–13.
23 Kirby, W., Chen, C., Desai, A. et al. (2011). Successful treatment of cosmetic mucosal tattoos via Q-switched laser. *Dermatol. Surg.* 37: 1767–1769.
24 Trotter, M.J., Tron, V.A., Hollingdale, J. et al. (1995). Localized chrysiasis induced by laser therapy. *Arch. Dermatol.* 131 (12): 1411–1414.
25 Yun, P.L., Arndt, K.A., and Anderson, R.R. (2002). Q-switched laser-induced chrysiasis treated with long-pulsed laser. *Arch. Dermatol.* 138 (8): 1012–1014.
26 Almoallim, H., Klinkhoff, A.V., Arthur, A.B. et al. (2006). Laser induced chrysiasis: disfiguring hyperpigmentation following Q-switched laser therapy in a woman previously treated with gold. *J. Rheumatol.* 33 (3): 620–621.
27 Geist, D.E. and Phillips, T.J. (2006). Development of chrysiasis after Q-switched ruby laser treatment of solar lentigines. *J. Am. Acad. Dermatol.* 55 (2 Suppl): S59–S60.
28 Pohl, L., Kaiser, K., and Raulin, C. (2013). Pitfalls and recommendations in cases of laser removal of decorative tattoos with pigmented lesions: case report and review of the literature. *JAMA Dermatol.* https://doi.org/10.1001/jamadermatol.2013.4901. [Epub ahead of print].
29 Zipser, M.C., Mangana, J., Oberholzer, P.A. et al. (2010). Melanoma after laser therapy of pigmented lesions – circumstances and outcome. *Eur. J. Dermatol.* 20 (3): 334–338. https://doi.org/10.1684/ejd.2010.0933. Epub 2010 Apr 27.
30 Anderson, R.R. (2003). Dermatologic history of the ruby laser: the long story of short pulses. *Arch. Dermatol.* 139 (1): 70–74.
31 Walgrave, S.E., Kist, D.A., Noyaner-Turley, A. et al. (2012). Minimally ablative resurfacing with the confluent 2,790 erbium: YSGG laser: a pilot study on safety and efficacy. *Lasers Surg. Med.* 44: 103–111.
32 Pfirrmann, G., Karsai, S., Roos, S. et al. (2007). Tattoo removal – state of the art. *JDDG* 5: 889–898.
33 Ross, V., Naseef, G., Lin, C. et al. (1998). Comparison of responses of tattoos to picosecond and nanosecond Q-switched neodymium: YAG lasers. *Arch. Dermatol.* 134: 167–171.
34 Zelickson, B.D., Mehregan, D.A., Zarrin, A.A. et al. (1994). Clinical, histologic, and ultrastructural evaluation of tattoos treated with three laser systems. *Lasers Surg. Med.* 15 (4): 364–372.
35 Leuenberger, M.L., Mulas, M.W., Hata, T.R. et al. (1999). Comparison of the Q-switched alexandrite, ND:YAG, and ruby lasers in treating blue-black tattoos. *Dermatol. Surg.* 25: 10–14.
36 Wenzel, S.M. (2010). Current concepts in laser tattoo removal. *Skin Therapy Lett.* 15 (3): 3–5.
37 Naversen, D.N. and Igelman, J.D. (2004). Q-switched laser management of an explosion tattoo. *J. Am. Acad. Dermatol.* 50 (3): 479–480.
38 Spicer, M.S., Goldberg, D.J., and Janniger, C.K. (1995). Lasers in pediatric dermatology. *Cutis* 55: 270–272, 278–80.
39 Riml, S., Larcher, L., Grohmann, M. et al. (2013). Second-degree burn within a tattoo after intense-pulsed-light epilation. *Photodermatol. Photoimmunol. Photomed.* 29 (4): 218–220. https://doi.org/10.1111/phpp.12039.
40 Kirby, W., Kartono, F., and Small, R. (2011). Tattoo removal with lasers. In: *Dermatologic and Cosmetic Procedures in Office Practice*, 1e (ed. R.P. Usatine, J.L.

Pfenninger, D.L. Stulberg, et al.), 267–376. Philadelphia, PA: Elsevier Saunders.

41 Tope, W.D. (1995). State and territorial regulation of tattooing in the United States. *J. Am. Acad. Dermatol.* 32 (5 Pt 1): 791–799.

42 McNichols, R.J., Fox, M.A., Gowda, A. et al. (2005). Temporary dermal scatter reduction: quantitative assessment and implications for improved laser tattoo removal. *Lasers Surg. Med.* 36: 289–296.

43 Graeme, L.M. and Anderson, R.R. (2003). Lasers in dermatology. In: *Fitzpatrick's Dermatology and General Medicine*, 6e (ed. E.N. Freedberg, A.Z. Eisen, K. Wolff, et al.), 2493–2509. New York: McGraw-Hill Professional.

44 Alster, T.S. and Lupton, J.R. (2001). Lasers in dermatology: an overview of types and indications. *Am. J. Clin. Dermatol.* 2: 291–303.

45 Kirby, W., Koriakos, A., Desai, A. et al. (2010). Undesired pigmentary alterations associated with quality-switched laser tattoo removal treatment: a retrospective study and review of the literature. *Skin Aging* 18 (8): 38–40.

46 Wu, J.J., Papajohn, N.G., Murase, J.E. et al. (2009). Generalized chrysiasis improved with pulsed dye laser. *Dermatol. Surg.* 35 (3): 538–542. https://doi.org/10.1111/j.1524-4725.2009.01092.x.

47 Anderson, R.R., Geronemus, R., Kilmer, S.L. et al. (1993). Cosmetic tattoo ink darkening. A complication of Q-switched and pulsed-laser treatment. *Arch. Dermatol.* 129: 1010–1014.

48 Swanson, V.S. (2002). Tattoo ink darkening of a yellow tattoo after Qswitched laser treatment. *Clin. Exp. Dermatol.* 27 (6): 461–463.

49 Chung, W.K., Yang, J.H., Lee, D.W. et al. (2009). Paradoxical darkening of unperceived tattoo ink after relatively low fluence from a Q-switched Nd:YAG (1064-nm) laser in the course of treatment for melisma. *Clin. Exp. Dermatol.* 34: 555–557.

50 Ross, E., Yashar, S., Michaud, N. et al. (2001). Tattoo darkening and nonresponse after laser treatment: a possible role for titanium dioxide. *Arch. Dermatol.* 137: 33–37.

51 Jimenez, G., Weiss, E., and Spencer, J.M. (2002). Multiple color changes following laser therapy of cosmetic tattoos. *Dermatol. Surg.* 28: 177–179.

52 Brauer, J.A., Reddy, K.K., Anolik, R. et al. (2012). Successful and rapid treatment of blue and green tattoo pigment with a novel picosecond laser. *Arch. Dermatol.* 148 (7): 820–823.

53 Izikson, L., Farinelli, W., Sakamoto, F. et al. (2010). Safety and effectiveness of black tattoo clearance in a pig model after a single treatment with a novel 758 nm 500 picosecond laser: a pilot study. *Lasers Surg. Med.* 42 (7): 640–646. https://doi.org/10.1002/lsm.20942.

54 Durkin, S.E. (2012). Tattoos, body piercing, and healthcare concerns. *J. Radiol. Nurs.* 31: 20–25.

55 Elsaie, M.L., Nouri, K., Vejjabhinanta, V. et al. (2009). Topical imiquimod in conjuction with Nd:YAG laser for tattoo removal. *Lasers Med. Sci.* 24: 871–875.

56 Kossida, T., Rigopoulos, D., Katsambas, A. et al. (2012). Optimal tattoo removal in a single laser session based on the method of repeated exposures. *J. Am. Acad. Dermatol.* 66 (2): 271–277. https://doi.org/10.1016/j.jaad.2011.07.024. Epub 2011 Oct 27.

57 Reddy, K.K., Brauer, J.A., Anolik, R. et al. (2013). Topical perfluorodecalin resolves immediate whitening reactions and allows rapid effective multiple pass treatment of tattoos. *Lasers Surg. Med.* 45 (2): 76–80. https://doi.org/10.1002/lsm.22106. Epub 2012 Dec 19.

24

Lasers for Hair Removal

Fleta Netter Bray[1], Leyre Falto-Aizpurua[1], Robert D. Griffith[1], Brian Simmons[1]
Ali Rajabi-Estarabadi[1], and Keyvan Nouri[2]

[1]Department of Dermatology & Cutaneous Surgery, University of Miami Miller School of Medicine, Miami, FL, USA
[2]Department of Dermatology, Ophthalmology, Otolaryngology & Surgery, University of Miami Leonard M. Miller School of Medicine, Miami, FL, USA

24.1 Introduction

- Laser hair removal (LHR) is the most commonly requested cosmetic procedure in the world, and there is increasing interest in application of LHR to adolescent populations.
- Few studies have been performed among pediatric populations, however current literature suggests LHR may be safe and well-tolerated.
- Selective photothermolysis is the means by which lasers target and destroy hair follicles. Lasers with wavelengths between 600 and 1064 nm have been successfully used to treat excessive hair.
- The ideal candidate for LHR is fair-skinned with dark hair; however, LHR can be successfully performed in all skin types.

Removal of unwanted body hair is an increasingly prevalent trend in our society, and interest in the application of LHR to the adolescent population has similarly amplified [1–4]. While LHR in adults is known to be well tolerated, there are fewer studies to date that have been performed within pediatric populations. However, excessive hair growth can have deep psychological consequences for children and adolescents, and treatment is warranted to improve quality of life [5, 6]. Currently available studies indicate that use of LHR in pediatric populations can be safe, effective, and promising.

With puberty, all individuals will experience increased hair growth, as follicles alter production from fine vellus hair, which is nonpigmented and has a diameter of roughly 30 μm, to thicker terminal hair, which is pigmented and ranges from 150 to 300 μm in diameter [7]. For some children and adolescents, however, hair growth may be excessive or occur outside of normal pubertal changes and can result in emotional discomfort and self-consciousness. This excessive hair growth has two broad classifications: hirsutism, which occurs in females and is defined as excessive growth of terminal hair in a male distribution, and hypertrichosis, which affects either gender and is defined as androgen-independent increased growth of hair anywhere on the body [8]. In either condition, excessive hair growth may be isolated in nature or related to underlying medical abnormalities [9]. Regardless of type or source of excessive hair growth, adolescent patients' perceptions of unwanted hair and its impact on quality of life is individual in nature and highly influenced by cultural preferences.

Pediatric Dermatologic Surgery, First Edition. Edited by Keyvan Nouri, Latanya Benjamin, Jasem Alshaiji, and Jan Izakovic.

It is important for medical practitioners to take concerns of excessive hair growth seriously and to provide these patients with emotional and therapeutic support [10].

Light Amplification by Stimulated Emission of Radiation (LASER) is one treatment modality that may be utilized to treat patients with excessive hair growth. Laser systems emit light of a single wavelength that is subsequently absorbed by a specific recipient color or chromophore. The laser medium determines the emitted wavelength and can be a solid (e.g. ruby, Nd:YAG and alexandrite), a liquid (e.g. dye), or a gas (e.g. argon, krypton and carbon dioxide). The skin contains several chromophores that selectively absorb light at certain wavelengths. These chromophores are water, melanin, and hemoglobin. Melanin has a broad range of peaks absorbing both infrared and visible wavelengths [5]. Once the light is absorbed, heat is generated and the tissue is selectively destroyed. This process is referred to as selective photothermolysis and is the means by which lasers are able to target and destroy hair follicles [5, 11]. Lasers with wavelengths between 600 and 1064 nm have been successfully utilized to treat excessive hair. These include ruby (694 nm), long-pulsed alexandrite (755 nm), diode (800–810 nm), and long-pulsed Nd-YAG (1064 nm) as well as intense pulse light (IPL) with output in 500–1000 nm range [1]. For hair removal to be permanent, the bulge and bulb regions of the hair must be destroyed (Figure 24.1) [12]. These cells are susceptible to damage during anogen phase, while the hair is growing. However, these cells are not destroyed by laser treatments during telogen phase, when the cells are resting [1]. Roughly 15–30% long-term hair loss may be seen with each treatment when optimal parameters are utilized [7].

LHR is best suited for darkly pigmented hair in light-skinned individuals. Importantly, darker skin may absorb emitted light along with the hair follicles and incur skin damage [13]. It is important to screen patients carefully. However, with careful choice of laser parameters including wavelength, pulse duration, energy fluence, spot size, and repetition rate, LHR may be safely and effectively utilized in darker skin types [1, 3].

24.2 Indications

- The indication for hair removal is subjective.
- Excessive hair may cause significant psychological distress for children and their parents, which may be alleviated by hair removal.
- LHR among pediatric populations is limited in the literature, though physicians may consider laser treatment on a per patient basis.

Children may experience substantial psychosocial distress due to excessive hair. In one retrospective study, enrolled children reported teasing at school, embarrassment during physical education, and embarrassment in public [6]. Patients who suffer with excessive hair may benefit from removal [14, 15]. A variety of nonpermanent solutions to treat excessive hair exist. These include shaving, waxing, plucking, and threading, among others. However, many of these hair removal solutions are inconvenient or undesirable for patients and are ultimately temporary. LHR has the potential to offer long-term reductions in unwanted hair [3]. The indications for LHR are subjective, and decision to pursue should be based on a thorough understanding of the benefits and risks of LHR.

24.3 Approach to the Patient and Patient Education

- Hirsutism may occur idiopathically or in association with underlying medical conditions; work-up for underlying disorders associated with hyperandrogenemia may be appropriate.
- Physical exam with classification of Fitzpatrick type should guide choice of laser and light source.

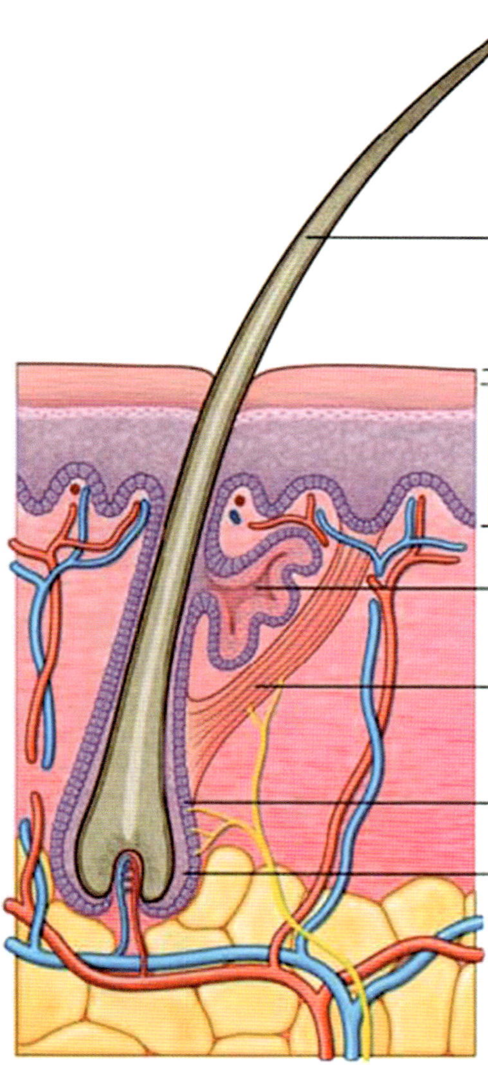

Figure 24.1 Each hair follicle consists of a permanent (upper) and nonpermanent (lower) portion. The follicular bulge forms the lowermost aspect of the permanent part. In periods of active growth (anagen phase), the bulbar matrix cells differentiate into the hair shaft and the hair lengths. The duration of each growth phase is dependent on body site. *Source:* Ibrahimi et al. 2011 [6]. Reprinted with permission of John Wiley & Sons.

- Benefits and risks of LHR should be reviewed with patients and their parents, and informed consent obtained.
- Patients should be educated that permanent and complete hair removal is not likely to be achieved, and hair regrowth does not constitute treatment failure.
- Instruct patients on pre- and post-LHR care. Redness and swelling in the treatment site may be expected for up to one week after treatment.

24.3.1 Approach to the Patient

Hirsutism and hypertrichosis may occur in isolation or in association with other underlying medical conditions. Because of this, a complete medical history and physical

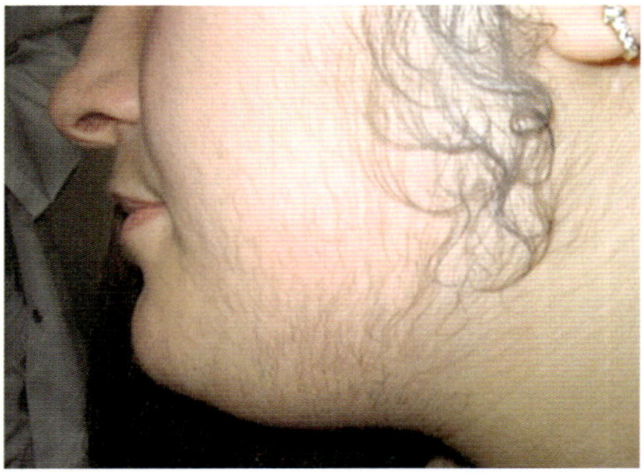

Figure 24.2 Hirsutism. *Source:* Gacaferri Lumezi et al. [16]. Reprinted with permission of Kowsar Corporation.

examination should be performed in these patients [7]. Approximately 5% of women of childbearing age currently suffer with hirsutism [10] (Figure 24.2). For those women with mild or moderate hirsutism and regular menstrual cycles, hirsutism is likely to be idiopathic in nature and hormonal testing is not necessary. However, all women with moderate to severe hirsutism, hirsutism in association with irregular menstrual cycles, or signs of virilization must undergo hormone testing to rule out androgen excess [10]. Conditions associated with hirsutism are listed in Table 24.1. The high frequency of polycystic ovarian syndrome

Table 24.1 Causes of hirsutism [17].

	Medication/Drug Use
• Idiopathic hirsutism	• Aripiprazole (Abilify)
• Androgen-secreting tumors	• Bimatoprost (Lumigan)*
• Adrenal	• Bupropion (Wellbutrin)
• Adenoma	• Carbamazepine (Tegretol)
• Adenocarcinoma (rare)	• Clonazepam (Klonopin)
• Ectopic adrenocorticotropic hormone-secreting tumor (rare)	• Corticosteroids (systemic)
• Gonadal stromal tumor	• Cyclosporine (Sandimmune)
• Thecoma	• Dantrolene (Dantrium)
• Lipoid tumor	• Diazoxide (Proglycem)
• Functional androgen excess	• Donepezil (Aricept)
• Adrenal enzyme deficiencies (congenital adrenal hyperplasia)	• Estrogens
• Early-onset 21 hydroxylase deficiency	• Eszopiclone (Lunesta)
• Late-onset 21 hydroxylase deficiency	• Fluoxetine (Prozac)
• 11β-hydroxylase deficiency	• Interferon alfa*
• 3β-ol dehydrogenase deficiency	• Isotretinoin
• Cushing syndrome	• Lamotrigine (Lamictal)
• Polycystic ovarian disease with or without adrenal contribution	• Leuprolide (Lupron)
	• Mycophenolate (Cellcept)*
	• Olanzapine (Zyprexa)
	• Paroxetine (Paxil)
	• Pregabalin (Lyrica)
	• Progestins
	• Selegiline (Eldepryl)
	• Tacrolimus (Prograf)*
	• Testosterones
	• Tiagabine (Gabitril)
	• Trazodone
	• Venlafaxine (Effexor)
	• Zonisamide (Zonegran)

* Cause of hirsutism.
Source: Hughes [18], Table 14.2.

Table 24.2 Work up for confirmed androgen excess [10].

- Pregnancy test
- Pelvic ultrasound (for suspected PCOS or ovarian neoplasm)
- Dehydroepiandrosterone sulfate and early morning 17-hydroxyprogesterone levels (for suspected congenital adrenal hyperplasia or adrenal neoplasm)
- Prolactin level
- Thyroid function testing, adrenocortical function testing, IGF-1 testing
- Dexamethasone suppression testing
  - If androgen excess not suppressible, consider Cushing's syndrome, neoplasm, PCOS
  - If androgen excess is suppressible, ACTH testing for CAH is indicated
- Further imaging studies if suspected undetected neoplasm
- Oxadiazolopyrimidine
- Fenoterol
- Porphyria
- Porphyria cutanea tarda
- Hepatoerythropoietic porphyria
- Variegate porphyria
- Erythropoietic porphyria
- POEMS (*p*olyneuropathy, *o*rganomegaly, *e*ndocrinopathy, *M* protein, and skin changes) syndrome
- Juvenile dermatomyositis
- Hypothyroidism
- Acrodynia
- Malabsorption syndromes
- Central nervous system-related problems or trauma
- After encephalitis
- Multiple sclerosis
- Schizophrenia
- Head injury
- Hyperostosis interna
- Anorexia nervosa

(PCOS) as a cause of hirsutism warrants special attention to signs of anovulation, obesity, metabolic syndrome, or insulin resistance [10]. Further workup for confirmed androgen excess is listed in Table 24.2. Of note, most androgenic drugs are not detectable by testosterone assays, so careful attention must be given to collecting the medication history [10].

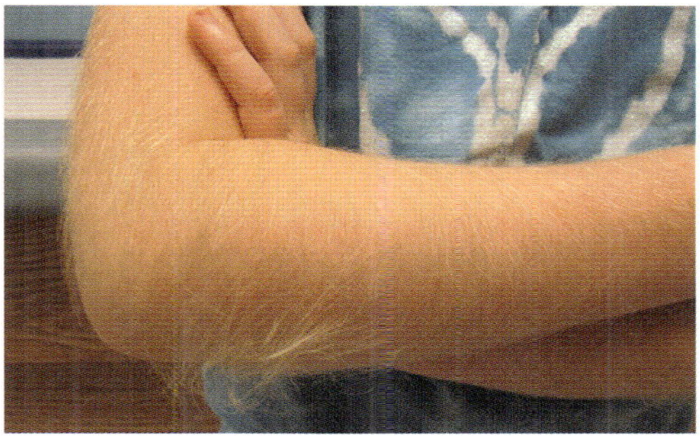

Figure 24.3 Hypertrichosis of the forearms in a female 8-year-old child. *Source:* CasteloSoccio [19]. Copyright 2012. Reprinted with permission of Elsevier.

Hypertrichosis is androgen-independent and causes generalized increased growth of hair on the body, which can be terminal or lanugo [10] (Figures 24.3 and 24.4). Hypertrichosis may be hereditary or acquired. Causes of hypertrichosis are listed in Table 24.3.

Other key elements of the history include: history of photosensitizing conditions, history of recurrent infections at or near the treatment site, and history of keloid or hypertrophic scar formation [7]. It is important to review past hair removal methods. Waxing and tweezing remove the target chromophore, and LHR will not be effective for at least two weeks, though some authors advocate waiting a minimum of six weeks [7]. Methods that do not remove the hair shaft, such as shaving, do not interfere with the efficacy of LHR.

On physical exam, the medical practitioners should note the severity and pattern of excess hair growth, Fitzpatrick skin type, presence of a tan, and hair color. Because patients may engage in various hair removal techniques, it may be prudent to also administer the Ferriman–Gallwey scale, which scores the degree of hirsutism based on patient responses (Figure 24.5) [20]. Fitzpatrick skin type determines which lasers and light sources are safe for use. Presence of a tan may warrant delay of LHR or careful adjustment of laser parameters for use on tanned skin. Finally, hair color should be noted. Dark hair contains melanin, which

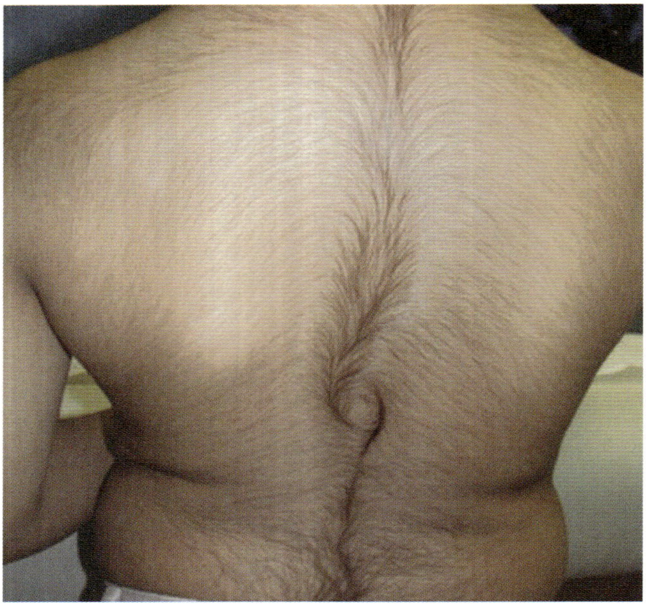

Figure 24.4 Hypertrichosis of the back in a 12-year-old male child. *Source:* CasteloSoccio [19]. Copyright 2012. Reprinted with permission of Elsevier.

Table 24.3 Causes of hypertrichosis [17].

Congenital/hereditary	Medication that causes hypertrichosis
• Congenital hypertrichosis lanuginose	• Acitretin (Soriatane)
• Ambras syndrome	• Azelaic acid (Finacea)
• Congenital generalized hypertrichosis	• Acetazolamide
• Congenital hypertrichosis with gingival fibromatosis	• Cetirizine (Zyrtec)
• Zimmermann-Laband syndrome	• Citalopram (Celexa)
• Ramon syndrome	• Corticosteroids (topical)
• Brachmann–de Lange syndrome	• Cyclosporine
• Wiedermann syndrome	• Diazoxide
• Cantu generalized hypertrichosis with osteochondrodysplasia	• Etonogestrel implant (Implanon)
• Hurler syndrome	• Phenytoin sodium (Dilantin)
• Reticular ichthyosiform erythroderma	• Psoralen and ultraviolet A light
• Donahue syndrome (leprechaunism)	• Minoxidil
• Buntinex syndrome	• Topical steroids
• Barbar–Say syndrome	• Streptomycin
• Pivnick syndrome	
• Jalili syndrome	
• Coffin–Siris syndrome	
• Gorlin syndrome	
• Hyperkinetic circulatory disorder	
• Schinzel–Giedion syndrome	
• Lawrence–Seip syndrome	
• Generalized smooth muscle hamartoma	
• Michelin tire syndrome	
• Schaap syndrome	
• Parme syndrome	
• Hemihypertrophy	
• Acquired	
• Acquired hypertrichosis lanuginosa (malignancy)	

Source: Otberg and Shapiro [10].

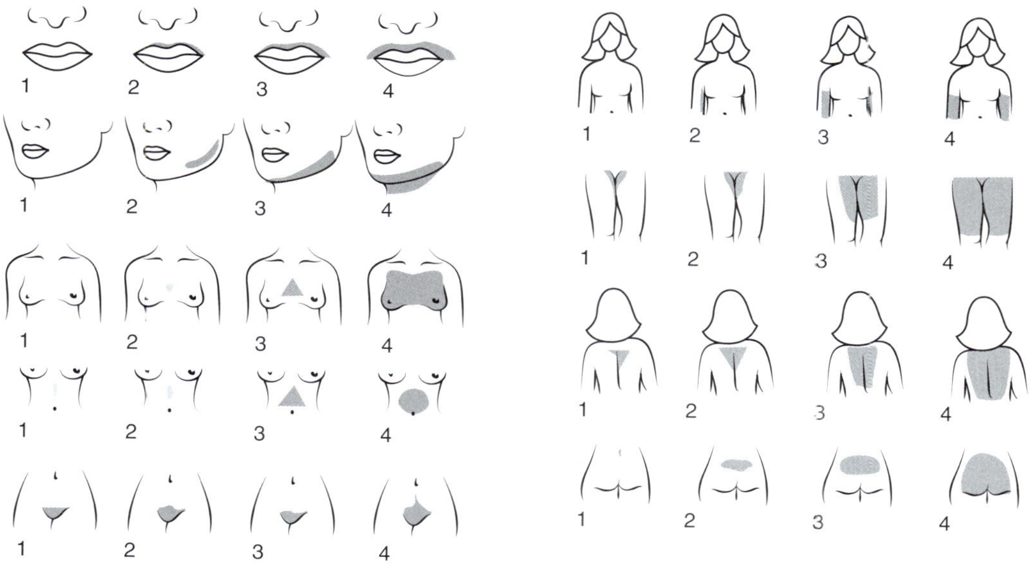

Figure 24.5 Ferriman–Gallwey hirsutism scoring system. Nine body areas sensitive to androgen are scored from 1 (no hair) to 4 (virilization). The sum indicates the degree of hirsutism. A score ≤ 7 is considered normal, a score of 8–15 indicates mild hirsutism, and a score > 15 indicates moderate or severe hirsutism [20, 21]. Copyright 2004. Reprinted with permission of Elsevier Limited. Adapted from [22].

serves as the chromophore for LHR. Blonde, red, white, and gray hair has less melanin and responds less favorably to LHR [7].

Finally, obtaining informed consent, including setting realistic expectations for treatment outcomes and potential risks, should be performed prior to instituting laser therapy [7]. Risks include hyperpigmentation that may be permanent, blistering, scarring, ulceration, hive-like response, bruising, infection, acne flare, and folliculitis. Patients of Fitzpatrick skin types IV–VI or those of Mediterranean, Middle Eastern, or Asian descent have a low, paradoxical risk of induced hypertrichosis [7]. The benefits and risks of treatment should be understood by the minor and the parents alike, and consent must be obtained from the parent.

We recommend patch testing prior to treatment of the entire affected area to assess tolerability of the procedure and need for anesthetic. When necessary, lidocaine, lidocaine/prilocaine, and other amide/ester anesthetic combinations should be applied 30 minutes to 1 hour prior to LHR under occlusion, with care taken to utilize non-toxic levels [7]. Some studies report need for general anesthesia in children, and this need should be assessed on a per patient basis [6]. Because the retina contains melanin and may be damaged by laser devices, protective eyewear is required for both patient and provider in all circumstances [7].

24.3.2 Patient Education

First and foremost, patients should be counseled on realistic expectations for LHR. Permanent and complete hair removal is not likely to be achieved. Generally, only about 15% of hairs are permanently removed with each laser treatment [7]. However, with multiple treatments patients may achieve significant reductions in unwanted hair. For some patients, maintenance treatments may be necessary [7]. Further, for women with moderate to severe hirsutism or androgen excess, counseling about the need for medical therapy in addition to hair removal is necessary

[10]. Comprehension of the risks and benefits of LHR should be ascertained for both the minor patient and their parent.

Prior to instituting LHR, patients and their parents should receive pre-treatment instructions. Patients should avoid the sun for six weeks prior to and after treatments. Ideally, waxing and plucking should also be avoided for the six weeks prior to treatment, though shaving is not contraindicated [7]. Instruct patients to discontinue photosensitizing medications prior to treatment and to discontinue topical retinoids used in the treatment area one to two days beforehand. Patients should also be instructed as to what to expect during LHR. Pain is expected with LHR, but may be minimized with topical anesthetics [7]. For post-treatment care, patients should again be instructed to avoid the sun for six weeks. The patient may expect redness and swelling in the area for up to one week after treatment. Ice and application of a topical corticosteroid may shorten the duration of these symptoms [7].

24.4 Laser Hair Technology

- Ruby (694 nm), long-pulsed alexandrite (755 nm), diode (800–810 nm), and long-pulsed Nd:YAG lasers and IPL in the 500–1000 nm range are capable of targeting hair follicles.
- Additional laser parameters include fluence, pulse duration, spot size, and skin cooling method.

Ruby, alexandrite, diode, and Nd:YAG lasers, as well as IPL devices, may successfully be utilized for LHR with careful attention to laser parameters. These device variables include wavelength, fluence, pulse duration, spot size, and skin cooling [7].

Wavelengths between 600 and 1064 nm are capable of successfully targeting the melanin chromophore of hair. These include ruby (694 nm), long-pulsed alexandrite (755 nm), diode (800–810 nm), and long-pulsed Nd:YAG (1064 nm) as well as IPL with output in 500–1000 nm range [1].

Fluence refers to the amount of energy delivered per unit area and is expressed in J/cm^2. While higher fluences may result in greater permanent hair removal, they are also more likely to result in treatment complications. Laser devices are often provided with recommendations for treatment parameters. However, Ibrahami et al. recommend finding the optimal treatment fluence for a given patient by evaluating for the appropriate clinical endpoint of erythema and edema [7, 13] (Figure 24.6).

Pulse duration is defined as the duration in seconds of laser exposure. By the theory of selective photothermolysis, the optimal pulse duration may be selected based on the thermal relaxation time (TRT) [7]. The calculated TRT of a terminal hair is roughly 100 ms. However, because there is spatial separation between the melanin chromophore and the stem cells which are the true target, the true optimal pulse duration is longer than the TRT [7].

The spot size is the diameter of the laser beam. Larger spot sizes are preferable, as photons are less likely to be scattered outside of the beam area. In a double-blind, randomized control trial of 17 women undergoing LHR with Alexandrite laser with either 18-mm

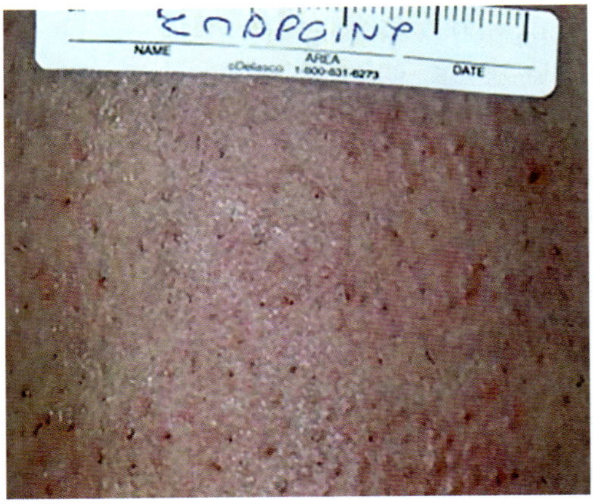

Figure 24.6 The optimal treatment fluence for a given patient may be found by evaluating for the appropriate clinical endpoint of erythema and edema. *Source:* Ibrahimi et al. [6]. Reprinted with permission of John Wiley & Sons.

versus 12-mm spot size, there was on average a 10.3% greater reduction in hair among those treated with 18-mm spot size at six-month follow-up [23]. Of further benefit, large spot sizes allow for faster treatment times [7].

Epidermal melanin, particularly in darker skin types, acts as a competing chromophore and creates risk of skin damage during LHR. Skin cooling is an important element of LHR that minimizes epidermal damage while allowing higher fluences to be used [24]. Most commercially available LHR systems have an included cooling device. These may consist of either contact cooling, usually with a sapphire tip, or cooling with a cryogen spray. Cooling creates a heat sink that draws heat from the skin surface, decreasing the risk of epidermal damage. Contact cooling is most useful for treatments with longer pulse duration (>10 ms), while cryogen spray cooling may be utilized for shorter pulse durations (<5 ms) [7].

24.5 Techniques

- Long-pulsed ruby, long-pulsed alexandrite, and diode lasers as well as IPL may be used for LHR among skin phototypes I–III.
- Long-pulsed Nd:YAG is generally considered safest for darker skin types, though efficacy may not be optimal. Long-pulsed alexandrite and diode lasers have also been used in patients with darker complexions.
- While long-pulsed ruby, long-pulsed alexandrite, and long-pulsed Nd:YAG laser use among pediatric populations has been reported upon in the literature, limited information exists for use of diode laser or IPL among children and adolescents.

24.6 Treatment of Skin Phototypes I–III

24.6.1 Long-Pulsed Ruby Laser

The long-pulsed ruby laser (694 nm) was the first device used for LHR with successful long-term hair loss (two-year follow-up) [25]. The long-pulsed ruby laser may be safely used in Fitzpatrick types I–III. In a multicenter trial enrolling 200 adult patients, most had over 75% hair loss on six-month follow-up after an average of four treatments [26]. In a later study assessing the efficacy of long-pulsed ruby laser in children under 16, 25 out of 28 children (mean age 9.2 years) experienced an average reduction in hair count of 63% at six-month follow-up [27]. No serious complications were noted. However, a substantial number of these children [15] required general anesthesia. In a small study of seven female patients (mean age 13 years) with lumbosacral hypertrichosis, patients were treated with long-pulsed ruby laser at three full treatments at two-month intervals [28]. Only two of the seven patients had notable change to hair density at six-month follow-up. However, though the efficacy in this patient population was low, no treatment complications were noted.

A limitation of these studies is that skin type of these children was not mentioned.

24.6.2 Long-Pulsed Alexandrite Laser

The long-pulsed alexandrite laser (755 nm) has been shown to be effective for hair removal in multiple studies and may be used in Fitzpatrick skin types I–III [29]. However, there are a few studies that demonstrate safety in darker skin types [30–32]. In a single-center randomized trial assessing efficacy and safety of long-pulsed alexandrite and Nd:YAG lasers, patients (aged 16–50 years with skin phototypes III–IV) were found to have 76–84% hair reduction at 18-month follow-up after four sessions at two-month intervals (12 and 18 mm spot size, 1.5 ms pulse duration and fluences of 20 or 40 J/cm^2) [33]. In a study of 24 children (mean age 12.3 years), patients with patients with Fitzpatrick types II–IV were treated with long-pulsed alexandrite with either continuous chilled-air cooling at fluences of 16–27 J/cm^2 or with cryogen cooling at fluences of 16–32 J/cm^2, while children with Fitzpatrick types IV–VI were treated with long-pulsed

Nd:YAG with a chilled contact sapphire tip [6]. These children had diagnoses ranging from idiopathic hirsutism, PCOS, congenital melanocytic nevus, and one with nevoid hypertrichosis. The authors found that when administered appropriately, LHR is safe and well-tolerated in children aged under 16 years [6]. The only recorded side effect in this study was intolerable discomfort reported by two children receiving treatment to the trunk and limbs that was managed with topical anesthesia. Only one child was reported to require general anesthesia, and this child was noted to have a learning disability and agitation. Of note, the youngest children in the study, ages five and six, tolerated the LHR treatments well [6].

24.6.3 Long-Pulsed Diode Laser

The long-pulsed diode laser (800–810 nm) has been extensively used for LHR and has demonstrated safety in Fitzpatrick types I–V [29, 34]. In a study of 50 adult volunteers with primarily skin types II–III treated with diode laser (800 nm, 10–40 J/cm^2, 5–30 ms, 9 mm spot size, and 5 °C chilled hand piece), hair reduction stabilized between 25 and 35% on follow-up an average of 20 months later [35]. A comparative study assessing efficacy of alexandrite laser (3 ms pulse width, cryogen spray-equipped) versus diode laser (variable pulse width, cooled sapphire window-equipped) in the axillae of 15 Fitzpatrick type I–V patients noted even greater results, with 85 and 84% hair reduction at one-year follow-up after four treatments [36]. In a study of 15 patients with hypertrichosis in Becker's nevus undergoing eight sessions of low-fluence, high- repetition-rate diode laser treatment, all patients experienced significant hair reduction at one-year follow-up without adverse events [37].

24.6.4 Intense Pulse Light (IPL)

IPL is composed of polychromatic light that ranges in wavelength. Various filters may be utilized to target specific chromophores, including melanin [7]. Wavelengths in the range of 500–1000 nm may be utilized in hair removal [1]. In a comparison study of diode lasers and IPL for axillary hair removal conducted in 30 patients with Fitzpatrick type II–III, both diode and IPL were found to result in effective reductions at one-year follow-up (69.2 and 52.7% respectively) [38]. However, two studies comparing IPL to long-pulsed alexandrite and Nd:YAG noted inferiority of IPL [39, 40]. IPL devices are also marketed for home use. In a multicenter study of 34 individuals tested with the Silk'n™ home IPL device, average hair clearance of 64% was reported after three treatments in a variety of anatomic locations. No long-term complications were reported [41]. Other studies demonstrate wide ranges of efficacy of home IPL devices, with reductions ranging from only 6 to 72% with repetitive treatments [42]. None of these studies have been performed among pediatric populations. Two children with faun-tail nevus treated with IPL (8–26 J/cm^2, pulse sequencing of 3–4, delay time of 20–35 ms) achieved 85% hair reduction with use of local anesthesia for one patient [43]. In general, there is a dearth of information relating to the safety, tolerability, and efficacy of IPL in pediatric populations.

24.7 Treatment of Skin Phototypes IV–VI

Patients with darker skin experience the highest rate of side effects with LHR [44]. Long-pulsed Nd:YAG is often considered safest for use in darker skin types. Depending on the source consulted, long-pulsed diode or long-pulsed alexandrite laser may also be suggested for use in darker skin types [32, 33].

24.7.1 Long-Pulsed Nd:YAG Laser

The long-pulsed Nd:YAG (1064 nm) is believed to offer the best combination of safety and efficacy for patients of darker skin types, however, there is variable evidence for efficacy [7]. In a trial of 20 women with Fitzpatrick types IV–VI and dark hair on the face, axillae, or legs, hair reduction of 70–90% was noted on 12-month follow-up [45]. However, later studies have not consistently shown the same degree of efficacy. In a comparison study of three treatments each of long-pulsed alexandrite laser, long-pulsed diode laser, and Nd:YAG laser in the axillae of 20 women, there was no difference in efficacy between alexandrite and diode lasers. However, both were more efficacious than Nd:YAG [46]. None of these studies, however, looked at pediatric populations. However, Rajpar et al. assessed long-pulsed Nd:YAG (chilled contact sapphire tip at fluences of 20–35 J/cm^2 versus cryogen cooling at fluences of 16–26 J/cm^2) for patients with Fitzpatrick type IV–VI in their study of 24 children [6]. The authors found that when administered appropriately, LHR with Nd:YAG was safe in children <16 years of age. However, efficacy was not assessed.

24.8 Treatment of Light Hair

- Light hair has little to no melanin, which serves as the target chromophore for LHR.
- Attempts to employ exogenous target chromophores for use with LHR have met with varying success in the literature, and none have been studied among pediatric populations.

Blonde, red, white, and gray hair has little to no melanin, which acts as the chromophore for LHR. Various attempts have been made to employ a topical chromophore for use in these patients, thereby making LHR more effective in these patients. However, these methods have met with varying success and some experienced authors look upon these methods with skepticism [7]. One recent randomized, controlled, double-blind study tested melanin-encapsulated liposomes as a chromophore for removal of blonde, white, and gray hair [47]. Sixteen patients were treated with liposomal melanin spray and 16 patients were treated with saline spray prior to each of three cycles of 800 nm diode laser treatments (28–40 J/cm^2). On six-month follow-up, there was a 14% reduction in terminal hair compared to baseline within the treatment group and 10% reduction in the control group. Although statistically significant, the authors argue against the routine use of this formulation as the results lacked clinical significance. In a 2014 study, authors tested the use of rose bengal loaded in liposomes (LRB) in a topical gel among patients with white and blonde hair [22]. Fifteen patients were given LRB to apply prior to each of three sessions of IPL while another 15 patients were given placebo gel prior to IPL. After six-month follow-up, average terminal hair count showed 40% reduction in the treatment group with a significant difference from the control group. No studies testing chromophore-delivering preparations have been tested among exclusively pediatric populations.

24.9 Complications

- Altered skin pigment is the most common complication following LHR, and may be temporary or permanent.
- Other complications include blistering, ulceration, hive-like response, bruising, infection, acne flare, and folliculitis.
- Although rare, patients of darker skin types have a risk of induced hypertrichosis with LHR.

The most common complication from LHR is altered skin pigmentation in the treatment area, which may become darker or lighter. While hyper- or hypopigmentation may occur due to operational error, such as selecting non-optimal wavelength, pulse duration, fluence, or cooling, altered pigment may also occur even when optimal parameters have been chosen [7]. Pigment changes can be temporary, but they can also be permanent and disfiguring (Figure 24.7). In addition to the risk of permanent hyperpigmentation

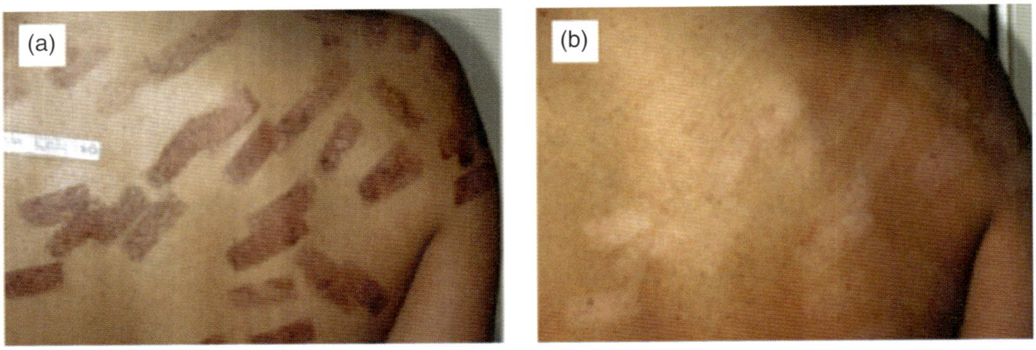

Figure 24.7 Post-LHR pigment changes. (a) Temporary hyperpigmentation after IPL, followed by (b) persisting hypopigmented patches. *Source:* Ibrahimi et al. 2011 [6]. Reprinted with permission of John Wiley & Sons.

seen with lasers, excess cryogen utilized in cooling may in itself cause hyperpigmentation in predisposed individuals [48]. Scarring is a much rarer possibility.

Other risks include blistering, ulceration, hive-like response, bruising, infection, acne flare, and folliculitis. Patients who undergo more treatment sessions to achieve greater hair reduction may experience an increased incidence in adverse effects [32]. Patients of Fitzpatrick skin types IV–VI or those of Mediterranean, Middle Eastern, or Asian descent have a low, paradoxical risk of induced hypertrichosis [7].

24.10 Conclusion and Future Directions

- Additional studies are needed to assess the safety, tolerability, and efficacy of LHR and IPL among pediatric populations.
- Additional studies are needed to investigate the appropriate use of anesthesia for children undergoing LHR.
- Unwanted hair has significant psychological burden for sufferers, and should be treated to improve QOL. When used appropriately, LHR may be a safe and effective means to provide long-lasting decreases in hair burden.

The vast majority of studies on LHR have been conducted in adult populations, with very few studying safety, tolerability, and efficacy among children. Those studies that have been conducted, however, indicate that LHR can be a viable option for children suffering with excessive hair when used appropriately [6, 27]. Additional studies conducted among pediatric populations are needed so that treatment guidelines may be suggested. Further, there appear to be significant discrepancies in the use of anesthesia among children with LHR procedures. While some study authors report no need for anesthesia, others report use of general anesthesia, which has inherent risks of its own. Further studies are needed so that guidelines for pain control in pediatric populations may be developed. In addition, there is a growing trend toward development of at-home LHR devices, none of which have been tested among pediatric populations. However, due to ease of access to these devices and greater affordability than professional care, it is possible that these devices have been used by children and adolescents within their homes. Studies are needed to assess the safety and efficacy of these for home devices.

In conclusion, excessive unwanted hair has a significant psychological effect for children and adolescents. When used appropriately, LHR may be a safe and effective means of offering long-lasting decreases in hair burden. Current knowledge of lasers for hair removal in the pediatric population is limited by a dearth of studies. Those that are currently available, however, have noted that lasers can be well tolerated among adolescent populations, even in children as young as five or six. LHR has the potential to decrease the emotional burden of children and adolescents suffering with hirsutism and hypertrichosis and should be considered where appropriate.

References

1 Dinulos, J.G. (2011). Cosmetic procedures in children. *Current Opinion in Pediatrics* 23 (4): 395–398.

2 Nouri, K., Vejjabhinanta, V., Patel, S.S. et al. (2008). Photoepilation: a growing trend in laser-assisted cosmetic dermatology. *Journal of Cosmetic Dermatology* 7 (1): 61–67.

3 Vejjabhinanta, V., Nouri, K., Singh, A. et al. (2011). *Lasers in Dermatology and Medicine* (ed. K. Nouri), 91–101. New York: Springer.

4 Crispin, M.K., Hruza, G.J., and Kilmer, S.L. (2017). Lasers and energy-based devices in men. *Dermatologic Surgery: Official Publication for American Society for Dermatologic Surgery [et al]* 43 (Suppl 2): S176–S184.

5 Cordisco, M.R. (2009). An update on lasers in children. *Current Opinion in Pediatrics* 21 (4): 499–504.

6 Rajpar, S.F., Hague, J.S., Abdullah, A. et al. (2009). Hair removal with the long-pulse alexandrite and long-pulse Nd:YAG lasers is safe and well tolerated in children. *Clinical and Experimental Dermatology* 34 (6): 684–687.

7 Ibrahimi, O.A., Avram, M.M., Hanke, C.W. et al. (2011). Laser hair removal. *Dermatologic Therapy* 24 (1): 94–107.

8 Rosenfield, R.L. (2005). Clinical practice. Hirsutism. *The New England Journal of Medicine* 353 (24): 2578–2588.

9 Trueb, R.M. (2002). Causes and management of hypertrichosis. *American Journal of Clinical Dermatology* 3 (9): 617–627.

10 Otberg, N. and Shapiro, J. (2012). Fitzpatrick's dermatology. In: *General Medicine*, 8e (ed. L.A. Goldsmith, S.I. Katz, B.A. Gilchrest, et al.). New York: McGraw-Hill.

11 Anderson, R.R. and Parrish, J.A. (1983). Selective photothermolysis: precise microsurgery by selective absorption of pulsed radiation. *Science* 220 (4596): 524–527.

12 Choudhary, S., Elsaie, M.L., and Nouri, K. (2009). Laser assisted hair-removal. *Giornale italiano di Dermatologia e Venereologia: Organo Ufficiale, Societa italiana di Dermatologia e Sifilografia* 144 (5): 595–602.

13 Alqubaisy, Y., McLeod, M.P., and Nouri, K. (2011). Laser hair removal pearls in skin of color. *Journal of Drugs in Dermatology: JDD* 10 (12 Suppl): s12–s13.

14 Loo, W.J. and Lanigan, S.W. (2002). Laser treatment improves quality of life of hirsute females. *Clinical and Experimental Dermatology* 27 (6): 439–441.

15 Maziar, A., Farsi, N., Mandegarfard, M. et al. (2010). Unwanted facial hair removal with laser treatment improves quality of life of patients. *Journal of Cosmetic and Laser Therapy: Official Publication of the European Society for Laser Dermatology* 12 (1): 7–9.

16 Gacaferri Lumezi, B., Goci, A. et al. (2014). Mixed form of hirsutism in an adolescent female and laser therapy. *Iranian Red Crescent Medical Journal* 16 (6): e9410.

17 Bode, D., Seehusen, D.A., and Baird, D. (2012). Hirsutism in women. *American Family Physician* 85 (4): 373–380.

18 Hughes, C.L. (1994). Hirsutism. In: *Disorders of Hair Growth: Diagnosis and Treatment* (ed. E.A. Olsen), 344. New York: McGraw-Hill.

19 Castelo-Soccio, L.A. (2012). Hair manifestations of systemic disease. *Current Problems in Pediatric and Adolescent Health Care* 42 (8): 198–203.

20 Ferriman, D. and Gallwey, J.D. (1961). Clinical assessment of body hair growth in women. *The Journal of Clinical Endocrinology and Metabolism* 21: 1440–1447.

21 Hatch, R., Rosenfield, R.L., Kim, M.H. et al. (1981). Hirsutism: implications, etiology, and management. *American Journal of Obstetrics and Gynecology* 140 (7): 815–830.

22 Samy, N. and Fadel, M. (2014). Topical liposomal rose bengal for photodynamic white hair removal: randomized, controlled, double-blind study. *Journal of Drugs in Dermatology: JDD* 13 (4): 436–442.

23 Nouri, K., Chen, H., Saghari, S. et al. (2004). Comparing 18- versus 12-mm spot size in hair removal using a gentlease 755-nm alexandrite laser. *Dermatologic Surgery: Official Publication for American Society for Dermatologic Surgery [et al]* 30 (4 Pt 1): 494–497.

24 Zenzie, H.H., Altshuler, G.B., Smirnov, M.Z. et al. (2000). Evaluation of cooling methods for laser dermatology. *Lasers in Surgery and Medicine* 26 (2): 130–144.

25 Grossman, M.C., Dierickx, C., Farinelli, W. et al. (1996). Damage to hair follicles by normal-mode ruby laser pulses. *Journal of the American Academy of Dermatology* 35 (6): 889–894.

26 Anderson, R.R., Burns, A.J., and Garden, J. (1999). Multicenter study of long-pulse ruby laser hair removal. *Lasers in Surgery and Medicine* 11 (Suppl): 14.

27 Morley, S. and Gault, D. (2000). Hair removal using the long-pulsed ruby laser in children. *Journal of Clinical Laser Medicine & Surgery* 18 (6): 277–280.

28 Mahendran, R. and Sheehan-Dare, R.A. (2003). Lumbosacral hypertrichosis treated with the normal-mode ruby laser. *Acta Dermato-Venereologica* 83 (2): 142–143.

29 Wanner, M. (2005). Laser hair removal. *Dermatologic Therapy* 18 (3): 209–216.

30 Garcia, C., Alamoudi, H., Nakib, M. et al. (2000). Alexandrite laser hair removal is safe for Fitzpatrick skin types IV–VI. *Dermatologic Surgery: Official Publication for American Society for Dermatologic Surgery [et al]* 26 (2): 130–134.

31 Galadari, I. (2003). Comparative evaluation of different hair removal lasers in skin types IV, V, and VI. *International Journal of Dermatology* 42 (1): 68–70.

32 Bouzari, N., Nouri, K., Tabatabai, H. et al. (2005). The role of number of treatments in laser-assisted hair removal using a 755-nm alexandrite laser. *Journal of Drugs in Dermatology: JDD* 4 (5): 573–578.

33 Davoudi, S.M., Behnia, F., Gorouhi, F. et al. (2008). Comparison of long-pulsed alexandrite and Nd:YAG lasers, individually and in combination, for leg hair reduction: an assessor-blinded, randomized trial with 18 months of follow-up. *Archives of Dermatology* 144 (10): 1323–1327.

34 Campos, V.B., Dierickx, C.C., and Farinelli, W.A. (2000). Hair removal with an 800-nm pulsed diode laser. *Journal of the American Academy of Dermatology* 43 (3): 442–447.

35 Lou, W.W., Quintana, A.T., Geronemus, R.G. et al. (2000). Prospective study of hair reduction by diode laser (800 nm) with long-term follow-up. *Dermatologic Surgery: Official Publication for American Society for Dermatologic Surgery [et al]* 26 (5): 428–432.

36 Eremia, S., Li, C., and Newman, N. (2001). Laser hair removal with alexandrite versus diode laser using four treatment sessions: 1-year results. *Dermatologic Surgery: Official Publication for American Society for Dermatologic Surgery [et al]* 27 (11): 925–929; discussion 9–30.

37 Lapidoth, M., Adatto, M., Cohen, S. et al. (2014). Hypertrichosis in Becker's nevus: effective low-fluence laser hair removal. *Lasers in Medical Science* 29 (1): 191–193.

38 Klein, A., Steinert, S., Baeumler, W. et al. (2013). Photoepilation with a diode laser vs. intense pulsed light: a randomized, intrapatient left-to-right trial. *The British Journal of Dermatology* 168 (6): 1287–1293.

39 McGill, D.J., Hutchison, C., McKenzie, E. et al. (2007). A randomised, split-face comparison of facial hair removal with the

alexandrite laser and intense pulsed light system. *Lasers in Surgery and Medicine* 39 (10): 767–772.

40 Goh, C.L. (2003). Comparative study on a single treatment response to long-pulse Nd:YAG lasers and intense pulse light therapy for hair removal on skin type IV to VI – is longer wavelengths lasers preferred over shorter wavelengths lights for assisted hair removal. *The Journal of Dermatological Treatment* 14 (4): 243–247.

41 Mulholland, R.S. (2009). Silk'n--a novel device using home pulsed light for hair removal at home. *Journal of Cosmetic and Laser Therapy: Official Publication of the European Society for Laser Dermatology* 11 (2): 106–109.

42 Thaysen-Petersen, D., Bjerring, P., Dierickx, C. et al. (2012). A systematic review of light-based home-use devices for hair removal and considerations on human safety. *Journal of the European Academy of Dermatology and Venereology: JEADV* 26 (5): 545–553.

43 Ozdemir, M., Balevi, A., Engin, B. et al. (2010). Treatment of faun-tail naevus with intense pulsed light. *Photomedicine and Laser Surgery* 28 (3): 435–438.

44 Lanigan, S.W. (2003). Incidence of side effects after laser hair removal. *Journal of the American Academy of Dermatology* 49 (5): 882–886.

45 Alster, T.S., Bryan, H., and Williams, C.M. (2001). Long-pulsed Nd:YAG laser-assisted hair removal in pigmented skin: a clinical and histological evaluation. *Archives of Dermatology* 137 (7): 885–889.

46 Rao, J. and Goldman, M.P. (2005). Prospective, comparative evaluation of three laser systems used individually and in combination for axillary hair removal. *Dermatologic Surgery: Official Publication for American Society for Dermatologic Surgery [et al]* 31 (12): 1671–1676; discussion 7.

47 Sand, M., Bechara, F.G., Sand, D. et al. (2007). A randomized, controlled, double-blind study evaluating melanin-encapsulated liposomes as a chromophore for laser hair removal of blond, white, and gray hair. *Annals of Plastic Surgery* 58 (5): 551–554.

48 Davidson, D., Ritacca, D., and Goldman, M.P. (2009). Permanent hyperpigmentation following laser hair removal using the dynamic cooling device. *Journal of Drugs in Dermatology: JDD* 8 (1): 58–69.

25

Lasers for Other Specific Dermatologic Disorders

Leyre Falto-Aizpurua[1], Mohammad-Ali Yazdani Abyaneh[1], Harleen Arora[2], Robert D. Griffith[1], Ali Rajabi-Estarabadi[1], and Keyvan Nouri[3]

[1] Department of Dermatology & Cutaneous Surgery, University of Miami Miller School of Medicine, Miami, FL, USA
[2] University of Miami, Coral Gables, FL, USA
[3] Department of Dermatology, Ophthalmology, Otolaryngology & Surgery, University of Miami Leonard M. Miller School of Medicine, Miami, FL, USA

25.1 Introduction

There are various dermatologic disorders that are common in the pediatric population for which laser and light therapy has become an alternate form of treatment. Mild presentations of disease usually respond to conventional treatment, but severe or atypical ones can become a treatment challenge for physicians. Unfortunately, the supporting evidence for laser and light therapies in children is limited.

In this chapter we will discuss some of the most common pediatric disorders for which laser or light therapy is a treatment option.

25.2 Alopecia Areata

Alopecia areata (AA) is a non-scarring form of alopecia, which commonly affects limited portions of the scalp. AA may progress to alopecia totalis, which affects the entire scalp or alopecia universalis, which affects the body [1]. The incidence of AA is equal in males and females and most commonly affects children and adolescents, although it can occur at any age [2]. The exact etiopathogenesis of AA remains unknown, but it is known to be an autoimmune disease with oxidative stress as a possible triggering factor [3]. The autoimmune nature of the disease is characterized by higher levels of autoantibodies, cytokine abnormalities, lymphocytic inflammatory infiltrate in the peribulbar area, and its linkage to select human leukocyte antigen class II alleles [2]. Histopathology reveals a higher number of terminal telogen and catagen follicles, especially in acute stages [4]. T lymphocytes take part in the mechanism of the disease, executing the autoimmune attack of the hair follicles and the consequential loss of hair [5] with possibly the accompanying characteristic nail changes. The diagnosis of AA can be done through biopsy, although clinical diagnosis is commonly performed. The hair follicle is not permanently damaged with this condition, allowing for possibility of hair regrowth. The treatment for AA, however, remains largely symptomatic, with none of the options being preventative or curative. Traditional methods include topical treatments such as corticosteroids and minoxidil [6], systemic corticosteroids, and intralesional injections [2]. Also immunotherapy with agents such as squaric acid dibutylester and diphenylcyclopropenone is commonly used as the

Pediatric Dermatologic Surgery, First Edition. Edited by Keyvan Nouri, Latanya Benjamin, Jasem Alshaiji, and Jan Izakovic.

second-line treatment for AA. The mechanism of action is unknown, but it is thought to cause antigenic competition, which distracts CD4 cells from attacking hair follicles [7].

Phototherapy and laser therapy are also possible treatments for AA. A universal treatment method cannot be prescribed and often physicians implement a cocktail method of several different treatments, followed by maintenance therapy if results are achieved.

The common laser treatment for AA is the use of 308 nm xenon-chloride excimer laser which emits all its energy at this wavelength, classifying it as a "super narrowband-UVB (NB-UVB) light source" [5, 8]. The excimer laser induces the apoptosis of T cells *in vitro* and does so more efficiently than other NB-UVB light sources [5, 9, 10]. The excimer laser has been used on children in particular with recalcitrant cases of AA and AA totalis. Controlled studies showed that regrowth of hair is observed with the use of this laser, with a small to no percentage of recurrence of AA, making the 308 nm excimer laser an appropriate treatment modality for AA, although often requiring several treatments over the span of several months [9, 10] (Figure 25.1). This laser, however, is inefficient in the treatment of patchy AA on the extremities [11]. A study

(a) (b)

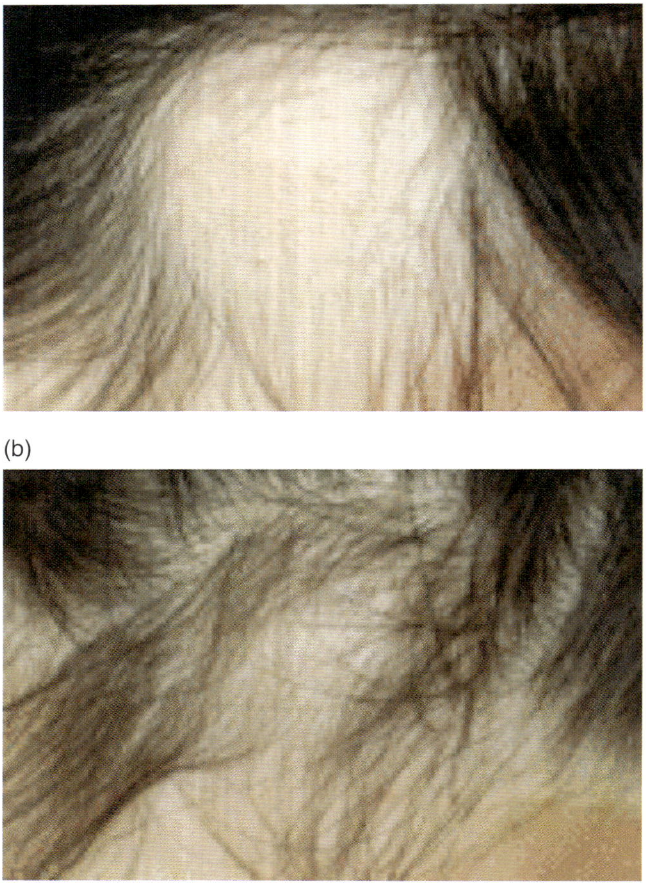

Figure 25.1 An oval region of hair loss (a) in the right occipital region of case 2, which was successfully treated (b) after eight sessions with a 308-nm excimer lamp. *Source:* Ohtsuki et al. [8] Reprinted with permission of John Wiley and Sons, Inc.

conducted by Ohtsuki et al. examined the use of the 308 nm lamp as opposed the laser, and the lamp was found to be a safe and effective treatment for AA as well, no side effects were observed other than erythema [12]. The lamp treatment should be considered for recalcitrant AA.

Other lasers have also been tested for AA treatment but are less established and require more research. Fractional photothermolysis laser has been studied for AA [13], as has low-level laser therapy (LLLT) (Figure 25.2). LLLT has been found to be safe and effective, with the mechanism being the stimulation of stem cells in the hair follicles of the epidermis and the modification of the cells into the anagen phase [14]. Furthermore, trials have been conducted on mice with low-level laser combs. The Hair Max Laser Comb (655 nm) showed hair growth in treated mice over a six-month period, making it an effective device needing human testing [1].

25.3 Vitiligo

Vitiligo is the most common disorder of depigmentation and affects approximately 0.1–2% of the population, and about half of patients present before the age of 20. While

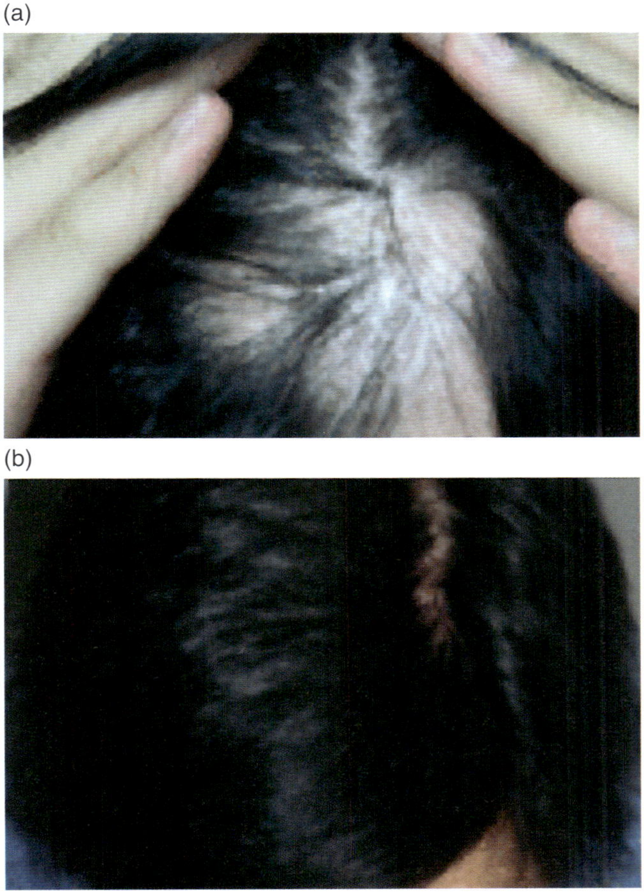

Figure 25.2 (a) A 35-year-old male with alopecia areata before treatment. (b) Regrowth of black hair after six months of treatment with fractional laser. *Source:* Yoo et al. [12]. Reprinted with permission of John Wiley and Sons, Inc.

NB-UVB phototherapy has become a first-line treatment option for generalized vitiligo, the xenon-chloride excimer laser has become an alternative treatment option for patients with localized disease. Since its introduction in the treatment of vitiligo in 2001, the excimer laser has been studied in a multitude of studies and has Food and Drug Administration approval for treatment of vitiligo. The laser offers the potential for targeted treatment of affected areas with limited adverse effects and lower cumulative radiation exposure [15].

The mechanism of action of the excimer laser in treating vitiligo is not completely understood, but it may mirror that of NB-UVB, with a combination of stimulatory effects on melanocytes in the outer root sheath of hair follicles and immunomodulation. Excimer light has actually been shown to be more effective at inducing T cell apoptosis than NB-UVB, which suggests other differences in their mechanisms of action may exist as well [16, 17].

In studies of the excimer laser, two to three treatments have been delivered for anywhere from 4 to 36 weeks. Results have varied widely across trials, with the percentage of patients achieving >75% repigmentation of lesions ranging from 12.5 to 61%. The face responds best to treatments, while the neck, axillae, and trunk respond well. Traditionally UVB-resistant regions of the body such as bony prominences and acral sites are the most resistant to the excimer laser as well. Moreover, greater total number of treatment sessions seems to improve outcomes given fixed treatment frequency. Follow-ups up to two years after treatment with the laser suggest stability of repigmentation and further improvement in some cases. The most common adverse effects of treatment are localized erythema, pain, pruritus, and blistering, which are all acute and self-limited [18].

Studies of the excimer laser for vitiligo, including randomized controlled trials, have demonstrated the safety and efficacy of the device for pediatric patients and adults of all skin types [18]. Studies specifically looking at pediatric patients suggest their response rates may be better than in adults [19, 20] (Figure 25.3). Additionally, the combination of excimer laser with pimecrolimus was statistically superior to laser therapy alone among children ages 6–14 in one study [20]. There is also evidence that laser dermabrasion of traditionally UV-resistant sites with the 2940-nm erbium laser or ablative fractional carbon dioxide laser before NB-UVB may increase response rates in these difficult to treat areas [21]. There is need for further study of the excimer laser in the pediatric population using standardized outcome measures, the use of excimer laser in combination with other conventional treatments, and the use of ablative lasers before NB-UVB for UVB-resistant sites.

25.3.1 Summary

- *Alopecia areata:* The 308 nm xenon-chloride excimer laser is commonly used to treat recalcitrant cases of AA and AA totalis.
- *Vitiligo:* The 308 nm xenon-chloride excimer laser has demonstrated to be safe and effective in the treatment of vitiligo. The face responds best to treatment while the neck, axillae and trunk respond well.

25.4 Psoriasis

Treatment for psoriasis is based on the severity of the disease. In children, psoriasis usually presents with a mild clinical course and responds well to conventional treatment. When children present with moderate to severe disease, or atypical presentations, treatment options are limited due to insufficient evidence of many of the agents used [22, 23]. Among the systemic therapies, UV radiation modalities are a good alternative in children and have minimal side effects [24]. It has been demonstrated that UV radiation has antiproliferative, anti-inflammatory and immunosuppressant effects [22]. Treatment modalities include phototherapy

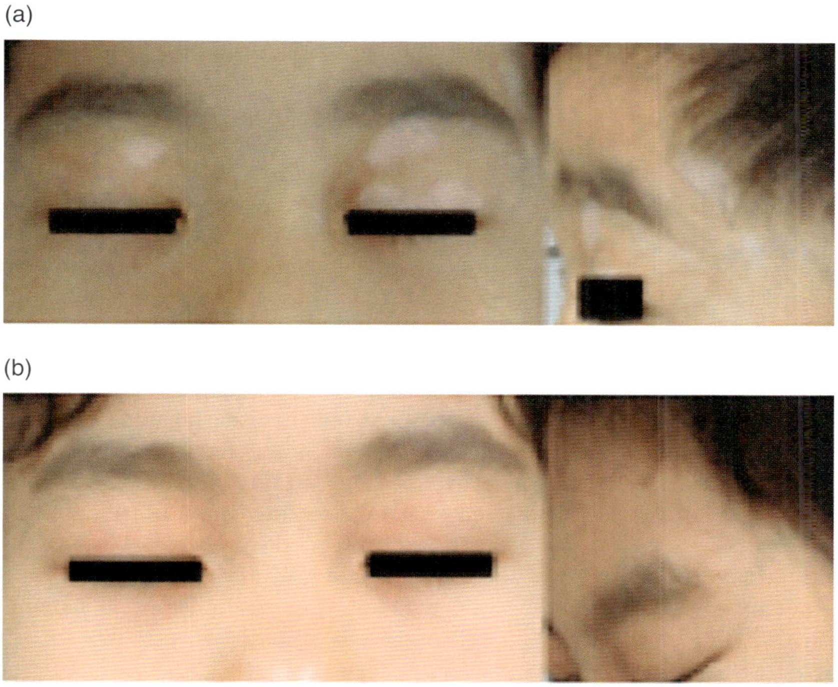

Figure 25.3 A 15-year-old male with two years of progressive facial vitiligo demonstrating marked improvement of lesions before (a) and after (b) one year of treatment with the excimer laser (total cumulative dose: 6.17 J/cm^2). *Source:* Cho et al. [17]. Reprinted with permission of John Wiley and Sons, Inc.

with broadband or NB-UVB, photochemotherapy, and excimer laser. Studies have shown that phototherapy works best when psoriasis plaques are small and thin, and involve large areas of the body or with guttate psoriasis [25].

Broadband UVB (290–320 nm) works by modulating the immune system [26, 27]. It is recommended for extensive disease, alone or combined with topical tar, and should be performed at least three times per week until remission and then continue with maintenance sessions.

NB-UVB (311 nm) is best tolerated and is more effective than broadband UVB, as it causes more apoptosis of T cells [25, 28]. Some studies have demonstrated good results in children [29, 30]. A systematic review concluded that plaque and guttate psoriasis respond well with comparatively minimal side effects [31]. Combination therapy with anthralin and vitamin D3 analogues has been suggested by some authors to reduce UVB exposure [32].

Photochemotherapy (PUVA) requires psoralen administration prior to UVA (320–400 nm) radiation. UVA exposure should be performed within two hours of the ingestion of the photosensitizer, and the patient should be advised of photoprotection afterwards. For bath PUVA, the medication is dissolved in water, and the area to be treated is soaked for 15–30 minutes prior to radiation. Treatments should be performed three times per week until remission and then once or twice per week for maintenance. PUVA can be considered for palmoplantar presentation of pustular psoriasis, using topical psoralen to avoid unnecessary photosensitivity and gastrointestinal side effects [24]. Due to the need for a photosensitizer, and UVA having better skin penetration when compared to UVB, PUVA is the one modality most highly associated with an increased risk of skin malignancy and patients should be monitored [25]. For this and other reasons, PUVA has been largely replaced by NB-UVB [33].

Home phototherapy has been proven to be safe, effective and cost-effective, minimizing absenteeism from school or work [34]. However, this is not a very popular option as some physicians have fears about its improper use.

Excimer (308 nm) laser allows the administration of a higher dose of UVB to a limited area [25]. Some studies have shown that results are seen even faster than with regular phototherapy (Figure 25.4) [36, 37]. A particular side effect of excimer laser is induced hyperpigmentation in the treated area that resolves after ceasing treatment.

The 585 or 595 nm pulsed dye laser (PDL) has been proven effective in treating nail psoriasis. PDL can effectively reach the nail bed through the nail plate, leading to microvessel destruction and destruction of T cells in the dermis and epidermis [38]. Unfortunately, there are no studies demonstrating this in pediatric patients.

Common side effects of phototherapy include erythema and burning. Children's anxiety while being inside the cabin and compliance issues are important limitations for this therapy that should be considered [33, 39]. There is a general concern of photodamage and increased risk of malignancy at an early age, but there are no studies observing long-term side effects in children to prove this. Due to this concern, some authors recommend treating only older children with widespread disease [32]. Besides the contraindications to any other light therapy, phototherapy is contraindicated in patients with melanoma or extensive NMSC.

(a)

(b)

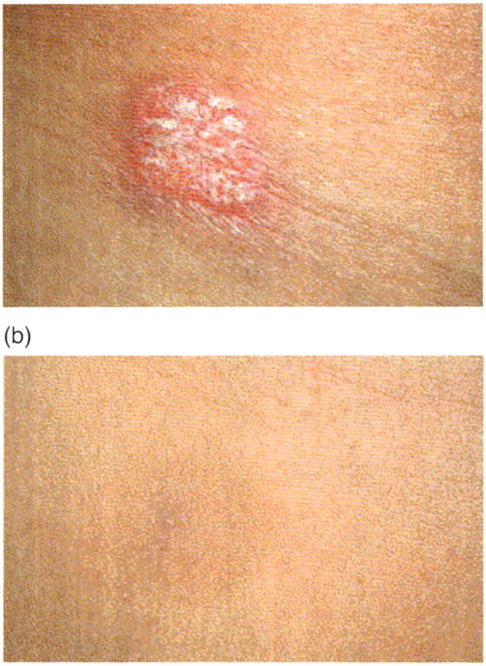

Figure 25.4 (a) Abdominal plaque of psoriasis, (b) one month after eight sessions of 308-nm excimer laser. Note the hyperpigmentation. *Source:* Passeron and Ortonne [35]. Reprinted with permission of Elsevier Limited, Inc.

25.5 Molluscum Contagiosum

Molluscum contagiosum (MC) is a benign viral skin infection that presents as smooth flesh-colored umbilicated papules, common among school age children. There are a great number of treatment options for MC including topical, intralesional, and systemic therapies with different efficacy rates and side effects [40].

Among the physically destructive methods, the PDL has been reported as a safe, well tolerated, quick, and highly effective treatment option for MC. PDL provides the advantage that is minimally painful when compared to other methods of destruction and it has no apparent permanent adverse effects. The exact mechanism of action remains unknown. Most likely nonspecific thermal damage produced by the treatment is responsible for clearing MC lesions.

Studies have shown that PDL has been well tolerated by children [41]. Topical anesthesia can be applied 30–60 minutes prior to therapy without altering efficacy. MC lesions can be treated at a rate of 1 every two to three

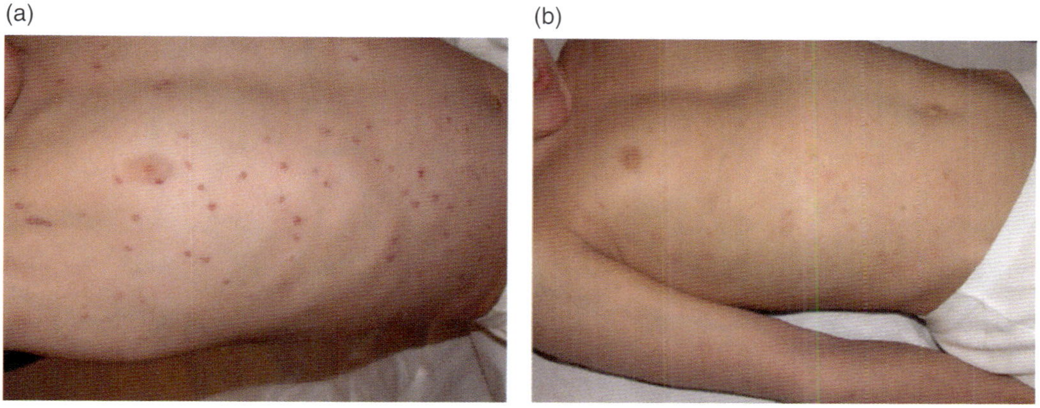

Figure 25.5 Molluscum contagiosum of the thorax resistant to local treatment with a 5% imiquimod cream, 595 nm pulsed dye laser treatment: 1 pass, pulse duration 0.25 ms; fluency from 2 to 4 J/cm^2; frequency 1 Hz; success at 15 days after a single treatment. *Source:* Michel et al. [42]. Reprinted with permission of Elsevier Limited, Inc.

seconds, making the physician able to treat multiple lesions in a short period of time (Figure 25.5). Adverse events include minimal pain during the procedure, transient post-operative purpura (lasting two to three weeks) and transient skin pigment change (lasting up to six months). No recurrence has been reported in studies with follow-up periods of 6–10 months.

25.5.1 Summary

- *Psoriasis:* NB-UVB is best tolerated and is more effective than BB-UVB. It has been proven to work best in plaque and guttate psoriasis. Combination therapy with anthralin and vitamin D3 analogues has been suggested to reduce UVB exposure, particularly in children.
- *Molluscum contagiosum:* PDL has been proven to be safe and highly effective and well tolerated by children.

25.6 Morphea

Morphea is a localized form of scleroderma that includes a spectrum of diseases affecting the skin, muscle and deeper structures. Localized scleroderma is the most common type of sclerosis in childhood, with approximately 1–3/100 000 children affected [43]. Linear morphea is the most common subtype and it is associated with a more progressive course and complications [44]. Other subtypes include circumscribed, generalized, bullous, deep, mixed morphea, as well as linear morphea with the *en coup de saber* subtype [43, 45]. The treatment and prognosis of morphea depends on the type and extent of disease. For some cases, the disease course is usually benign and may resolve spontaneously within three to five years [46]. Monitoring and symptomatic treatment for more superficial or single lesions is usually sufficient. Treatment options include emollients, topical steroids or calcipotriene. Phototherapy has also been demonstrated beneficial in a various studies in children, but it may not be accessible to everyone and is time-consuming [47]. Untreated morphea that is active or at particular locations represent a major problem as it may lead to movement and developmental disorders.

Phototherapy has anti-inflammatory effects and reduces collagen deposition in the dermis by different mechanisms [48]. NB-UVB, PUVA (Figure 25.6) and UVA1 (Figure 25.7) phototherapies benefit morphea. NB-UVB

(a)

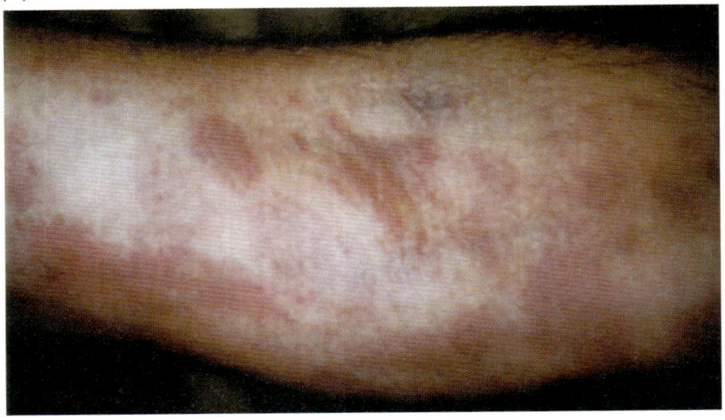

(b)

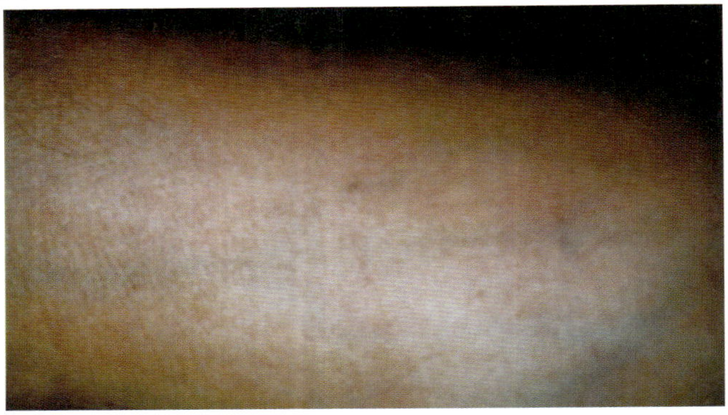

Figure 25.6 (a) Erythematous lesions on right arm before treatment. (b) Normal appearance at end of treatment with PUVA. *Source:* Morrison [49]. Reprinted with permission of Elsevier Limited, Inc.

(a)

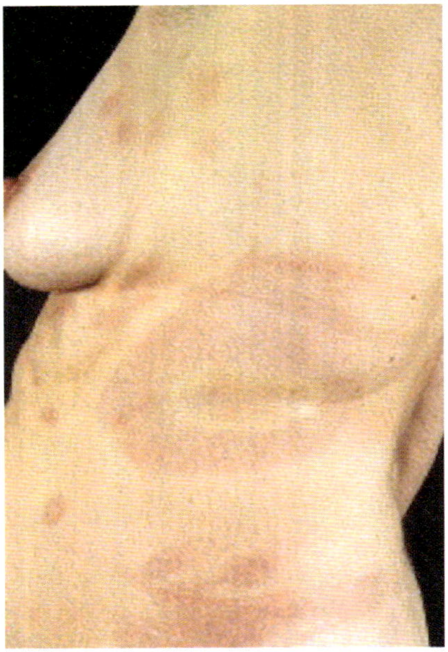

(b)

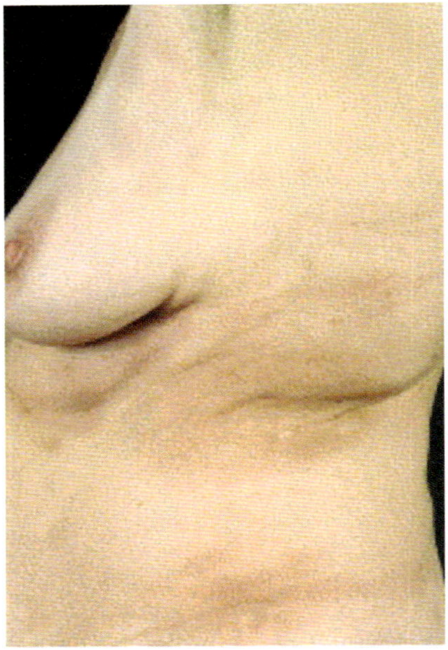

Figure 25.7 (a) Clinical presentation of patient with active morphea before treatment with low-dose UVA1. (b) Complete clearance of all signs of active disease. Residual postinflammatory hyperpigmentation. *Source:* Kreuter et al. [50]. Reprinted with permission of Elsevier Limited, Inc.

has been effective in different childhood diseases including morphea [51]. In different prospective studies, 80% of the patients receiving PUVA and 77% receiving broadband UVA showed improvement [52]. Treatments ranged from 5 to 20 J/cm^2 per treatment with a total of up to 400 J/cm^2 of irradiation with no statistical significance between these groups.

UVA1 (340–400 nm) is also an effective option as it penetrates deeper into the skin when compared to NB-UVB, PUVA or broadband UVA with diminished side effects [48, 53]. Various dosing regimens with low, medium and high doses of UVA have been studied with all of them decreasing to some degree skin thickness and firmness [48]. Unfortunately, there is no consensus on the optimal dose but some studies have demonstrated that a low dose can be as effective as high dose, minimizing exposure to radiation. Limitations of this therapy are that it is more expensive, not widely available in the United States, and it is time-consuming, as it requires 30–60 minutes' exposure time per treatment. The main acute adverse reactions of phototherapy are erythema, pruritus, tanning, polymorphic light eruption, xerosis cutis, and herpes simplex infection outbreaks [53].

Based on the studies reviewed above, phototherapy is now considered by many authors a first-line treatment for localized scleroderma. It has the advantage that stops inflammation rapidly and consistently, halting lesion progression, as it also reverts skin sclerosis and these effects may continue after treatment cessation [48].

25.7 Atopic Dermatitis

There are numerous available topical treatments for atopic dermatitis, however, phototherapy can be considered as an adjuvant treatment or as an alternate option to classical treatment. Two different extensive literature reviews suggest that in children, NB-UVB phototherapy should be considered as first-line therapy [54] due to its safety, efficacy and ease of administration whereas the second review suggests it as a second line therapy due to potential, theoretical long-term adverse effects [55]. A prospective study treated 29 patients with moderate to severe atopic dermatitis with NB-UVB, which improved their mean six area six sign atopic dermatitis (SASSAD) score by 61%, compared to the untreated group (26 patients), whose mean SSASD score increased by 6%.

A pilot study performed with 18 patients, six of which were children, found that monochromatic excimer light provided complete remission in 12/18 patients with atopic dermatitis [56]. On a mouse model, the excimer lamp was shown to have antihyperinnervative effects and reduced DNA damage when used with a cutoff excimer filter, improving pruritus [57].

25.7.1 Summary

- *Morphea:* Phototherapy is now being considered by many authors as first-line treatment for localized scleroderma.
- *Atopic dermatitis:* Although NB-UVB is currently considered an adjuvant treatment for atopic dermatitis, two extensive literature reviews suggest that this should be first or second line treatment option in children as it is safe, effective and easily administered. However, long-term safety remains a concern.

25.8 Lichen Planus

Lichen planus is uncommon in the pediatric population. There is no consensus or defined protocol for treating LPP in children. Recommended drugs includes topical and systemic corticosteroids and immunomodulators, oral antibiotics, phototherapy, and systemic immunosuppressants [58, 59].

However, different reports have described symptomatic relief and disease remission upon NB-UVB therapy [60]. A retrospective study reported complete response for 70% of the treated patients (n = 50, ages 12–77) after NB-UVB therapy [61].

25.9 Pityriasis Lichenoides Chronica

Pityriasis lichenoides is an acquired cutaneous disease spectrum than can present as pityriasis lichenoides et varioliformis acuta (PLEVA) to pityriasis lichenoides chronica (PLC). PLC is a clinical diagnosis, but characteristic histopathologic features confirm the diagnosis. PLEVA is characterized by a vacuolar interface dermatitis with a wedge-shaped superficial and deep perivascular lymphocytic infiltrate and transepidermal extravasation of erythrocytes [58].

PL often follows a waxing and waning path, and spontaneous resolution can occur. There are no standard guidelines for the treatment of PL in children. Topical corticosteroids and immunomodulators, oral antibiotics, phototherapy, and systemic immunosuppressants are recommended therapies [58].

Phototherapy, particularly NB-UVB, has been proven effective in children resistant to common therapies [62, 63].

25.9.1 Summary

- NB-UVB may provide symptomatic relief and disease remission in patients with lichen planus and has been proven effective in children with PLC resistant to common therapies.

25.10 Conclusion

Lasers and lights have shown promise in treating the above-mentioned disorders. NB-UVB and excimer laser appear to be safer than other modalities of phototherapy, offering benefit with few adverse events. However, further studies in the pediatric population are required to establish their efficacy and long-term safety. Additionally, cost-effectiveness and school absenteeism need to be assessed.

References

1 Wikramanayake, T.C., Rodriguez, R., Choudhary, S. et al. (2012). Effects of the Lexington LaserComb on hair regrowth in the C3H/HeJ mouse model of alopecia areata. *Lasers in Medical Science* 27 (2): 431–436.

2 Papadopoulos, A.J., Schwartz, R.A., and Janniger, C.K. (2000). Alopecia areata. Pathogenesis, diagnosis, and therapy. *American Journal of Clinical Dermatology* 1 (2): 101–105.

3 Shah, A.A. and Sinha, A.A. (2013). Oxidative stress and autoimmune skin disease. *European Journal of Dermatology: EJD.* 23 (1): 5–13.

4 Dy, L.C. and Whiting, D.A. (2011). Histopathology of alopecia areata, acute and chronic: why is it important to the clinician? *Dermatologic Therapy* 24 (3): 369–374.

5 McMichael, A.J. (2013). Excimer laser: a module of the alopecia areata common protocol. *The Journal of Investigative Dermatology Symposium proceedings/The Society for Investigative Dermatology, Inc [and] European Society for Dermatological Research.* 16 (1): S77–S79.

6 Hon, K.L. and Leung, A.K. (2011). Alopecia areata. *Recent Patents on Inflammation & Allergy Drug Discovery* 5 (2): 98–107.

7 Darwin, E., Arora, H., Hirt, P.A. et al. (2017). A review of monochromatic light devices for the treatment of alopecia areata. *Lasers in Medical Science* 33 (2): 435–444.

8 Swanson, A. and Canty, K. (2013). Common pediatric skin conditions with protracted courses: a therapeutic update. *Dermatologic Clinics* 31 (2): 239–249.

9 Ohtsuki, A., Hasegawa, T., and Ikeda, S. (2010). Treatment of alopecia areata with 308-nm excimer lamp. *The Journal of Dermatology* 37 (12): 1032–1035.

10 Gundogan, C., Greve, B., and Raulin, C. (2004). Treatment of alopecia areata with the 308-nm xenon chloride excimer laser: case report of two successful treatments with the excimer laser. *Lasers in Surgery and Medicine* 34 (2): 86–90.

11 Al-Mutairi, N. (2007). 308-nm excimer laser for the treatment of alopecia areata. *Dermatologic Surgery: Official Publication for American Society for Dermatologic Surgery [et al].* 33 (12): 1483–1487.

12 Ohtsuki, A., Hasegawa, T., Komiyama, E. et al. (2013). 308-nm excimer lamp for the treatment of alopecia areata: clinical trial on 16 cases. *Indian Journal of Dermatology* 58 (4): 326.

13 Yoo, K.H., Kim, M.N., Kim, B.J. et al. (2010). Treatment of alopecia areata with fractional photothermolysis laser. *International Journal of Dermatology* 49 (7): 845–847.

14 Avci, P., Gupta, G.K., Clark, J. et al. (2014). Low-level laser (light) therapy (LLLT) for treatment of hair loss. *Lasers in Surgery and Medicine* 46 (2): 144–151.

15 Nicolaidou, E., Antoniou, C., Stratigos, A., and Katsambas, A.D. (2009). Narrowband ultraviolet B phototherapy and 308-nm excimer laser in the treatment of vitiligo: a review. *Journal of the American Academy of Dermatology* 60 (3): 470–477.

16 Ozawa, M., Ferenczi, K., Kikuchi, T. et al. (1999). 312-nanometer ultraviolet B light (narrow-band UVB) induces apoptosis of T cells within psoriatic lesions. *The Journal of Experimental Medicine* 189 (4): 711–718.

17 Esmat, S., Hegazy, R.A., Shalaby, S. et al. (2017). Phototherapy and combination therapies for vitiligo. *Dermatologic Clinics* 35 (2): 171–192.

18 Park, K.K., Liao, W., and Murase, J.E. (2012). A review of monochromatic excimer light in vitiligo. *The British Journal of Dermatology* 167 (3): 468–478.

19 Cho, S., Zheng, Z., Park, Y.K., and Roh, M.R. (2011). The 308-nm excimer laser: a promising device for the treatment of childhood vitiligo. *Photodermatology, Photoimmunology & Photomedicine* 27 (1): 24–29.

20 Hui-Lan, Y., Xiao-Yan, H., Jian-Yong, F. et al. (2009). Combination of 308-nm excimer laser with topical pimecrolimus for the treatment of childhood vitiligo. *Pediatric Dermatology* 26 (3): 354–356.

21 Yazdani Abyaneh, M., Griffith, R.D. et al. (2014). Narrowband ultraviolet B phototherapy in combination with other therapies for vitiligo: mechanisms and efficacies. *Journal of the European Academy of Dermatology and Venereology: JEADV* 28 (12): 1610–1622.

22 Lara-Corrales, I., Ramnarine, S., and Lansang, P. (2013). Treatment of childhood psoriasis with phototherapy and photochemotherapy. *Clinical medicine insights Pediatrics* 7: 25–33.

23 Zhang, P. and Wu, M.X. (2017). A clinical review of phototherapy for psoriasis. *Lasers in Medical Science* 33 (1): 173–180.

24 Sen, B.B., Rifaioglu, E.N., Ekiz, O. et al. (2014). Narrow-band ultraviolet B phototherapy in childhood. *Cutaneous and Ocular Toxicology* 33 (3): 189–191.

25 Rahman, M., Alam, K., Ahmad, M.Z. et al. (2012). Classical to current approach for treatment of psoriasis: a review. *Endocrine, Metabolic & Immune Disorders Drug Targets* 12 (3): 287–302.

26 Cooper, K.D., Oberhelman, L., Hamilton, T.A. et al. (1992). UV exposure reduces immunization rates and promotes tolerance to epicutaneous antigens in humans: relationship to dose, CD1a-DR+ epidermal macrophage induction, and Langerhans cell depletion. *Proceedings of the National Academy of Sciences of the United States of America* 89 (18): 8497–8501.

27 Matos, T.R., Ling, T.C., and Sheth, V. (2016). Ultraviolet B radiation therapy for psoriasis: pursuing the optimal regime. *Clinics in Dermatology* 34 (5): 587–593.

28 Walters, I.B., Burack, L.H., Coven, T.R. et al. (1999). Suberythemogenic narrow-band UVB is markedly more effective than conventional UVB in treatment of psoriasis

vulgaris. *Journal of the American Academy of Dermatology* 40 (6 Pt 1): 893–900.
29 Al-Fouzan, A.S. and Nanda, A. (1995). UVB phototherapy in childhood psoriasis. *Pediatric Dermatology* 12 (1): 66.
30 Jain, V.K., Aggarwal, K., Jain, K. et al. (2007). Narrow-band UV-B phototherapy in childhood psoriasis. *International Journal of Dermatology* 46 (3): 320–322.
31 de Jager, M.E., de Jong, E.M., van de Kerkhof, P.C. et al. (2010). Efficacy and safety of treatments for childhood psoriasis: a systematic literature review. *Journal of the American Academy of Dermatology* 62 (6): 1013–1030.
32 Benoit, S. and Hamm, H. (2007). Childhood psoriasis. *Clinics in Dermatology* 25 (6): 555–562.
33 Veith, W., Deleo, V., and Silverberg, N. (2011). Medical phototherapy in childhood skin diseases. *Minerva Pediatrica* 63 (4): 327–333.
34 Koek, M.B., Buskens, E., van Weelden, H. et al. (2009). Home versus outpatient ultraviolet B phototherapy for mild to severe psoriasis: pragmatic multicentre randomised controlled non-inferiority trial (PLUTO study). *BMJ* 338: b1542.
35 Passeron, T. and Ortonne, J.P. (2006). Use of the 308-nm excimer laser for psoriasis and vitiligo. *Clinics in Dermatology* 24 (1): 33–42.
36 Feldman, S.R., Mellen, B.G., Housman, T.S. et al. (2002). Efficacy of the 308-nm excimer laser for treatment of psoriasis: results of a multicenter study. *Journal of the American Academy of Dermatology* 46 (6): 900–906.
37 Gerber, W., Arheilger, B., Ha, T.A. et al. (2003). Ultraviolet B 308-nm excimer laser treatment of psoriasis: a new phototherapeutic approach. *The British Journal of Dermatology* 149 (6): 1250–1258.
38 Yin, N., Choudhary, S., and Nouri, K. (2013). Pulsed dye laser for the treatment of nail psoriasis. *Cutis* 92 (3): 129–135.
39 Pasic, A., Ceovic, R., Lipozencic, J. et al. (2003). Phototherapy in pediatric patients. *Pediatric Dermatology* 20 (1): 71–77.
40 Griffith, R.D., Yazdani Abyaneh, M.A., Falto-Aizpurua, L. et al. (2014). Pulsed dye laser therapy for molluscum contagiosum: a systematic review. *Journal of drugs in dermatology: JDD.* 13 (11): 1349–1352.
41 Binder, B., Weger, W., Komericki, P. et al. (2008). Treatment of molluscum contagiosum with a pulsed dye laser: pilot study with 19 children. *Journal der Deutschen Dermatologischen Gesellschaft = Journal of the German Society of Dermatology: JDDG* 6 (2): 121–125.
42 Michel, J.-L., Le Pillouer-Prost, A., and Misery, L. (2006). Lasers and viral tumors in children. *Medical Laser Application* 21 (3): 149–158.
43 Peterson, L.S., Nelson, A.M., and Su, W.P. (1995). Classification of morphea (localized scleroderma). *Mayo Clinic Proceedings* 70 (11): 1068–1076.
44 Weibel, L. (2012). Localized scleroderma (morphea) in childhood. *Der Hautarzt; Zeitschrift fur Dermatologie, Venerologie, und verwandte Gebiete* 63 (2): 89–96.
45 Rossi, P., Fossaluzza, V., and Gonano, L. (1985). Localized scleroderma evolving into systemic sclerosis. *The Journal of Rheumatology* 12 (3): 629–630.
46 Christianson, H.B., Dorsey, C.S., Kierland, R.R. et al. (1956). Localized scleroderma; a clinical study of two hundred thirty-five cases. *A.M.A. Archives of Dermatology* 74 (6): 629–639.
47 Torok, K.S. (2012). Pediatric scleroderma: systemic or localized forms. *Pediatric Clinics of North America* 59 (2): 381–405.
48 Pereira, N., Santiago, F., Oliveira, H. et al. (2012). Low-dose UVA(1) phototherapy for scleroderma: what benefit can we expect. *Journal of the European Academy of Dermatology and Venereology: JEADV* 26 (5): 619–626.
49 Morison, W.L. (1997). Psoralen UVA therapy for linear and generalized morphea. *Journal of the American Academy of Dermatology* 37 (4): 657–659.
50 Kreuter, A., Hyun, J., Stucker, M. et al. (2006). A randomized controlled study of low-dose UVA1, medium-dose UVA1, and

narrowband UVB phototherapy in the treatment of localized scleroderma. *Journal of the American Academy of Dermatology* 54 (3): 440–447.

51 Tan, E., Lim, D., and Rademaker, M. (2010). Narrowband UVB phototherapy in children: a New Zealand experience. *Australian Journal of Dermatology* 51 (4): 268–273.

52 Fett, N. and Werth, V.P. (2011). Update on morphea: part II. Outcome measures and treatment. *Journal of the American Academy of Dermatology* 64 (2): 231–242; quiz 243–234.

53 Su, O., Onsun, N., Onay, H.K. et al. (2011). Effectiveness of medium-dose ultraviolet A1 phototherapy in localized scleroderma. *International Journal of Dermatology* 50 (8): 1006–1013.

54 Sidbury, R., Davis, D.M., Cohen, D.E. et al. (2014). Guidelines of care for the management of atopic dermatitis: section 3. Management and treatment with phototherapy and systemic agents. *Journal of the American Academy of Dermatology* 71 (2): 327–349.

55 Dogra, S. and Mahajan, R. (2015). Phototherapy for atopic dermatitis. *Indian Journal of Dermatology, Venereology and Leprology* 81 (1): 10–15.

56 Nistico, S.P., Saraceno, R., Capriotti, E. et al. (2008). Efficacy of monochromatic excimer light (308 nm) in the treatment of atopic dermatitis in adults and children. *Photomedicine and Laser Surgery* 26 (1): 14–18.

57 Kamo, A., Tominaga, M., Kamata, Y. et al. (2014). The excimer lamp induces cutaneous nerve degeneration and reduces scratching in a dry-skin mouse model. *The Journal of Investigative Dermatology* 134 (12): 2977–2984.

58 Geller, L., Antonov, N.K., Lauren, C.T. et al. (2015). Pityriasis lichenoides in childhood: review of clinical presentation and treatment options. *Pediatric Dermatology* 32 (5): 579–592.

59 Góes, H.F.O. (2017). Lichen planopilaris developed during childhood. *Anais Brasileiros de Dermatologia* 92 (4): 543–545.

60 Sharma, A., Bialynicki-Birula, R., Schwartz, R.A. et al. (2012). Lichen planus: an update and review. *Cutis* 90 (1): 17–23.

61 Pavlotsky, F., Nathansohn, N., Kriger, G. et al. (2008). Ultraviolet-B treatment for cutaneous lichen planus: our experience with 50 patients. *Photodermatology, Photoimmunology & Photomedicine* 24 (2): 83–86.

62 Brazzelli, V., Carugno, A., Rivetti, N. et al. (2013). Narrowband UVB phototherapy for pediatric generalized pityriasis lichenoides. *Photodermatology, Photoimmunology & Photomedicine* 29 (6): 330–333.

63 Park, J.M., Jwa, S.W., Song, M. et al. (2013). Is narrowband ultraviolet B monotherapy effective in the treatment of pityriasis lichenoides? *International Journal of Dermatology* 52 (8): 1013–1018.

26

Medical Ethics and Bioethics in Pediatric Dermatology

Katlein França[1], Tulsie Narendra Patel[2], Shailee Bipin Patel[1], and Keyvan Nouri[3]

[1] *Department of Dermatology & Cutaneous Surgery, University of Miami Miller School of Medicine, Miami, FL, USA*
[2] *University of Miami Miller School of Medicine, Miami, FL, USA*
[3] *Department of Dermatology, Ophthalmology, Otolaryngology & Surgery, University of Miami Leonard M. Miller School of Medicine, Miami, FL, USA*

> *"I swear by Apollo the physician, and Aesculapius, and Health, and All-heal, and all the gods and goddesses, that, according to my ability and judgment, I will keep this Oath and this stipulation..."*
>
> Hippocrates, 5th century BCE

Since the beginning of the history of medicine, ethics has been the foundation of medical practice [1]. Hippocrates of Cos, considered one of the most outstanding figures in the history of medicine, was the founder of the "Hippocratic oath" [2, 3]. Still mentioned today at medical graduations, this requires a new physician to swear upon healing gods that he will follow a number of professional ethical standards [1, 4]. His contribution in clinical medicine was so important that many clinical and ethical terms used today have their origins in Hippocrates [4]. Other documents, decrees and laws were created afterwards to regulate medical conduct in different societies. Different countries and cultures have their health care system and own regulations that have to be followed by physicians and other health professionals [5, 6].

Medical ethics can be defined as the moral principles that apply moral, judgments, values and conduct to the medical practice [7]. The study of these principles is part of the basic medical formation and is a scholarly discipline in medical schools [8]. Present in all medical specialties, medical ethics is an upcoming field of study in the dermatology practice. The term "dermatoethics", constantly present in the recent literature, was only incorporated into medical vocabulary in the past decade [9]. The study of medical ethics in pediatric dermatology is recent and the peculiarities of this age group make this an interesting challenge [10].

Bioethics refers to the study of controversial ethical issues in the field of medicine, biology and law. It also involves the studies of philosophical, social, and legal issues arising in medicine and the life sciences [11]. The study of bioethics and applied ethics have been present since ancient times, but they are considered recent and upcoming sciences [12].

This chapter will present and discuss the most important topics related to medical ethics and bioethics in pediatric dermatology. The reader should be able to understand the concepts of ethics and bioethics, learn about the peculiarities of informed consent for children, understand the *off-label* use of medications in pediatric dermatology, comprehend the importance of the doctor–patient relationship and the definition and value of an ethics committee.

Pediatric Dermatologic Surgery, First Edition. Edited by Keyvan Nouri, Latanya Benjamin, Jasem Alshaiji, and Jan Izakovic.

26.1 Ethics and Bioethics

Dermatology is the branch of medicine concerned with the physiology and pathology of the skin [13]. Pediatric dermatologists are a group of dermatologists who are specialists in the evaluation and management of skin diseases that occur in children and adolescents [14]. Like all other specialists, this group faces numerous ethical and professional issues throughout their work day [15]. Pediatric dermatologists constantly have to decide on the best treatment for the patient in a matter of moments. These decisions can impact the patient's immediate and long-term health [10, 15, 16].

All decision-making process and procedures require ethical behavior and professional conduct [8, 15] Most dermatology residency programs do not have ethics classes incorporated in their curriculums and young dermatologists are not specifically trained to deal with certain medical dilemmas [15]. On the other hand, many dermatology societies have their own ethics committee. The American Academy of Dermatology has developed a "Code of Medical Ethics for Dermatologists" that is constantly revised by a board of directors. This code emphasizes the essentials of honorable behavior for these professionals. It also mentions the fact that dermatologists are models for other health professionals and dermatologists in training and should comply with this Code [17].

Bioethics, or biomedical ethics, is the discipline that explores the ethical questions arising in the health care setting [18]. The field encompasses decision-making issues related to patient care, covering health policy, health care delivery, and biomedical research [19, 20]. Ethics is the pursuit of providing a rationale to support the course of action one should take when dealing with a medically related predicament [21]. Thus bioethics is an applied form of ethics centered on health care provider behaviors and the ways of thinking to promote an environment to uphold the dignity of the patient [21].

The moral issues of bioethics are the rights, responsibilities, choices, and well-being of the patient, family, and care team. Bioethics is considered to be the ability to reach a social consensus about what should and should not be done in health care. This is achieved by philosophical analysis of new medical technologies and legal cases studied by health care providers, lawyers, and scientists. Combined with discussion about innovative biomedical knowledge and personal experiences, the multidisciplinary nature of bioethics helps people make informed and relevant decisions about their behavior and plan of action [18].

The ongoing change in medicine has had ripple effects within the field of dermatology. In the past decade, this specialty has seen major advancements in methods of diagnosis and management. Due to these developments, the risk-to-benefit ratio and potential conflicts of interests need thorough assessment [22].

Studying dermatoethics can help provide basic tools to deal with daily medical ethics, and learning in a group setting allows for open dialog about shared controversial cases. Following a curriculum allows for exposure to most of the realities of the clinical issues, such as the ethics of dermatologic genetics, drug pricing, and medical errors. The expectation of instilling this training during residency is that these individuals will gain the knowledge base and analytical skills to evaluate predicaments early in their professional career and thereafter will uphold the integrity of dermatology as a specialty [9, 15].

26.2 Bioethical Principles

In application, bioethics can be complicated by the difficulty of coming to a consensus about which principles should be applied based on the specifics of the situation at hand. Despite these complexities, four principles of biomedical ethics have been outlined by Beachamp and Childress, which include beneficence, nonmaleficence, justice,

Figure 26.1 Bioethical principles.

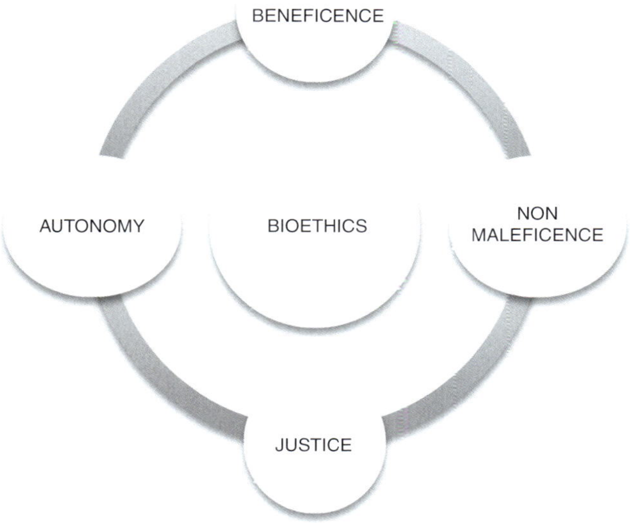

and autonomy [23]. These basic moral tenets provide the analytical platform to reflect on moral issues as they arise and to weigh them against one another while considering the scope of their application [24].

26.2.1 Beneficence and Nonmaleficence

Beneficence is the responsibility to act in ways that promote patient welfare [23]. Every health intervention has the potential to harm, so the physician must consider the risk-to-benefit ratio and act only after determining that the benefits outweigh the risks. This principle is often paired with nonmaleficence, which is the obligation that physicians should do no harm [23]. While beneficence is the active duty to help patients, nonmaleficence is the passive act to ensure not to inflict harm and the physician must balance these competing principles to produce the net benefit over harm.

26.2.2 Justice

The principle of justice describes equal and fair allocation of resources [23]. In terms of health care, it refers to evenly distributing access to care, irrespective of ability to pay. Justice involves keeping individual and collective costs in mind while providing health care [24]. It can be a challenge for a physician to determine this while personally treating a patient due to the possible conflict of interest; thus, the principle is ideally implemented at the institutional level [16]. Justice ensures that people in like situations are treated the same.

26.2.3 Autonomy

Autonomy describes the patient's privilege to make decisions about their own health, while taking into account that the patient is free from external influences and without specific impediments like incomplete comprehension to make a decision [23]. Autonomy is contingent on the patient's ability to make decisions and being provided with what they need to make informed consent. The patient must be able to remember, understand, communicate, and evaluate the issues in order to be considered to have the ability to form a decision [25]. Informed consent consists of the explanation of the procedure; alternatives to the intervention; risks, benefits, and uncertainties for each feasible option; an evaluation of patient comprehension; and voluntary approval of the health intervention by the patient [16, 23–26]. The patient's presence within a hospital does not imply that he or she is prepared to undergo every procedure, treatment, and imaging suggested by the patient health care team [26]. Many procedures require signed consent and, furthermore, physicians should also discuss and record potential important side effects for medications [25].

Autonomy also includes fulfilling patient confidentiality. The exception to this rule is when the physician believes that the duty to warn and the duty to protect take priority [26]. Confidentiality provides for the sanctity of the patient-physician relationship by allowing the patient to share sensitive and possibly convicting information to physicians without the worry that the information will be passed on to a third party. Nevertheless, a physician has the responsibility to breach confidentiality when others may be harmed, such as with sexually transmitted diseases or child, elder, or domestic partner abuse [27].

In dealing with an adult of full capacity, autonomy can be upheld in a relatively effortless manner. However, when caring for a pediatric patient, the physician will often rely on one or both of the parents to make decisions for the child. The rights of children in health care decision-making are equivocal, and physicians and parents will frequently supersede the autonomy of a child when a specific intervention is considered in the child's best interest [28]. Children are not legally autonomous, with a few exceptions; however, as they mature their decision-making capacity is more valued by the physician and their parents, in a process known as assent. The minor must be mature enough to comprehend the information and weigh the factors to establish a decision in order to be granted significant assent [28]. Each case is looked at individually based on the child's cognitive developmental and emotional maturity as well as the magnitude and potential consequences of the decision.

The origin of assent is from the concept of "respect for persons" expressed in the Belmont Report and was meant to acknowledge the child's budding autonomy and decision-making capacity [29]. In the clinical setting, there is no recommended process for minor assent. In contrast, when dealing with minors in non-therapeutic research, a maturity-based assent is mandated for children older than eight. The American Academy of Pediatrics Committee on Bioethics has outlined obtaining developmentally appropriate assent "to the greatest extent feasible" as including the minor in decision-making [30]. Regardless of whether in a clinical or a research setting, it is imperative to make the decision-making process a collaboration that interconnects the child, the parents, and the health care professional. The Committee on Bioethics also suggested that if medical intervention is going to be pursued despite the child's dissent, the health care provider should be open and inform the child [28].

The American Academy of Pediatrics Committee on Bioethics promotes using the term "informed permission" instead of "informed consent" to refer to the process of pediatric decision-making. This is to highlight the fact that the autonomous choices of the minor do not create the platform of substituted judgment [30]. Parents serve as a proxy decision-maker and typically choose options that they deem to be in the best interest of their child and the family parallel to their value system. In most cases courts have respected the legal authority of the parents to make a decision as long as there was no risk to the child's well-being [31]. Maintaining ethical practice necessitates the physician to be aware and respectful of the cultural, religious, educational, and other personal views that can influence the patient's and the proxy's outlook on the consent process. In cases where the parents and physician disagree, the physician should politely take note of their perspective and try to reach a cooperative reasonable agreement [28]. In situations where this is not possible, the physician has a moral duty to promote for the best interests of the child, while also being aware of the parent's legal authority.

26.3 Informed Consent or Informed Permission in Pediatric Dermatology

Determining the treatment for a child is radically different than for an adult [32, 33]. When treating an adult, the physician is able to logically explain the entire treatment plan to the patient [32, 34]. The patient then undergoes the treatment if he/she consents [32]. Children, however, are considered vulnerable with respect to their treatment and how it is decided, as their understanding and decision-making process is not developed enough to provide true consent [32–34].

Although they are granted their basic human rights, their ability to make decisions about their medical care is more complex [10]. For the most part, the decision of the physician or parent is considered more highly until the child reaches the age at which he/she is thought to be capable of making his/her own decision [10, 33]. Because children are so different in their maturity and development, there is no one age at which this transition becomes official [10, 33, 34]. This transition is known as "assent" [32].

The "informed permission" term was created to better explain a system that allows for the child's parents to make decisions about the child's medical care, in association with their physician [30, 32]. This permission is granted as long as it is judged to be in the patient's best interest and for the best interest of his/her family and the cultural and religious values they uphold [30, 32]. This responsibility is allotted to a child's parents, specifically, because they are assumed to know and understand the child the best [32].

A child is given the ability to take over the control of their care when they have undergone assent and are therefore able to rationally make these decisions by and for themselves [32]. This autonomy is encouraged through the introduction of the child into the medical decision-making process earlier in their care [32, 33]. As children grow older, they become more aware of their bodies and medical conditions and should be encouraged to be involved in their treatment by their parents and physicians [31]. However, the time at which this occurs varies by child [32–34].

There are some exceptions to parental consent [32, 33]. The three major ones include decisions for a mature minor, an emancipated minor, and emergency treatment for a child [32]. Mature minors are individuals who have taken legal action to prove that they are mature enough to handle making their own medical decisions [32, 34]. Emancipated minors include individuals who are older than 16 who are self-sufficient and live separately from their parents, or are part of the armed services, are pregnant or already have a child, or are married [32]. Emergency situations allow for a child to be treated when necessary as it is assumed that a parent would approve of the treatment if they were present at the time [32, 35]. Other exceptions include access to testing and treatment for sexually transmitted diseases, access to outpatient drug/alcohol counseling, and access to treatment for sexual abuse [32]. Most states also allow access to contraceptives and family planning services without parental consent as well [32, 36]. Abortion, however, requires parental consent in most states [32].

With assent and the development of a child into an independent young adult, the importance of confidentiality also arises [32–34]. While a child is under parental consent, the parents are given access to all of their child's medical reports so that they can make an informed decision [32]. However, as children become more aware, such as when they reach adolescence, the physician may choose to grant the child greater confidentiality, when possible and safe [32, 33]. This is important in developing a better relationship between the patient and the physician for all future care [32].

Overall, informed consent plays a major role in the dermatological treatment of a child [10, 32]. Parents and physicians ideally work together to provide the best possible care for the child until he/she reaches an age where he/she can not only be involved in the patient-parent-physician dynamic but also eventually take ownership of the patient-physician relationship [32].

26.4 Use of Off- Label Medications in Pediatric Dermatology

The use of off-label medications, drugs that have not been officially approved for treatment of a specific condition, has become more common in the field of pediatric dermatology as the Food and Drug Administration (FDA) has yet to approve medications for patients younger than the standard, 12 years old, for numerous conditions [37, 38]. Studies have shown that nearly 12% of off-label use in children is to treat dermatological conditions [10]. These drugs include nystatin, mupirocin, and pimecrolimus, to name a few [10, 39, 40]. However, this practice is lawful, and most importantly, ethical, when the patient's best interest is the top priority [10, 37] The acceptance of this practice has come about most notably through need; for example, as even younger children are struggling with acne vulgaris as puberty is undergone earlier [41–43]. Further, many pediatric dermatological cases are rare and must therefore be treated using the experience and personal knowledge of the physician, as research may not have been completed on every special condition [10, 37, 38].

Many off-label drugs have shown their efficacy in and application toward this new patient population [41]. Physicians are most often drawn to use off-label medications because there are only a few FDA-approved drugs for preadolescents [41, 44]. As of 2002, nearly 75% of prescription medications did not contain information regarding use in pediatrics [10]. This is due to the fact that clinical trials are more complicated and expensive when conducted on children [10, 45]. Therefore, physicians must often take into account small studies as reference for possible outcomes and thus assess the benefits-to-risks ratio using their own judgment [44]. For example, physicians have effectively prescribed off-label medications such as tacrolimus and pimecrolimus for the treatment of atopic dermatitis in patients as young as two years old [44, 46, 47]. The gold standard in topical therapies, topical retinoids, has recently been shown to be successful in treating acne vulgaris in patients as young as seven years old and minocycline, an oral antibiotic, is often prescribed to patients as young as eight years old to treat acne [41, 42, 48]. Another important consideration in the use of off-label medications in pediatric dermatology is the way in which different specialties treat conditions, such as acne vulgaris [41]. Studies have shown that general pediatricians tend to prescribe oral antibiotics, whereas pediatric dermatologists most often choose to treat patients with a topical treatment [1–43]. This is important because it indicates that there are numerous treatment options for these children and that further research will help to better develop and distinguish drugs that are not only effective but also truly suited for this population [41]. Thus, the use of off-label medications has been shown to not only be effective in the treatment of pediatric dermatology, but also necessary, until further studies are done and approval is granted by the FDA for their use, or the use of new drugs, on preadolescents [10].

26.5 Doctor-Patient Relationship in Pediatric Dermatology

A solid and long-lasting doctor-patient relationship is critically important in any field of medicine. However, a great deal of importance is placed on the relationship that a pediatric dermatologist has with his/her patient [49, 50]. These relationships are not only important in discerning what is necessary to care for the patient but also to enhance the patient's and parents' experience and compliance [51].

Numerous factors must be taken into consideration when treating a patient, in dermatology and in all other fields of medicine [10]. Most importantly, the physician must maintain an outlook of acting in the best interest of patient through a balanced approach [10, 49]. Further, the physician must always account for the personal, religious, and cultural preferences of the patient, where possible [10].

At different stages in a patient's life, they require different attention from their dermatologist [51]. For example, patients in their infancy are soothed most often through attention that the physician provides the accompanying parents [51]. Parents of an ill child often assume responsibility for what is occurring and must therefore be taken care of along with the infant patient [10, 51]. Once a child enters early childhood, he/she is more cognizant of their environment and body [51]. Simple explanations must be offered for treatment and procedures to ensure that the child is comfortable [51]. School-aged children are greatly focused on acceptance by their peers and are even more capable of understanding their condition [51, 52]. This is a great time for a dermatologist to include the child in the treatment considerations, along with his/her parent [51]. Adolescents are focused on body image and rapid results [51]. Therefore, in order to ensure compliance, physicians must create an alliance with their adolescent patients, most often stemming from the idea of trust and confidentiality [51–53].

In pediatric dermatology, an important balance must be maintained in that a patient's care may evolve from a patient-parent-physician relationship to one in which the patient becomes more involved and vocal over time [10]. It is important for the physician to understand this transition and to help it come about smoothly and safely [10, 52, 53]. The true foundation of medical care is trust and it is important to maintain that value in all relationships [51]. For example, a patient, once an adolescent, may no longer wish to discuss everything with their parent present, such as sexually transmitted conditions [51]. In order to provide the patient with the best care, physicians must establish a new sense of confidentiality, stemming from a good understanding with the whole family [51, 53]. Thus the nature of these doctor-patient relationships is not only ever-changing but also vital to ensuring that the proper care is attained [51, 52].

26.6 Ethics Committee: A Help for Medical Dilemmas

Predecessors of modern-day Hospital Ethics Committees (HECs) in the United States began as groups to discuss morals in medicine around the 1960s [54]. Around that time abortion review committees and kidney dialysis selection committees were propping up around the country [55]. The initial published recommendation to form HECs was in the early 1970s by Pediatrician Karen Teel, who suggested creating HECs to allow dialog for professionals in specific clinical situations [56]. Thereafter in 1992, the Joint Commission for the Accreditation of Healthcare Organizations mandated that hospitals have a means to address ethical disputes, which led to several states requiring their hospitals to have ethics committees [57].

The role of an Ethics Committee can vary between hospitals and regions; however, three functions are agreed upon, which include case review, policy advice, and staff education [58]. These committees are encouraged to be a multidisciplinary group including bioethicists, physicians, residents, nurses, social workers, clergy, administrators, and lay members. The diversity, including gender, ethnicity, political viewpoints, and professional background, of the group is important in providing a variety of different perspectives to address the intricacies of the case at hand [59]. The main functions outlined by the Universal Draft

Declaration on Bioethics and Human Rights [54] are: counsel on ethical issues in the clinical setting [55]; evaluating technological and scientific developments and formulate recommendations [56]; and encouraging debate, education, and public awareness of bioethics [59]. In addition, the group promotes resolution of conflict in an appropriate manner while influencing institutional policies to be of highest ethical standards [60].

Ethical issues can be hard to decipher, as there is not necessarily a right or a wrong answer but only a scaffold of bioethical principles. Dermatology as a field has significantly evolved in the recent years, requiring vigilant evaluation of the risk-to-benefit ratio and also possible conflicts of interests. With changes including electronic communication, social networking, medical spas, and dermatologic genetics, it is important to consider utilizing the advice of HECs to help maneuver physicians through these intricate dilemmas [15]. Furthermore, when dermatologists stay informed about how to avoid ethical conundrums and resolve issues in a sound way, the specialty can maintain its integrity and professionalism.

26.7 Conclusion

The medical profession is entirely based on ethical statements that focus on the benefit of the patient. Ethical and bioethical principles are the standards of medical conduct and a guide for the honorable behavior expected from a physician. Pediatric dermatologists are constantly exposed to conflicting situations and medical dilemmas in their practice. The particularities of the informed consent for this age population as well as the doctor–patient relationship that has to be extended to parents are important topics presented in this chapter. The off-label use of medications in pediatric dermatology was also discussed by the authors, since new medications are proving to be effective in this population. Solving medical dilemmas and getting right answers for ethical questions can be a challenge in medical practice. Consulting an ethics committee may be important to clarify controversial issues and treat patients accordingly. The study of ethical and bioethical issues in pediatric dermatology is an evolving field. The new challenges, behaviors and values of the coming generations will require the physician to be constant updated on ethics and bioethics subjects.

References

1 Cunningham, B. and Wagner, A.M. (2011). Surgical techniques. In: *Pediatric Dermatology* (ed. L.A. Schachner and R.C. Hansen), 222. Philadelphia, PA: Elsevier Mosby.

2 Bujalkova, M. (2001). Hippocrates and his principles of medical ethics. *Bratisl. Lek. Listy* 102 (2): 117–120.

3 Imran, M., Samad, S., Maaz, M. et al. (2013). Hippocratic oath and conversion of ethico-regulatory aspects onto doctors as a physician, private individual and a clinical investigator. *J. Midlife Health* 4 (4): 203–209.

4 Yapijakis, C. (2009). Hippocrates of Kos, the father of clinical medicine, and Asclepiades of Bithynia, the father of molecular medicine. Review. *In Vivo* 23 (4): 507–514.

5 Jones, P., Seoane, L., Deichmann, R. et al. (2011). Differences and similarities in the practice of medicine between Australia and the United States of America: challenges and opportunities for the University of Queensland and the Ochsner clinical school. *Ochsner J.* 11 (3): 253–258.

6 Corallo, A., Croxford, R., Goodman, D. et al. (2014). A systematic review of medical practice variation in OECD countries. *Health Policy* 114 (1): 5–14. https://doi.org/10.1016/j.healthpol.2013.08.002.

7 Clarke, D.D. and Clarke, D.M. (1977). Analysis: an introduction to ethical concepts. Definition and ethical decisions. *J. Med. Ethics* 3 (4): 186–188.

8 Mills, S. and Bryden, D.C. (2010). A practical approach to teaching medical ethics. *J. Med. Ethics* 36 (1): 50–54. https://doi.org/10.1136/jme.2009.031153.

9 Bercovitch, L. and Long, T.P. (2007). Dermatoethics: a curriculum in bioethics and professionalism for dermatology residents at Brown Medical School. *J. Am. Acad. Dermatol.* 56 (4): 679–682.

10 Kelly, J.B. 3rd and Makkar, H.S. (2012). Ethics in pediatric dermatology. *Clin. Dermatol.* Patients' rights 30 (5): 471–475. https://doi.org/10.1016/j.clindermatol.2011.06.014.

11 Dell'Oro, R. (2013). Why bioethics? On the anamnesis of meaning in medicine. *Med. Law* 32 (2): 163–176.

12 Encyclopaedia Britannica Online (2014) Bioethics. www.britannica.com/EBchecked/topic/65851/bioethics (accessed 5 January 2014).

13 Encyclopaedia Britannica Online (2014) Dermatology. www.britannica.com/EBchecked/topic/158586/dermatology (accessed 6 January 2014).

14 American Academy of Dermatology (2014) What is a pediatric dermatologist? American Academy of Dermatology. www.aad.org/dermatology-a-to-z/about-dermatology/what-is-a-pediatric-dermatologist (accessed 6 January 2014).

15 Bercovitch, L. and Long, T.P. (2009). Ethics education for dermatology residents. *Clin. Dermatol.* 27 (4): 405–410. https://doi.org/10.1016/j.clindermatol.2009.02.015.

16 Hansra, N.K., Shinkai, K., and Fox, L.P. (2012). Ethical issues in inpatient consultative dermatology. *Clin. Dermatol.* 30 (5): 496–500. https://doi.org/10.1016/j.clindermatol.2011.06.019.

17 American Academy of Dermatology (2014) Code of medical ethics for dermatologists. www.aad.org/Forms/Policies/Uploads/AR/AR%20Code%20of%20Medical%20Ethics%20for%20Dermatologists.pdf (accessed 6 January 2014).

18 McWhirter, R.E. (2012). The history of bioethics: implications for current debates in health research. *Perspect. Biol. Med.* 55 (3): 329–338.

19 Beauchamp, T.L. and Childress, J.F. (1979). *Principles of Biomedical Ethics*. New York: Oxford University.

20 Veatch, R. (1997). *Medical Ethics: An Introduction*. Sudbury, MA: Jones and Barlett.

21 NIH Staff (2010). *Exploring Bioethics*. Newton, MA: Education Development Center.

22 Carroll, K.A. (2006). Dermatology and the changing face of medicine, virtual mentor. *Am. Med. Assoc. J. Ethics* 8 (8): 493–494.

23 Beauchamp, T.L. and Childress, J.F. (2008). *Principles of Biomedical Ethics*, 432. Oxford: Oxford University Press.

24 Vevaina, J.R., Nora, L.M., and Bone, R.C. (1993). Issues in biomedical ethics. *Dis. Mon. Dec.* 39 (12): 869–925.

25 Lepping, P. (2009). Consent and capacity for dermatologists: an ethical review and update. *Clin. Exp. Dermatol.* 34: 655–657.

26 Rajput, V. and Bekes, C.E. (2002). Ethical issues in hospital medicine. *Med. Clin. North Am.* 86: 869–886.

27 Pantilat, S., Alpers, A., and Wachter, R. (1999). A new doctor in the house: ethical issues in hospitalist systems. *JAMA* 281: 171–174.

28 Berkovitch, L. and Clifford, P. (eds.) (2012). *Dermatoethics: Contemporary Ethics and Professionalism in Dermatology*. London: Springer.

29 The National Commission for the Protection of Human Subjects of Biomedical and Behavioral Research (2014). *The Belmont Report: Ethical Principles and Guidelines for the Protection of Human Subjects of Research*. New York: Office of the Secretary Department of Health, Education, and Welfare.

30 Committee on Bioethics, American Academy of Pediatrics (1995). Informed consent, parental permission, and assent in pediatric practice. *Pediatrics* 95: 314–317.

31 Diekema, D.S. (2009). Boldt v. boldt: a pediatric ethics perspective. *J. Clin. Ethics* 3: 251–257.

32 Bloom, K. and Bercovitch, L. (2012). "Who Speaks for the Child?" Consent, assent, and confidentiality in pediatric dermatology. In: *Dermatoethics: Contemporary Ethics and Professionalism in Dermatology* (ed. L. Berkovitch and P. Clifford), 25–31. London: Springer.

33 Kaushik, J.S., Narang, M., and Agarwal, N. (2010). Informed consent in pediatric practice. *Indian Pediatr.* 47 (12): 1039–1046.

34 Bartholome, W.G. (1995). Informed consent, parental permission, and assent in pediatric practice. *Pediatrics* 96 (5 Pt 1): 981–982.

35 Thewes, J., FitzGerald, D., and Sulmasy, D.P. (1996). Informed consent in emergency medicine: ethics under fire. *Emerg. Med. Clin. North Am.* 14 (1): 245–254.

36 Thompson, H.A. (1989). Consent requirements for treatment of minors. *Tex. Med.* 85 (8): 56–59.

37 Hsu, B. and Brazelton, T. (2009). Off-label medication use in an academic hospital pediatric critical care unit. *WMJ* 108 (7): 343–348.

38 Gavrilov, V., Lifshitz, M., Levy, J. et al. (2000). Unlicensed and off-label medication use in a general pediatrics ambulatory hospital unit in Israel. *Isr. Med. Assoc. J.* 2 (8): 595–597.

39 Manthripragada, A.D., Pinheiro, S.P., MaCurdy, T.E. et al. (2013). Off-label topical calcineurin inhibitor use in children. *Pediatrics* 132 (5): e1327–e1332. https://doi.org/10.1542/peds.2013-0931. Epub 2013 Oct 14.

40 Lepainteur, M., Royer, G., Bourrel, A.S. et al. (2013). Prevalence of resistance to antiseptics and mupirocin among invasive coagulase-negative staphylococci from very preterm neonates in NICU: the creeping threat? *J. Hosp. Infect.* 83 (4): 333–336. https://doi.org/10.1016/j.jhin.2012.11.025. Epub 2013 Feb 13.

41 Davis, S.A., Sandoval, L.F., Gustafson, C.J. et al. (2013). Treatment of preadolescent acne in the United States: an analysis of nationally representative data. *Pediatr. Dermatol.* 30 (6): 689–694. https://doi.org/10.1111/pde.12201. Epub 2013 Jul 22.

42 Schnopp, C. and Mempel, M. (2011). Acne vulgaris in children and adolescents. *Minerva Pediatr.* 63 (4): 293–304.

43 Bergfeld, W.F. (2004). The pathophysiology of acne vulgaris in children and adolescents, part 2: tailoring treatment. *Cutis* 74 (3): 189–192.

44 Sidbury, R. (2004). What's new in pediatric dermatology: update for the pediatrician. *Curr. Opin. Pediatr.* 16 (4): 410–414.

45 Khan-Boluki, J. and Hundt, F. (2008). Children in clinical trials: survey on the current situation in pediatric university clinics in Germany. *Ger. Med. Sci.* 6: Doc01.

46 Remitz, A., Harper, J., Rustin, M. et al. (2007). Long-term safety and efficacy of tacrolimus ointment for the treatment of atopic dermatitis in children. *Acta Derm. Venereol.* 87 (1): 54–61.

47 Fowler, J., Johnson, A., Chen, M. et al. (2007). Improvement in pruritus in children with atopic dermatitis using pimecrolimus cream 1%. *Cutis* 79 (1): 65–72.

48 Brecher, A.R. and Orlow, S.J. (2003). Oral retinoid therapy for dermatologic conditions in children and adolescents. *J. Am. Acad. Dermatol.* 49 (2): 171–182; quiz 183–6.

49 Poot, F. (2009). Doctor-patient relations in dermatology: obligations and rights for a mutual satisfaction. *J. Eur. Acad. Dermatol. Venereol.* 23 (11): 1233–1239. https://doi.org/10.1111/j.1468-3083.2009.03297.x. Epub 2009 May 19.

50 França, K. (2012). *A Dermatologia e o Relacionamento Médico-Paciente-Aspectos Psicossociais e Bioéticos.* Curitiba: Editora Juruá.

51 Rauch, P. and Jellinek, M.S. (1986). Developmental and psychosocial considerations in pediatric dermatology practice. *Pediatr. Dermatol.* 3 (5): 380–383.

52 Tates, K., Elbers, E., Meeuwesen, L. et al. (2002). Doctor-parent-child relationships: a 'pasde trois'. *Patient Educ. Couns.* 48 (1): 5–14.

53 Tates, K. and Meeuwesen, L. (2001). Doctor-parent-child communication. A (re)view of the literature. *Soc. Sci. Med.* 52 (6): 839–851.

54 McGee, G., Spanogle, J.P., Caplan, A.L. et al. (2002). Success and failures of hospital ethics committees: a national survey of ethics committee chairs. *Camb. Q. Healthc. Ethics* 11: 87–93.

55 Sanders, J. (2004). Developing clinical ethics committees. *Clin. Med.* 4: 232–234.

56 Teel, K. (1975). The physician's dilemma, a doctor's view: what the law should be. *Bayl. Law Rev.* 27: 6–9.

57 Joint Commision for the Accreditation of Healthcare Organizations (1992). *Accreditation Manual of Hospitals*. Chicago, IL: JCAHO.

58 Moreno, J.D. (2010). Ethics Committees and Ethics Consultants. In: *A Companion to Bioethics*, 2e (ed. H. Kuhse and P. Singer), 573–583. Oxford: Wiley-Blackwell.

59 UNESCO (2005). *Explanatory Memorandum on the Elaboration of the Preliminary Draft Declaration on the Universal Norms of Bioethics*. Paris: UNESCO.

60 Fletcher, J.C. and Siegler, M. (1996). What are the goals of ethics consultation? A consensus statement. *J. Clin. Ethics* 7: 122–126.

Index

a

AA *see* alopecia areata
ablative lasers 199–200
absorbable staples 121
absorbable sutures 117, 118, 154
ACC *see* aplasia cutis congenita
acetaminophen 144–146
acne
  intra-lesional injections 88
  laser therapy 207–221
    complications 218–219
    indications 208–209
    infrared diode 209–212, 217–218
    intense pulsed light 216
    narrowband light 209–210, 217
    photodynamic therapy 212, 218, 219
    potassium titanyl phosphate 216–217
    pulsed-dye laser 212–216
acquired nevi 173
actinobacteria colonization 18
adaptation, at birth 13–14
adhesives 102, 121–122
adipose tissue, differentiation 5
adolescents
  anxiety 29
  diagnosis 25–26
  skin structure and function 19–21
adrenarche 19
Adson forceps 40, 43
advancement flaps 112
adverse events
  chemosurgery 81
  cryosurgery 75–77
  curettage 79
  electrosurgery 84–85
  general anesthesia 57–58
  local anesthetics 53
  see also complications
5-ALA *see* 5-aminolevulinic acid
alexandrite lasers
  hair removal 281–282
  pigmented lesion laser therapy 243, 246–248, 250
  tattoo removal 258–259
alginate dressings 128–129
alopecia areata (AA)
  intra-lesional injections 86
  laser therapy 289–291
aluminum chloride 41
American College of Surgeons and Center of Disease Control classifications of wounds 129
5-aminolevulinic acid (5-ALA) 236
AMPs *see* antimicrobial peptides
analgesics
  postoperative 35
  preoperative preparation 33
anesthesia 49–61
  explanation of 33–34
  general 56–58
  injectable 52–56
  injection pain reduction 53–54
  laser therapies 193
  local 49–56
  local excision trays 42–43
  nail surgery 132
  nerve blocks 55–56
  topical 49–52, 147–148

Pediatric Dermatologic Surgery, First Edition. Edited by Keyvan Nouri, Latanya Benjamin, Jasem Alshaiji, and Jan Izakovic.

antibiotics 152–154
anti-inflammatories, non-steroidal 33
antimicrobial peptides (AMPs), infants 19
anxiety 27–29, 32–34, 147–148
aplasia cutis congenita (ACC) 176–177
apocrine glands 20
appendage formation 6–7
argon lasers 189–190
assessment, pain 143–144
A-T flaps 111–112
atopic dermatitis 297
atrophic scars 199–206
autonomy 305
avulsion of nails 133–136
axillary hyperhidrosis 88–89

b

bacteria
  adolescent skin 20
  childhood skin 20
  infants 16, 17–18
  neonates 15
  postoperative infections 151–154
bandaging of nails 138–139
barrier function
  adolescents 20–21
  childhood skin 20
  infantile skin 18
  neonates 14, 15
basal cell carcinoma (BCC) 80, 179
basal cell nevus syndrome (BCNS) 179
basal cells
  morphogenesis 4
  specification 2
basic wound dressings 125–126
BCC *see* basal cell carcinoma
BCNS *see* basal cell nevus syndrome
Beaver blade handles 43
Becker's nevi 242, 248–249
beneficence 305
bioethics 303–313
  doctor–patient relationships 308–309
  Hospital Ethics Committees 309–310
  informed consent 307–308
  off-label medications 308
  principles 304–306
biopsies 63–71
  complications 69–70
  excisional 69
  general principles 37–38
  incisional 69
  nails 136–137
  preparation 63–64
  punch 38–41, 64–65, 136–137
  scissors 67–69
  shave 39, 44, 65–67, 137
  surgical trays 37–41
bipolar electrosurgery 82, 83–84
Bishop–Harmon forceps 43, 44
bleeding, postoperative 148–149
Botox *see* botulinum toxin injections
botulinum toxin (Botox) injections 88–89
Brown–Adson forceps 40
bupivacaine 52–53
buried vertical mattress sutures 97–99
burns, prevention, electrosurgery 84

c

café au lait macules (CALMs) 242–244, 246–248
camouflage, wound closure 108
capillarity of sutures 116
carbon dioxide (CO_2) lasers
  onychomycosis 231
  scars and striae 199, 202–203
  vascular lesions 189–190
  verrucae 224–226
carcinoembryonic antigen (CEA) 6–7
Castroviejo forceps 43
CDC *see* Center for Disease Control
CEA *see* carcinoembryonic antigen
cell proliferation, infants 19
Center for Disease Control (CDC) wound classifications 150
chalazion clamps 43, 44
characteristics of sutures 115–120
chemical nail surgery 133
chemosurgery 79–81
children
  anxiety 29
  developmental evaluation 32
  diagnosis 25
  medical evaluation 31–32
  as patients 23–29
  skin structure and function 19–21
  treatment plan discussion 32–33
chorionic villus sampling 1–2

classifications
  hirsutism 279
  vascular lesions 190–191
  wounds 129, 150
clean-contaminated wounds 129
cleansing agents 44
clean wounds 129
CMN *see* congenital melanocytic nevi
codeine 146–147
coefficients of friction 116
CO_2 lasers *see* carbon dioxide lasers
collagens
  differentiation 5
  specification 2–3
combination laser therapies
  scarring 203
  verrucae 225–226
common procedures 73–91
  chemosurgery 79–81
  cryosurgery 73–77
  curettage 77–79
  electrosurgery 81–85
  intra-lesional injections 85–89
complications 143–159
  biopsies 69–70
  bleeding and hematoma 148–149
  botulinum toxin injections 89
  chemosurgery 81
  cryosurgery 75–77
  curettage 79
  dehiscence of wounds 155–157
  electrosurgery 84–85
  general anesthesia 57–58
  infections 150–154
  laser therapies
    acne 218–219
    hair removal 283–284
    onychomycosis 237
    pigmented lesions 250–251
    scars and striae 202–203
    tattoo removal 266–267
    vascular lesions 195
  local anesthetics 53
  medical evaluation 31–32
  nail surgery 140
  non-opiod analgesics 144–145
  opiod analgesics 146–147
  pain 143–148
  postoperative care 35–36
  scarring 157
  seroma 150
  suture reactions 154–155
  wound closure 113, 122–123
components
  biopsy trays 37–41
  local excision trays 41–44
  nail trays 45–47
  punch biopsy trays 38–41
  shave biopsy trays 39, 44
  suture removal trays 44–45
composition
  adolescent skin 19–20
  childhood skin 19–20
  infantile skin 16, 17
  neonatal skin 14
congenital melanocytic nevi (CMN) 78, 172–173, 241, 245–246
consent 307–308
contaminated wounds 129
continuous wave (CW) lasers 189–190
contraindications
  chemosurgery 80
  cryosurgery 75
  curettage 78
  intra-lesional injections 165–166
  laser scar reduction therapy 167
  onychomycosis laser therapy 230
  pigmented lesion laser therapy 243–244
  scar massage 163
  silicone scar reduction products 163
  tattoo removal 258–259
corneocytes
  infants 16–17
  neonatal skin 15
corticosteroids 86–87, 164–166
cosmetics, wound closure 108
crescentic excisions 109–110
cryosurgery 73–77
curettage 77–79
curettes 39, 44
Cushing's syndrome 166
cutaneous nerves, specification 2–3
CW *see* continuous wave
cyanoacrylates 121

d

Davis and Geck needles 120
DC *see* dermoid cysts

deep sutures 97–100
dehiscence, postoperative 155–157
DEJ *see* dermoepidermal junction
depth classifications of wounds 129
DermaBlade 41
dermatofibrosarcoma protuberans (DFSP) 80, 179
dermis
  differentiation 5
  morphogenesis 4
  specification 2–3
dermoepidermal junction (DEJ)
  differentiation 5
  morphogenesis 4
  specification 3
dermoid cysts (DC) 177
dermosubcutaneous vascular plexus 4
design principles, wound closure 107–108
desmopressin 140
developmental evaluation 32
DFSP *see* dermatofibrosarcoma protuberans
diagnosis
  correct procedures 24–26
  developmental evaluation 32
  medical evaluation 31–32
differentiation 1, 4–5
digital nerve block 55
digits
  nail surgery 133–141
  nerve blocks 55
  scissor biopsies 68–69
  sweat gland formation 6–7
diode lasers
  acne treatment 209–212, 217–218
  hair removal 282
  onychomycosis 233, 235
dirty wounds 129
discussions
  anesthesia 33–34
  anxiety management 27–29
  further evaluations 26–27
  hirsutism 275–280
  parent education 26
  treatment modalities 27
  treatment plans 32–33
doctor–patient relationships 308–309
dog ears 107–108
dorsal hands, scissor biopsies 69
double-action nail splitters 45
dressings 125–130
  basic 125–126
  nails 138–139
  occlusive 126–129
  wound classifications 129

e

EB *see* epidermolysis bullosa
eccrine sweat glands
  adolescent skin 20
  embryogenesis 6–7
education of parents 26, 274–275
EDV *see* epidermodysplasia verruciformis
EGA *see* estimated gestational age
ELA-Max 85
elasticity of sutures 116, 118–119
elastin, specification 2
electrocautery 41, 43, 81–83
electrocoagulation 82, 84
electrodessication 82, 83
electrofulguration 82, 83
electrosection 82–84
electrosurgery 81–85
embryogenesis 1–12
  appendage formation 6–7
  differentiation 1, 4–5
  eccrine sweat glands 6–7
  keratinization 4, 6
  morphogenesis 1, 3–4
  nail formation 4, 6
  periderm 5–8
  pilosebaceous apparatus 7–8
  regionalization 6
  specification 1, 2–3
embryonic development 1–3
embryonic-fetal transition 3–4
EMLA *see* Eutectic Mixture of Local Anesthetics
EN *see* epidermal nevus
English anvil-action nail splitters 136
epidermal nevus (EN) 176
epidermis
  differentiation 4–5
  layers of 15
  morphogenesis 3–4
  neonatal 14
  specification 2
epidermodysplasia verruciformis (EDV) 78
epidermolysis bullosa (EB) 178

erbium-doped yttrium-aluminum-garnet (Er:YAG) lasers 200, 202–203, 243–251
estimated gestational age (EGA) 1
Ethicon needles 120
ethics 303–313
  committees 309–310
  doctor–patient relationships 308–309
  informed consent 307–308
  off-label medications 308
  principles 304–306
Eutectic Mixture of Local Anesthetics (EMLA) 50, 85
evaluation
  developmental 32
  nail surgery 132
  wound gaps 99–100
excessive sweating *see* hyperhidrosis
excisional biopsies 69
excisions, nails 137–138
explanation
  of anesthesia 33–34
  of procedure 34
  of treatment plan 32–33
  see also discussion

f

facial lesions, nerve blocks 55–56
feet, scissor biopsies 69
Ferriman–Gallwey hirsutism scoring system 279
fetal development 1–12
  appendage formation 6–7
  differentiation 1, 4–5
  eccrine sweat glands 6–7
  keratinization 4, 6
  nail formation 4, 6
  periderm 5–8
  pilosebaceous apparatus 7–8
  regionalization 6
  specification 1, 2–3
fetal skin biopsy 2
fibrillin, specification 2
film dressings 126
fingers
  nail surgery 131–141
  nerve blocks 55
  scissor biopsies 68–69
firmicutes, infantile skin 17
fluorouracil (5-FU) 203
foam dressings 126–127
forceps 40, 41, 43, 44, 95
forehead, nerve blocks 55
Freer septum elevators 134
freezing *see* cryosurgery
frequency-doubled Q-switched lasers 190
friction coefficients 116
5-FU *see* fluorouracil
full nail avulsion 133
full-thickness wounds 129
functions
  childhood/adolescent skin 20–21
  infantile skin 16, 18–19
  neonatal skin 14–15
fungal nails *see* onychomycosis
further evaluations, discussion of 26–27

g

GCMN *see* giant congenital melanocytic nevus
general anesthesia 34, 56–58
genitalia, scissor biopsies 68
gestation, estimated age 1
giant congenital melanocytic nevus (GCMN) 78, 172–173
giant juvenile xanthogranuloma 178
Gradle tissue scissors 43
granulomas 154–155
greater occipital nerve block 56
guiding sutures 111

h

hair removal 273–274, 280–287
  Ferriman–Gallwey scoring 279
  laser therapies 273–274, 280–287
  light hair 283
  parental education 274–275
  patient-centered care 275–280
  thermal relaxation time 280
half-buried vertical mattress sutures 101
Halsey needle drivers 40
Halsted hemostats 133, 134–135
handles for scalpels 43
handling characteristics of sutures 116–119
Healy forceps 44
hemangiomas of infancy *see* infantile hemangiomas
hematomas, postoperative 148–149
hemidesmosome differentiation 5
hemoglobin, light absorbtion 189

hemostatic agents 47, 69–70
hemostats 43, 46, 133
herpes labialis 32
hirsutism 273–287
  causes 276
  Ferriman–Gallwey scoring 279
  laser hair removal 273–274, 280–287
  light hair removal 283
  parental education 274–275
  patient-centered care 275–280
home care, post nail surgery 139
horizontal mattress sutures 101
Hospital Ethics Committees (HECs) 309–310
HTS *see* hypertrophic scars
hydrocodone 146–147
hydrocolloid dressings 128
hydrogel dressings 127–128
hyperhidrosis 88–89
hypertrichosis 273–287
  causes 278
  laser hair removal 273–274, 280–287
  light hair removal 283
  parental education 274–275
  patient-centered care 275–280
hypertrophic scars (HTS) 161–169, 197–206
  formation 198
  intra-lesional injections 86–87, 164–166
  laser therapies 197–206
  laser therapy 166–167
  massage 163
  silicone products 164
  topical therapies 167
hypodermis *see* subcutis

i

IH *see* infantile hemangiomas
IL-TAC *see* intralegional triamcinolone
immune regulation
  childhood skin 20
  infant skin 19
improvement of scars 161–169
incisional biopsies 69
indications
  acne laser therapies 208–209
  chemosurgery 80
  cryosurgery 74–75
  curettage 77–78
  general anesthesia 56–57
  intra-lesional injections 86–89
  local anesthesia 49
  onychomycosis laser therapy 230
  pigmented lesion laser therapy 243–244
  tattoo removal 258–259
  verruca laser therapies 223–224
infantile hemangiomas (IH) 87–88, 174–175, 191–192
infants
  anxiety 29
  developmental evaluation 32
  diagnosis 25
  medical evaluation 31–32
  as patients 23–29
  skin characteristics 15–19
  treatment plan discussion 32–33
infections
  biopsies 70
  electrosurgery 85
  nail surgery 140
  postoperative 150–154
  postoperative avoidance 35–36
inflamed cysts, intra-lesional injections 88
informed consent/permission 307–308
infraorbital nerve block 55–56
infrared 1450nm diode lasers 209–212, 217–218
initial consultations 23–24
injectable local anesthesia 52–56
innate immunity, infants 19
Insorb staples 121
instrument ties 95–96
intense pulsed light (IPL)
  acne 216
  hair removal 282
  pigmented lesions 243–246
  tattoo removal 262
  vascular lesions 190
interrupted sutures 100
intralegional triamcinolone (IL-TAC) 86–88
intra-lesional injections 85–89, 164–166
iontophoresis 51
IPL *see* intense pulsed light
iris tissue scissors 43, 134
ischemia, tourniquets 133

j

justice 305
juvenile xanthogranuloma (JXG) 178
JXG *see* juvenile xanthogranuloma

k

keloids 161–169, 197–206
- formation 198
- intra-lesional injections 86–87, 164–166
- laser therapies 197–206
- laser therapy 165–167
- massage 163
- silicone products 164
- topical therapies 167

keratinization, fetal development 4, 6
keratinocytes
- differentiation 4
- infants 19
- morphogenesis 3
- specification 2

keratins, eccrine sweat gland formation 7
knots 95
knot strength and security of sutures 116, 118–119
KTP lasers *see* potassium titanyl phosphate lasers

l

lamina densa/lucida 3
Langerhans cells
- differentiation 4
- morphogenesis 3
- specification 2

Langer's lines 107
large lesions, wound closure 112–113
laser hair removal (LHR) 273–274, 280–287
lasers
- concepts 189
- *see also types of laser…*

laser therapies 189–301
- acne 207–221
- alopecia areata 289–291
- anesthesia 193
- atopic dermatitis 297
- Becker's nevi 242, 248–249
- café au lait macules 242–244, 246–248
- congenital melanocytic nevi 241, 245–246
- hair removal 273–274, 280–287
- infantile hemangiomas 191–192
- lichen planus 297–298
- lymphatic malformations 193
- molluscum contagiosum 294–295
- morphea 295–297
- Nevus of Ito/Ota 242, 249–250
- onychomycosis 229–240
- pigmented lesions 241–256
- pityriasis lichenoides chronica 298
- port-wine stains 191
- psoriasis 292–294
- pyogenic granulomas 193, 194
- scars and striae 165–167, 197–206
- spider angiomas 192–193
- tattoo removal 257–272
- vascular lesions 189–196
- verrucae 223–228
- vitiligo 292
- *see also* light therapy; *types of laser…*

lateral longitudinal nail excisions 137–138
lateral nail plate avulsion 134
layers of the epidermis 15
lazy S closure 110
LET *see* liposome-encapsulated tetracaine
lichen planus, light therapy 297–298
lidocaine
- 4% cream (LMX) 50–51, 73
- injections 52
- iontophoresis 51

light hair, laser removal 283
light therapy
- acne treatment 209–210, 217
- alopecia areata 289–291
- atopic dermatitis 297
- lichen planus 297–298
- morphea 295–297
- onychomycosis 237
- pityriasis lichenoides chronica 298
- psoriasis 292–294
- vitiligo 292
- *see also* laser therapies

limitations
- injectable local anesthetics 54–55
- topical anesthetics 52

lipids
- childhood/adolescent skin 20
- infantile skin 18

liposome-encapsulated tetracaine (LET) 51
lips
- nerve blocks 56
- scissor biopsies 67

liquid adhesives 122
LLLT *see* low-level laser therapy
LMX *see* lidocaine, 4% cream
loading of sutures 94–95

local anesthesia 49–56
  indications 49
  injectable 52–56
  injection pain reduction 53–54
  nail surgery 132
  nerve blocks 55–56
  side effects 53
  topical 49–52
local excision trays 41–44
localized hyperhidrosis, botulinum toxin injections 88–89
locking the knot 98
long-pulsed alexandrite lasers 281–282
long-pulsed diode lasers 282
long-pulsed neodymium-doped yttrium-aluminum-garnet (Nd:YAG) lasers 194–195, 231–232, 282–283
low-level laser therapy (LLLT) 291
lymphatic malformations 193

m

MAL *see* methyl ester methylaminolevulate
malformations, vascular 175–176
massage 163
Mastisol adhesive 122
matrix shaves 137
mattress sutures 97–99, 101–102
medial cheek, nerve blocks 55–56
medical evaluation 31–32, 132, 275–279
melanin, infantile skin 18
melanocytes
  differentiation 4
  morphogenesis 3
  specification 2
memory of sutures 116
mental nerve block 56
Merkel cells
  differentiation 4
  morphogenesis 3–4
  specification 2
mesenchymal cells
  differentiation 5
  morphogenesis 4
  specification 2
methicillin-resistant *Staphylococcus aureus* (MRSA) 151
methyl ester methylaminolevulate (MAL) 236
Metzenbaum scissors 43
microbiome
  adolescent skin 20
  childhood skin 20
  infants 16–18
  neonates 15
minor's starch iodine test 88
Mohs micrographic surgery (MMS) 79–81
molluscum contagiosum (MC) 294–295
monofilament sutures 115, 118–119
monopolar electrosurgery 82, 83
morphea, light therapy 295–297
mosquito hemostats 134–135
M-plasty 110
MRSA *see* methicillin-resistant *Staphylococcus aureus*
mucosal surfaces, topical anesthetics 51–52
multifilament sutures 115, 118–119

n

nail elevators 45
nail-pulling forceps 45
nails
  anatomy 131
  formation 4, 6
  onychomycosis 229–240
nail splitters 45, 134–136
nail surgery 131–141
  avulsion 133–136
  complications 140
  excisions 137–138
  home care 139
  postoperative management 138–139
  punch biopsy 136–137
  replacement 136
  shave biopsies 137
nail trays 45–47
narrowband light, acne treatment 209–210, 217
natural moisturizing factor (NMF) 17
nausea, postoperative 35
Nd:YAG lasers *see* neodymium-doped yttrium-aluminum-garnet lasers
near-infrared diode lasers, onychomycosis 233, 235
needle drivers 40, 43, 47, 94
needle points 120
needles 120–121
neodymium-doped yttrium-aluminum-garnet (Nd:YAG) lasers

  - hair removal 280–283
  - onychomycosis 231–232
  - pigmented lesions 243–251
  - scars and striae 201–203
  - tattoo removal 258–269
  - vascular lesions 191–195
  - verrucae 225
- neonatal skin 13–15
- neonates, diagnosis 25
- nerve blocks 55–56
- neurodevelopment, general anesthesia 34, 57–58
- nevus flammeus 191
- Nevus of Ito 242, 249–250
- Nevus of Ota 242, 249–250
- nevus sebaceus (NS) of Jadassohn 171–172
- NMF *see* natural moisturizing factor (NMF)
- non-ablative lasers 200–201
- non-absorbable staples 121
- non-absorbable sutures 119
- nonmaleficence 305
- non-opiod analgesics 144–146
- non-pharmacological pain management 144
- non-steroidal anti-inflammatory drugs (NSAIDs) 33, 35, 144–146
- NS *see* nevus sebaceus
- NSAIDs *see* non-steroidal anti-inflammatory drugs

o

- occlusive dressings 126–129
- off-label medications 308
- onychomycosis
  - laser therapy 229–240
  - light therapy 237
  - photodynamic therapy 236, 237
- oxycodone 147

p

- pain management 143–148
  - assessment 143–144
  - nerve blocks 55–56
  - non-opiod analgesics 144–146
  - non-pharmacological 144
  - opiod analgesics 146–147
  - topical anesthetics 147–148
  - *see also* analgesics; anesthesia
- palmar hyperhidrosis 89
- parents
  - anxiety 29
  - education 26, 274–275
  - treatment plan discussion 32–33
- partial distal plate avulsion 134
- partial nail avulsion 133
- partial proximal nail plate avulsion 135–136
- partial-thickness wounds 129
- partial wound closure 110–111
- patient-centered care 23–29
  - anesthesia discussion 33–34
  - anxiety 27–29, 32–34
  - diagnosis 24–26
  - doctor–patient relationships 308–309
  - ethics 303–313
  - further evaluations 26–27
  - hematomas 148–149
  - hirsutism 275–280
  - infection control 150–154
  - informed consent 307–308
  - initial consultations 23–24
  - injection pain reduction 53–54
  - medical evaluation 31–32
  - off-label medications 308
  - pain management 143–148
  - postoperative 35–36, 143–159
  - preoperative 31–35
  - procedures, timing of 27
  - suture reactions 154–155
  - treatment discussion 27, 32–34
  - wound dehiscence 155–157
- PCOS *see* polycystic ovarian syndrome
- PDL *see* pulsed-dye laser therapy
- PDT *see* photodynamic therapy
- perfect ellipse 108–109
- periderm 2, 5–8
- permission, informed 307–308
- personal comfort items 33
- PG *see* pyogenic granulomas
- pH, infant skin 16, 18–19
- phenol 47
- photochemotherapy (PUVA)
  - morphea 295–297
  - psoriasis 293–294
- photodynamic therapy (PDT)
  - acne 212, 218, 219
  - molluscum contagiosum 294–295
  - onychomycosis 236, 237
  - verrucae 225
- pigmented lesions, laser therapy 241–256

pilomatricoma 177–178
pilosebaceous apparatus, fetal development 7–8
pityriasis lichenoides chronica (PLC) 298
placement of sutures 95
plasticity of sutures 116, 118–119
PLC *see* pityriasis lichenoides chronica
pliability of sutures 116
poles, electrosurgery 83–84
polycystic ovarian syndrome (PCOS) 276–277
port-wine stains 191
posterior scalp, nerve blocks 56
postoperative care 35–36
  bleeding and hematoma 148–149
  dehiscence of wounds 155–157
  infections 150–154
  onychomycosis 234
  pain 143–148
  seroma 150
  suture reactions 154–155
  vascular lesion laser therapy 195
potassium titanyl phosphate (KTP) lasers
  acne 216–217
  vascular lesions 190, 195
preoperative care 31–35
  anesthesia discussion 33–34
  dehiscence prevention 156
  developmental evaluation 32
  medical evaluation 31–32
  nails 132–133
  preparation for procedure 33
  treatment discussion 32–34
preparation
  preoperative 33
  sutures 94
preschool children, anxiety 29
pressure dressings 125
preterm children 15
primary intention of wound closure 106–107, 129
procedures *see* laser therapies; surgical procedures
proliferation, infant skin 19
Proximate staples 121
psoriasis, light therapy 292–294
puberty 19–21
pulley stitch 100
pulsed-dye laser (PDL) therapy
  acne 212–216
  fluorouracil combination therapy 203
  scarring 165–167
  scars and striae 200–203
  tattoo removal 258–269
  vascular lesions 189–194
  verrucae 224–225
pulsed lasers 190
punch biopsies 38–41, 64–65
punches, surgical trays 38–40, 46
purse string closures 110–111
PUVA *see* photochemotherapy
pyogenic granulomas (PG) 175, 193, 194

q

Q-switched (QS) lasers 190
  onychomycosis 232
  pigmented lesions 243–251
  tattoo removal 258–269
quasi-continuous wave lasers 189–190
Q.U.E.S.T. assessment 143–144

r

RDEB *see* recessive dystrophic epidermolysis bullosa
reactions to sutures 154–155
recessive dystrophic epidermolysis bullosa (RDEB) 178
reef knots 95–96
regionalization, embryogenesis 6
replacement of nails 136
ring blocks 55, 132
risk factors
  non-opiod analgesics 144–145
  opiod analgesics 146–147
  postoperative infections 150
rotation flaps 112
ruby lasers
  hair removal 280–283
  pigmented lesions 243, 245–246, 249–250
  tattoo removal 258–269
rulers 44
running sutures 101

s

safety considerations, general anesthesia 57–58
scalp
  nerve blocks 56
  scissor biopsies 69

scalpel blades 44
scalpels
  biopsy trays 41
  local excision trays 43
  nail trays 46
scarring 161–169, 197–206
  electrosurgery 85
  intra-lesional injections 86–87
  laser therapies 197–206
  laser therapy 165–167
  massage 163
  postoperative formation 157
  silicone products 164
  topical therapies 163, 167
SCC *see* squamous cell carcinoma
school-age children 29
scissors
  biopsies 67–69
  surgical trays 40, 43, 44–45, 46
  see also suture scissors; tissue scissors
sebaceous glands, development 19–20
secondary intention of wound closure 106, 129
selection of sutures 117–120
septum elevators 134
seroma 150
shanks 94, 120
sharps containers 44
shave biopsies 39, 44, 65–67, 137
short-pulsed neodymium-doped yttrium-aluminum-garnet lasers 232
side effects
  intra-lesional injections 167
  laser scar reduction therapy 167
  local anesthetics 53
  non-opiod analgesics 144–145
  opiod analgesics 146–147
  scar massage 163
  silicone scar reduction products 165–166
Siegel handles 43
silver-impregnated dressings 129
simple flaps 111–112
simple interrupted sutures 100
simple running sutures 101
size of sutures 116
skin closure tapes 102–103, 122
skin hooks 43, 46, 95
specification 1, 2–3
Spencer stitch scissors 44
spider angiomas 192–193
Spitz nevi 173–174
squamous cell carcinoma (SCC) 80, 178
square knots 95–96
staged excisions 112–113
staples 102, 121
sterile draping 42
steroids, intra-lesional injections 86–88, 165
striae, laser therapies 197, 199–206
structure
  childhood/adolescent skin 19–20
  infantile skin 16–17
  nails 131
  neonatal skin 14
  skin 14–15
sub-cuticular sutures 101
subcutis (hypodermis)
  differentiation 5
  morphogenesis 4
  specification 3
superficial sutures 100–102
superficial wounds 129
super narrow-band-UVB (NB-UVB) light
  alopecia areata 290–291
  atopic dermatitis 297
  lichen planus 297–298
  morphea 295–297
  pityriasis lichenoides chronica 298
  psoriasis 293–294
  vitiligo treatment 292
supplies
  punch biopsies 64
  scissor biopsies 67
  shave biopsies 65
supraorbital nerve block 55
supratrochlear nerve block 55
surgeon's knot 95–96
surgical blades, local excision trays 43
surgical needles 120–121
surgical procedures
  acquired nevi 173
  anxiety 27–29
  aplasia cutis congenita 176–177
  basal cell nevus syndrome 179
  biopsies 63–71
  chemosurgery 79–81
  common 73–91
  complications 143–159
  congenital melanocytic nevi 172–173

surgical procedures (*cont'd*)
cryosurgery 73–77
curettage 77–79
deep sutures 97–100
dehiscence prevention 156
dermatofibrosarcoma protuberans 179
dermoid cysts 177
discussion of 27, 32–34
electrosurgery 81–85
epidermal nevus 176
epidermolysis bullosa 178
excisional biopsies 69
incisional biopsies 69
infantile hemangiomas 174–175
intra-lesional injections 85–89
juvenile xanthogranuloma 178
nails 131–141
nevus sebaceus of Jadassohn 171–172
pilomatricoma 177–178
preparation 33
punch biopsies 38–41, 64–65, 136–137
pyogenic granulomas 175
scissor biopsies 67–69
shave biopsies 39, 44, 65–67, 137
special 171–187
Spitz nevi 173–174
superficial sutures 100–102
sutures 93–104
timing of 27
vascular malformations 175–176
see also laser therapies; techniques
surgical trays 37–48
biopsy 37–41
local excision 41–44
nails 45–47
punch biopsy 38–41
shave biopsy 39, 44
suture removal 44–45
suture removal trays 44–45
sutures 93–104
alternative materials 102–103
biopsy trays 40–41
characteristics 115–120
deep 97–100
guiding 111
instrument ties 95–96
loading 94–95
local excision trays 43–44
nail trays 46
needles 120–121
placement 95
preparation 94
principles 94–100
reactions to 154–155
selection 117–120
superficial 100–102
techniques 96–102
tissue stabilization 95
suture scissors 44
sweat glands, fetal development 6–7

t

TAC *see* tetracaine, adrenaline and cocaine
Tanner stages 20
tapes, skin closure 102–103, 122
tattoo removal 257–272
complications 266–267
contra-/indications 258–259
laser types 259–263
techniques 263–266
techniques
acne laser therapy 217–218
chemosurgery 80–81
cryosurgery 75
curettage 78–79
deep sutures 97–100
injection pain reduction 53–54
intra-lesional injections 85–86
nail surgery 133–141
onychomycosis laser therapy 233–234
superficial sutures 100–102
sutures 96–102
tattoo removal 263–266
see also surgical procedures
tendon damage from nail surgery 140
tensile strength of sutures 115, 118–119
tension, wound closure 107–108
tetracaine 51
tetracaine, adrenaline and cocaine (TAC) 51
TEWL *see* transedipermal water loss
TGF-β *see* transforming growth factor-β
thermal relaxation time (TRT), hair removal 280
threads, sutures 94
timing of procedures 27
tiredness, postoperative 35
tissue adhesives 102, 121–122
tissue destruction, electrosurgery 85

tissue expansion 113
tissue reactivity of sutures 117–119
tissue scissors 43
tissue stabilization, sutures 95
titanium sapphire lasers, onychomycosis 232–233
toddlers, anxiety 29
toes
  nail surgery 131–141
  nerve blocks 55
  scissor biopsies 68–69
tongues, scissor biopsies 67–68
topical anesthesia 34, 49–52, 147–148
  formulations 50–51
  intra-lesional injections 85
  iontophoresis 51
  limitations 52
  mucosal surfaces 51–52
topical therapies, scarring 167
tourniquets 47, 133, 140
transedipermal water loss (TEWL)
  infants 18
  neonates 14, 15
transforming growth factor-β (TGF-β) 203
transglutaminase 5
trapdoor nail avulsion 134
trays *see* surgical trays
treatment modalities, discussion of 27
treatment plans, discussion 32–33
triamcinolone 86–88
triangular needles 120
T ring tourniquets 133

u
ultraviolet (UV) therapy
  alopecia areata 290–291
  atopic dermatitis 297
  lichen planus 297–298
  morphea 295–297
  onychomycosis 237
  pityriasis lichenoides chronica 298
  psoriasis 292–294
  vitiligo treatment 292
urethral swabs 47
UV *see* ultraviolet

v
vascular lesions
  anesthesia 193
  classifications 190–191
  infantile hemangiomas 87–88, 174–175, 191–192
  laser therapies 189–196
  lymphatic malformations 193
  Nd:YAG lasers 190, 194–195
  port-wine stains 191
  postoperative care 195
  pulsed-dye lasers 189–194
  pyogenic granulomas 175, 193, 194
  spider angiomas 192–193
vascular malformations (VM) 175–176
  see also vascular lesions
vasculogenesis 5
verrucae, laser therapies 223–228
vertical mattress sutures 101–102
vimectin, eccrine sweat gland formation 7
viral warts, laser therapies 223–228
vitiligo, light therapy 291–292
VM *see* vascular malformations
von Willebrand's disease 140

w
water handling
  infantile skin 18
  neonates 14, 15
Webster needle holders 40, 43
weight-based dosing 145
Westcott tissue scissors 43
window nail plate avulsion 134
wing blocks 132
Wong–Baker-FACES 143–144
Woods lamps 236
wound classifications 129, 150
wound closure 105–114
  A-T flaps 111–112
  complications 113, 122–123
  cosmetic considerations 108
  crescentic excisions 109–110
  design principles 107–108
  dog ears 107–108
  guiding sutures 111
  indications 105–106
  large lesions 112–113
  lazy S closure 110
  materials 115–124
  M-plasty 110
  needles 120–121
  partial 110–111

wound closure (*cont'd*)
  perfect ellipse 108–109
  primary intention 106–107
  principles 106–108
  purse string 110–111
  secondary intention 106
  simple flaps 111–112
  skin closure tapes 102–103, 122
  staged excisions 112–113
  staples 102, 121
  suture materials 115–120
  suturing 93–104, 111
  tissue adhesives 102, 121–122
  tissue expansion 113
wound dehiscence 155–157
wound dressings 125–130
  basic 125–126
  occlusive 126–129
  wound classifications 129
wound gaps, sutures 99–100